Additional Praise for *The Heart-Healthy Handbook*

"Knowledge is power," and T*he Heart-Healthy Handbook* gives you the *knowledge* to understand and manage your heart health. This important book contains critical information about the prevention and treatment of heart disease. It gives you the power to create and sustain a heart-healthy lifestyle. This wonderful book has lifesaving messages for us all.

—Kathy Berra, MSN, NP, Cardiovascular Nurse Practitioner; Co-Director of the LifeCare Company, Stanford Prevention Research Center (Retired), Palo Alto, CA

I am very impressed with this outstanding book by Drs. Franklin and Dixon. They collaborated with a very talented and knowledgeable team of expert authors who provided many chapters that will be very useful for individuals who want to lead a healthy life. The chapters provide important and accurate information for all areas of heart health. I enthusiastically support the book and encourage people to read it and become informed about how to promote their health.

—Steven N. Blair, PED, Retired Professor, Arnold School of Public Health, University of South Carolina, Columbia, SC

This state-of-the-art book is simply outstanding. Once I started reading it, I could not put it down. It is a "must read" for anyone interested in preventing or managing cardiovascular disease. Although the book is intended for the lay public, cardiologists and other healthcare providers will also find it to be an invaluable resource.

—Neil F. Gordon, MD, PhD, MPH, FACC, CEO and Medical Director, INTERVENT International, Savannah, GA

I highly recommend this book as required educational reading for all patients with cardiovascular heart disease. The book is an outstanding team effort of delivering the most current and comprehensive professional information offered by a foremost heart hospital for the benefit of all heart patients.

—Murray Low, EdD, MAACVPR, FACSM, FAACVPR, Past President, AACVPR; Program Director, Cardiac Rehabilitation Deparement, Stamford Hospital, Stamford, CT

Patients, their families, and healthcare providers alike will be immediately engaged by this beautifully illustrated, precise, and easy-to-read and -understand *Heart-Healthy Handbook*.

—Nanette K. Wenger, MD, MACC, MACP, FAHA, Professor of Medicine (Cardiology) Emeritus, Emory University School of Medicine; Consultant, Emory Heart and Vascular Center, Atlanta, GA

All royalties for this book will be directed to the Cardiac Rehabilitation Enhancement Fund, Beaumont Hospital, Royal Oak, Michigan.

The information and recommendations appearing in this book are research-based and appropriate in most instances, but they are not a substitute for medical diagnosis and counseling. This information is intended to be a resource to guide additional discussion, with your physician, regarding your personal medical condition and cardiovascular risk reduction program.

ISBN: 978-1-60679-373-2
Library of Congress Control Number: 2016960650
Book layout: Cheery Sugabo
Cover design: Cheery Sugabo
Front cover photo: bai1ran/iStock/Thinkstock
Text photos: Thinkstock

Healthy Learning
P.O. Box 1828
Monterey, CA 93942
www.healthylearning.com

THE HEART-HEALTHY HANDBOOK

Editors:
Barry A. Franklin
Simon R. Dixon

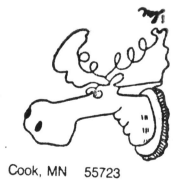
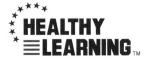

ACKNOWLEDGMENTS

The Heart-Healthy Handbook was prepared by a highly skilled and dedicated medical writing team of Beaumont Health professionals, with representative expertise in clinical and interventional cardiology, cardiovascular surgery, electrophysiology, nursing, pharmacology, exercise physiology, geriatrics, psychosocial issues, diagnostic testing, cardiac imaging, nutrition, obesity, diabetes and metabolism, and women's heart issues. Our acknowledgments begin with Brenda White, the managing editor of the *State of the Heart* newsletter since its inception. She bore the atlas of transcription, word processing, serial revisions, and editing of the articles, laboriously checking references and factual information with patience, endurance, and a unique sense of responsibility.

We would also like to express our sincerest appreciation and gratitude to Robert Levin, MD, a cardiologist par excellence, for his clinical insights and regular outstanding contributions to the newsletter over the years, many of which have been reproduced herein (see Chapter 12, Ask the Cardiologist). Special thanks are also extended to a talented graphic designer, Paul Murch, for his extraordinary expertise in orchestrating the layout and design of our quarterly newsletter, as well as the enormous help he provided with complementary artwork and consolidation of the selected columns via extensive archived InDesign files for processing by the publisher.

In addition, we would like to extend a debt of gratitude to Delynn Meyer and Jennifer Carbary, administrative staff in Beaumont's Marketing Department, for their support of this herculean endeavor. Finally, appreciation is extended to Jim Peterson, Aaron Huffman, and Kristi Huelsing, our "dream team" at Healthy Learning, for their tireless attention to detail, unflagging endurance, pioneering vision, and organizational wizardry in bringing this contemporary "cardiovascular compendium" to fruition.

Barry A. Franklin, Ph.D.
Simon R. Dixon, MBChB

CONTENTS

PREFACE

Despite impressive recent medical advances, cardiovascular disease (CVD), which includes atherosclerotic coronary heart disease (partially or completely obstructed coronary arteries), stroke, angina pectoris (chest pain/pressure), and congestive heart failure (the heart's inability to pump effectively causing reduced blood flow to body tissues), remains the leading cause of death in the United States, as well as in most developed countries. According to the American Heart Association (AHA), CVD causes approximately one out of every four U.S. deaths each year. In fact, nearly 2,300 Americans die of CVD each day, corresponding to one death every 37 seconds! In 2012, an estimated 785,000 and 470,000 Americans had a first or recurrent heart attack, respectively. Moreover, one third of all heart attacks are fatal, killing as many women as men. Furthermore, survivors are at increased risk for a second, potentially more serious heart attack.

Atherosclerosis and CVD: The New View

Investigations begun more than three decades ago have since refuted the traditional view of atherosclerosis that cholesterol simply accumulates on the inner lining of the coronary arteries, forming plaque, which can ultimately obstruct blood flow. Contemporary research currently points to arterial inflammation playing a key role in the development and progression of atherosclerosis (*Scientific American*, May 2002), which can be triggered by excess levels of low-density lipoprotein cholesterol (LDL-C), a plasma protein also referred to as the "bad" cholesterol. This new view highlights the importance of interventions to not only improve cardiovascular health, but also to reduce risk factors that may heighten or exacerbate arterial inflammation.

Cardiovascular health is generally defined in three categories—ideal, intermediate, and poor. This classification is undertaken on the basis of seven simple health factors and modifiable behaviors (i.e., lose weight, get physically active, control cholesterol, manage blood pressure, reduce blood sugar, quit smoking, improve dietary habits), as detailed in the American Heart Association's My Life Check assessment tool that can be reviewed at http://mylifecheck.heart.org.

It is interesting to note that numerous studies have shown that most heart attacks (~86 percent) occur at mild-to-moderate coronary artery blockages (< 70 percent obstruction) (*Circulation*, Aug. 1995), not the severe obstructions that are being treated with bypass surgery or balloon angioplasty. These findings suggest a new treatment plan for preventing and managing heart disease (Table 1), highlighting the synergistic role of lifestyle modification and cardioprotective medications, both of which provide independent and additive benefits. As such, several mechanisms may contribute to the improved clinical outcomes, including partial (albeit small) anatomic regression of coronary artery stenosis, a reduced incidence of coronary inflammation, platelet aggregation, plaque rupture, and enhanced coronary artery vasomotor function.

Focus	Definition	Intervention
Traditional view:		
A simple plumbing problem	The degree of coronary artery obstruction determines the risk of acute coronary events.	Balloon angioplasty or coronary artery bypass surgery are the only effective approaches to improving prognosis associated with atherosclerotic coronary heart disease.
The new view:		
Focus is on arterial inflammation	The nature of plaque determines the risk of acute coronary events.	Inflammation, plaque rupture, and thrombosis (blood clots) represent the final common pathway for acute cardiac events. The goals of therapy are plaque stabilization and normalization of coronary artery function—best achieved through lifestyle modification and cardioprotective medications.

Table 1. Heart Disease: Changing Treatment Approaches

Disease Prevention: Comprehensive Approaches to Risk Reduction

Unfortunately, patients, as well as the medical community, often rely on coronary revascularization interventions (coronary angioplasty or bypass surgery) and/or cardioprotective medications as a *first-line strategy* to either stabilize or favorably modify established risk factors and the course of coronary disease. On the other hand, these palliative therapies do not address the underlying problem, that is, the most proximal risk factors for heart disease, including poor dietary habits, physical inactivity, and cigarette smoking/secondhand smoke (Figure 1) (*Circulation*, June 2008). Accordingly, it's time to change our emphasis from disease management to disease prevention, increasingly focusing on the foundational causes of CVD.

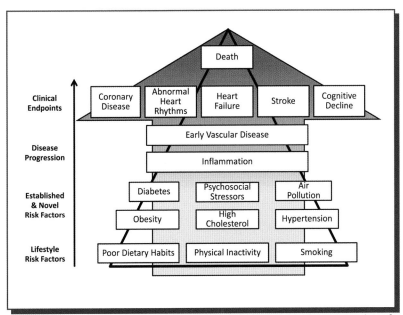

Figure 1. Unhealthy lifestyle habits lead to risk factors, the progression of cardiovascular disease, and ultimately, adverse outcomes or clinical endpoints. Thus, the *first-line* strategy to prevent heart disease (or recurrent cardiac events) is to favorably modify poor lifestyle habits or practices, including suboptimal dietary habits, physical inactivity, and cigarette smoking.

The question arises concerning how the likelihood of initial and recurrent cardiac events can be reduced. In a nutshell, the response dictates that interventions should be undertaken that can decrease the potential for coronary artery injury, inflammation, plaque rupture, and blood clotting in the heart's arteries. This objective can be achieved by behavior modification and adopting a heart-healthy lifestyle that includes such factors as engaging in regular moderate-to-vigorous aerobic exercise, refrains from cigarette smoking, avoiding secondhand smoke, decreasing excess body weight and fat stores, getting adequate sleep, making healthier dietary choices (Table 2) (Circulation, June 2011), and taking adjunctive cardioprotective medications (e.g., aspirin, statins, beta-blockers, angiotensin-converting enzyme inhibitors), if appropriate. Moreover, cardiorespiratory fitness, expressed as metabolic equivalents (METs; 1 MET = 3.5 ml O_2/kg/min), appears to be one of the strongest prognostic indicators in persons with and without heart disease (*Mayo Clinic Proceedings*, Sept. 2009).

Consume More ...	Consume Less ...
• Fish and shellfish	• Potatoes
• Whole grains	• Refined grains
• Fruits	• Processed meats
• Vegetables	• Sugars, sweetened beverages, diet sodas
• Nuts & legumes	• Grain-based deserts and bakery goods
• Low-fat or no-fat dairy products	• Fats, oils, or foods with partially hydrogenated vegetable oils
• Vegetable oils*	• Salt
• Water	• Alcohol+
*Examples include flaxseed, canola and soybean oil	• +For adults who drink alcohol, no more than moderate consumption (up to two drinks/day for men, one drink/day for women), ideally with meals.

Other Lifestyle Recommendations: Stop cigarette smoking and avoid secondhand smoke, reduce food portion sizes, limit prolonged sitting and computer interactions, increase daily physical activity, and get enough quality sleep.

Table 2. Dietary and Lifestyle Priorities Associated With Cardioprotective Benefits

The aforementioned lifestyle modifications can favorably impact high blood pressure (hypertension), overweight/obesity, elevated blood cholesterol, diabetes, and chronic stress. In fact, one widely-cited review of published research studies demonstrated that 75 to 90 percent of all heart attacks are explained by these conventional risk factors (*American Journal of Cardiology*, Feb. 2009). Consequently, modifying these risk factors via lifestyle changes and prescribed medications is critical to reducing the risk of future cardiac events.

Some Good News, But a Disturbing Trend

Between 1980 and 2000, death rates from heart disease fell by more than 40 percent. In a landmark report, researchers found that approximately half the decline in cardiovascular deaths could be attributed to reductions in conventional risk factors (obesity and diabetes mellitus were notable exceptions), while the other half would be ascribed to contemporary medical therapies (e.g., cardioprotective medications, exercise-based cardiac rehabilitation, and initial treatments for heart attacks). In contrast, emergent and elective coronary revascularization (i.e., angioplasty and bypass surgery) accounted for only 7 percent of the overall decline in deaths from coronary heart disease (*New England Journal of Medicine*, June 2007). Similar results were reported in a Canadian study that evaluated the decrease in cardiovascular mortality between 1994 and 2005 (*Journal of the American Medical Association*, May 2010).

From 2000 to 2010, mortality rates for CVD in the United States decreased by an additional 25 percent (*Circulation*, Feb. 2010). Although there were also impressive reductions in the prevalence of uncontrolled high blood pressure, elevated blood cholesterol, and, to a lesser extent, cigarette smoking, there were concomitant increases in the prevalence of obesity and diabetes mellitus, and little or no change in those individuals who engaged in regular moderate-to-vigorous physical activity, despite continued reductions in work-related and domestic energy expenditure (*PLoS One*, May 2011). Unfortunately, after more than three decades of declining cardiovascular mortality, there has been a recent increase in the death rate from CVD, suggesting challenges ahead, unless patients more aggressively embrace the aforementioned interventions.

Moving From a Reactive Sick Care System to Proactive Healthcare

Numerous studies have now shown that the single most important contributor to premature death in the U.S., as well as most countries worldwide, are *health behaviors*, that is, the lifestyle choices people make on a day-to-day basis, which account for 40 to 50 percent of all deaths, and approximate the influence of genetics, environmental factors, and access to medical care combined (*New England Journal of Medicine*, Sept. 2007). Accordingly, in recent years, there has been increasing interest to change our emphasis from disease management to disease prevention, focusing, instead, on the foundational or lifestyle-related causes of chronic disease. A just-published study found that bad genes can double the risk of heart disease, but that a healthy lifestyle cuts it in half. Just as important, researchers found that an unhealthy lifestyle erases about half the benefits of good genetics (New England Journal of Medicine, Nov. 2016).

Currently, the dominant form of healthcare financing in the U.S. supports a reactive, visit-based model, in which patients are seen when they become ill, typically during hospitalizations and at outpatient visits. That particular care model falls short not just because it is expensive and often fails to proactively improve health, but also because so much of health is explained by individual health behaviors, most of which occur outside healthcare encounters (5,000+ waking hours each year) (*New England Journal of Medicine*, July 2012). An accompanying editorial emphasized that a readily accessible, culturally sensitive prevention model, focused on forestalling the development of risk factors for initial and recurrent cardiovascular events, is the best solution to the current crisis. Accordingly, the prevention of atherosclerotic CVD can be categorized into three types: primordial (prevention of risk factors); primary (treatment of existing risk factors); and secondary (prevention of recurrent cardiovascular events) (*Circulation*, May 2011). In reality, much of the success in reducing CVD, in recent years, has been through primary and secondary prevention.

Additional emphasis on primordial prevention is needed to sustain and enhance our efforts in combating CVD.

The bottom line? As healthcare providers, we need to become proponents of achieving healthy lifestyle overhauls in the patients we serve, well beyond the acute and palliative care provided in our emergency centers, surgical suites, cardiac catheterization laboratories, hospital rooms, and physician offices. The "paradigm shift" needs to move from not only helping patients when they are ill, injured, or sick, to "helping patients help themselves (24/7)." This change will be further championed by contemporary healthcare insurers who will increasingly provide their hospitals and patient subscribers with financial incentives for achieving certain performance metrics, lifestyle habits, and risk factor goals.

Evolution of *The Heart-Healthy Handbook*

For more than a decade, we've successfully published Beaumont's *State of the Heart* educational newsletter, geared to "helping patients help themselves." The underlying goal has been to help them improve their overall health and well-being, with specific reference to favorably modifying their risk factor profiles and, as a result, preventing inital and recurrent cardiovascular events. Our goal was to develop an attractive, informative, timely, entertaining, high-quality, reader-friendly quarterly newsletter, dedicated to improving the cardiovascular health of the patients we serve.

The newsletter has a number of unique features, including a multidisciplinary approach to the prevention and treatment of CVD, brief articles, liberal use of subtitles, color graphics, boxed information, self-assessment tests, cartoons, frequently asked questions, and accompanying citations (journal, month, year) for anyone who desires additional information. The newsletter also includes brief "snippets" peppered throughout the text that highlight practical heart-healthy tips and/or just published, groundbreaking relevant studies. Regular columns in the newsletter are complemented by invited submissions, authored by preeminent Beaumont physicians, including clinical/interventional cardiologists, cardiovascular surgeons, internal medicine specialists, and allied health professionals.

An extensive array of topics is covered in the newsletter. Collectively, the topics address such areas as preventive cardiology, lifestyle medicine, cardioprotective medications, heart-healthy nutrition, obesity/weight control, exercise/physical activity, hazards of cigarette smoking/secondhand smoke, conventional and psychosocial risk factors, diabetes mellitus, common heart rhythm disturbances, congestive heart failure, triggers of acute cardiac events, adjunctive anti-anginal therapies (i.e., enhanced external counterpulsation therapy), exercise prescription and proscription, high-risk activities (e.g., hazards of snow removal), sexual activity and the cardiac patient, conventional and minimally invasive cardiovascular surgery, coronary revascularization, and common questions/answers. This book represents a compilation of outstanding, timely articles, selected from previous editions of our *State of the Heart* newsletter and accompanying snippets.

Beaumont

Contributor	Title
Barry A. Franklin, PhD	Director, Preventive Cardiology and Cardiac Rehabilitation Beaumont Hospital, Royal Oak Professor, Department of Internal Medicine Oakland University William Beaumont School of Medicine
Simon R. Dixon, MBChB	Chair, Department of Cardiovascular Medicine Dorothy Susan Timmis Endowed Chair of Cardiology Beaumont Hospital, Royal Oak Professor, Department of Internal Medicine Oakland University William Beaumont School of Medicine
Amr Abbas, MD	Director, Interventional Cardiology Research Co-Director, Echocardiography Lab Beaumont Hospital, Royal Oak Associate Professor, Department of Internal Medicine Oakland University William Beaumont School of Medicine
Steven Ajluni, MD	Interventional Cardiologist Beaumont Hospital, Royal Oak Assistant Professor, Department of Internal Medicine Oakland University William Beaumont School of Medicine
Samuel Allen, DO	Medical Director, Pulmonary Hypertension Center Beaumont Hospital, Troy Associate Professor, Department of Internal Medicine Oakland University William Beaumont School of Medicine
Steven Almany, MD	Director, Cardiac Catheterization Laboratory Beaumont Hospital, Troy Associate Professor, Department of Internal Medicine Oakland University William Beaumont School of Medicine
Jeffrey Altshuler, MD	Cardiovascular Surgeon Beaumont Hospital, Royal Oak Assistant Professor, Department of Internal Medicine Oakland University William Beaumont School of Medicine
Emily Balagna, BS	Exercise Physiologist Preventive Cardiology and Cardiac Rehabilitation Beaumont Hospital, Royal Oak
Aaron Berman, MD	Clinical Chief, Cardiology Associate Physician-in-Chief Beaumont Hospital, Royal Oak Associate Professor, Department of Internal Medicine Oakland University William Beaumont School of Medicine
A. Neil Bilolikar, MD	Clinical Cardiologist Beaumont Hospital, Royal Oak Assistant Professor, Department of Internal Medicine Oakland University William Beaumont School of Medicine

CONTRIBUTORS

Megan Bowdon, BS	Exercise Specialist Preventive Cardiology and Cardiac Rehabilitation Beaumont Hospital, Royal Oak
Terry Bowers, MD	Director, Vascular Medicine Beaumont Hospital, Royal Oak Assistant Professor, Department of Internal Medicine Oakland University William Beaumont School of Medicine
Jacqueline Brewer, RN	Nurse Clinician Heart and Vascular Clinics Beaumont Hospital, Troy
Jenna Brinks, MS	Manager, Preventive Cardiology and Cardiac Rehabilitation Beaumont Hospital, Royal Oak
O. William Brown, MD	Section Head, Vascular Surgery Beaumont Hospital, Royal Oak Professor, Department of Internal Medicine Oakland University William Beaumont School of Medicine
Kavitha Chinnaiyan, MD	Director, Cardiovascular Imaging Education Beaumont Hospital, Royal Oak Associate Professor, Department of Internal Medicine Oakland University William Beaumont School of Medicine
David R. Cragg, MD	Clinical Cardiologist Beaumont Hospital, Troy Associate Professor, Department of Internal Medicine Oakland University William Beaumont School of Medicine
Anne Davis, RN	Nurse Clinician Preventive Cardiology and Cardiac Rehabilitation Beaumont Hospital, Royal Oak
William Devlin, MD	Director, Coronary Care Unit Beaumont Hospital, Troy Assistant Professor, Department of Internal Medicine Oakland University William Beaumont School of Medicine
Kathy Faitel, RN	Nurse Clinician Preventive Cardiology and Cardiac Rehabilitation Beaumont Hospital, Royal Oak
Angela Fern, MS	Senior Exercise Physiologist Preventive Cardiology and Cardiac Rehabilitation Beaumont Hospital, Royal Oak
David H. Forst, MD	Clinical Cardiologist Beaumont Hospital, Troy Professor, Department of Internal Medicine Oakland University William Beaumont School of Medicine
Amy Fowler, BS	Senior Exercise Physiologist Preventive Cardiology and Cardiac Rehabilitation Beaumont Hospital, Royal Oak

Harold Friedman, MD	Director, Cardiac Rehabilitation Beaumont Hospital, Royal Oak Associate Professor, Department of Internal Medicine Oakland University William Beaumont School of Medicine
Michael Gallagher, MD	Director, Advanced Cardiac Imaging Beaumont Hospital, Troy Director, Cardiovascular Disease Fellowship Beaumont Hospital, Royal Oak Associate Professor, Department of Internal Medicine Oakland University William Beaumont School of Medicine
Georges Ghafari, MD	Clinical Chief, Cardiology Beaumont Hospital, Grosse Pointe Assistant Professor, Department of Internal Medicine Oakland University William Beaumont School of Medicine
James A. Goldstein, MD	Director, Research and Education Director, Cardiomyopathy Clinic Beaumont Hospital, Royal Oak Professor, Department of Internal Medicine Oakland University William Beaumont School of Medicine
Stephen Gunther, MD	Clinical Cardiologist Beaumont Hospital, Royal Oak
Sue Haapaniemi, MS	Exercise Physiologist Non-Invasive Cardiology Beaumont Hospital, Royal Oak
Dana Haddad, RN	Nurse Clinician Preventive Cardiology and Cardiac Rehabilitation Beaumont Hospital, Royal Oak
David E. Haines, MD	Director, Heart Rhythm Center Beaumont Hospital, Royal Oak Professor, Department of Internal Medicine Oakland University William Beaumont School of Medicine
Susan Halley, RN	Nurse Clinician Preventive Cardiology and Cardiac Rehabilitation Beaumont Hospital, Royal Oak
Joyce Said Hansen, MS	Exercise Physiologist Preventive Cardiology and Cardiac Rehabilitation Beaumont Hospital, Royal Oak
Ivan Hanson, MD	Interventional Cardiologist Beaumont Hospital, Royal Oak Assistant Professor, Department of Internal Medicine Oakland University William Beaumont School of Medicine
George S. Hanzel, MD	Director, Cardiac Catheterization Laboratory Director, Structural Heart Disease Beaumont Hospital, Royal Oak Associate Professor, Department of Internal Medicine Oakland University William Beaumont School of Medicine

Cindy Haskin-Popp, MS	Exercise Specialist Preventive Cardiology and Cardiac Rehabilitation Beaumont Hospital, Royal Oak
Andrew Hauser, MD	Clinical Cardiologist Beaumont Hospital, Royal Oak Associate Professor, Department of Internal Medicine Oakland University William Beaumont School of Medicine
Kirk Hendrickson, MS	Exercise Physiologist Preventive Cardiology and Cardiac Rehabilitation Beaumont Hospital, Royal Oak
Jenna M. Holzhausen, PharmD, BCPS	Clinical Pharmacy Specialist, Critical Care Cardiac Intensive Care Unit Beaumont Hospital, Royal Oak
Monica Jiddou-Patros, MD	Interventional Cardiologist Beaumont Hospital, Royal Oak Course Director, Oakland University William Beaumont School of Medicine Assistant Professor, Department of Internal Medicine Oakland University William Beaumont School of Medicine
Kaylee Kaeding, BS	Exercise Physiologist Preventive Cardiology and Cardiac Rehabilitation Beaumont Hospital, Royal Oak
Nathan Kerner, MD	Co-Director, Echocardiography Lab Beaumont Hospital, Royal Oak Assistant Professor, Department of Internal Medicine Oakland University William Beaumont School of Medicine
Kristen Kubert, BS	Exercise Specialist Preventive Cardiology and Cardiac Rehabilitation Beaumont Hospital, Royal Oak
Robert N. Levin, MD	Clinical Cardiologist Beaumont Hospital, Royal Oak Associate Professor, Department of Internal Medicine Oakland University William Beaumont School of Medicine
Pam Marcovitz, MD	Director, Ministrelli Women's Heart Center Beaumont Hospital, Royal Oak Associate Professor, Department of Internal Medicine Oakland University William Beaumont School of Medicine
Wendy Miller, MD	Section Head, Nutrition and Prevention Medicine Beaumont Hospital, Royal Oak Corporate Medical Director, Weight Control Centers Professor, Department of Internal Medicine Oakland University William Beaumont School of Medicine

Heidi Pillen, PharmD	Senior Assistant Director, Clinical Services & Quality Program Director PGY-2 Health-System Pharmacy Administration Bwell Wellness Ambassador Beaumont Hospital, Royal Oak
Phillip Robinson, MD	Cardiovascular Surgeon Beaumont Hospital, Troy Assistant Professor, Department of Internal Medicine Oakland University William Beaumont School of Medicine
Daniel Rothschild, MD	Cardiology Fellow Beaumont Hospital, Royal Oak
Roger Sacks, BS	Exercise Physiologist Preventive Cardiology and Cardiac Rehabilitation Beaumont Hospital, Royal Oak
Robert D. Safian, MD	Director, Center for Innovation and Research in Cardiovascular Disease Director, Interventional Cardiology Fellowship Beaumont Hospital, Royal Oak Professor, Department of Internal Medicine Oakland University William Beaumont School of Medicine
Marc Sakwa, MD	Chief, Cardiovascular Surgery Beaumont Hospital, Royal Oak Professor, Department of Internal Medicine Oakland University William Beaumont School of Medicine
Lisa Schornak, MS	Exercise Physiologist Non-Invasive Cardiology Beaumont Hospital, Royal Oak
Alan J. Silverman, DO	Clinical Cardiologist Beaumont Hospital, Royal Oak Assistant Professor, Department of Internal Medicine Oakland University William Beaumont School of Medicine
Troy Silverthorn, BS	Cardiovascular Medical Technician Preventive Cardiology and Cardiac Rehabilitation Beaumont Hospital, Royal Oak
Daniel Stettner, PhD	Psychologist Eastwood Clinic – Royal Oak Adjunct Graduate Professor Counseling Psychology Wayne State University
James R. Stewart, MD	Director, Pacemaker Clinic Beaumont Hospital, Royal Oak
Rachel Sumner, MPH, RD	Dietitian Ministrelli Women's Heart Center Beaumont Hospital, Royal Oak

Nicholas Tepe, MD	Cardiovascular Surgeon Beaumont Hospital, Royal Oak Assistant Professor, Department of Internal Medicine Oakland University William Beaumont School of Medicine
Steven B.H. Timmis, MD	Director, Coronary Care Unit Beaumont Hospital, Royal Oak Assistant Professor, Department of Internal Medicine Oakland University William Beaumont School of Medicine
Justin Trivax, MD	Interventional Cardiologist Director, Cardiovascular Performance Clinic Beaumont Hospital, Royal Oak Assistant Professor, Department of Internal Medicine Oakland University William Beaumont School of Medicine
Silvia Veri, RD	Nutrition Supervisor Weight Control Centers Beaumont Hospital, Royal Oak
Kerstyn C. Zalesin, MD	Bariatric Medical Director Division of Nutrition and Prevention Medicine Beaumont Hospital, Royal Oak Assistant Professor, Department of Internal Medicine Oakland University William Beaumont School of Medicine

CHAPTER

1

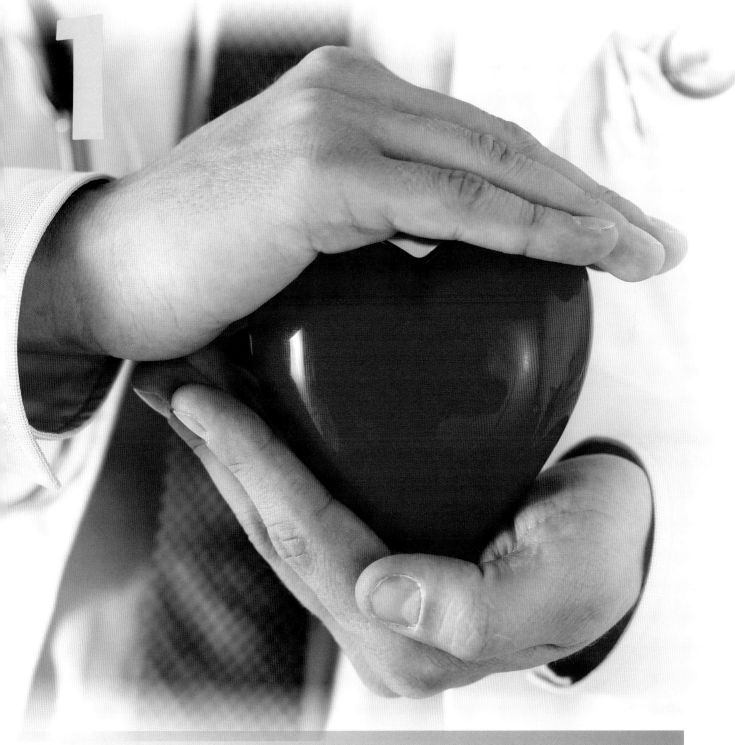

HEART HEALTH:
UNDERSTANDING
THE BASICS

Understanding Coronary Artery Disease

Harold Friedman, M.D.

"My blocked artery is fixed with a stent, my symptoms are gone, I'm totally fine." I often hear these words spoken by patients treated for coronary artery disease. Unfortunately, to believe that this statement is true is to misunderstand the nature of the disease.

To fully understand coronary disease, one needs to re-examine the biology (or behavior) of the cells that comprise the blood vessel wall. Our medical knowledge about what exactly causes cell damage and subsequent thickening of the arterial wall is incomplete. We do know that this process, called atherosclerosis, never attacks the thin-walled and low pressure veins in the body—only arteries. It has a predilection for the heart (coronary), brain (carotid) and leg (femoral) arteries.

Atherosclerosis within the heart arteries, or coronary artery disease, is a process that starts slowly and gradually progresses over decades. It involves a transformation of cells within the artery wall into macrophages, cells that function like a sponge absorbing cholesterol. Eventually the macrophages die, releasing their contents within the artery wall. Over time, this debris accumulates, leading to thickening of the artery wall by a waxy substance called cholesterol and localized inflammation caused by release of macrophage digestive enzymes. As the artery wall thickens, it begins to attract calcium and forms a plaque or outcropping that can obstruct blood flow within the central channel or lumen. This build up can culminate in a narrowing or stenosis severe enough to restrict blood flow and oxygen delivery to the heart muscle itself, causing a variety of signs and symptoms including electrocardiographic abnormalities, chest pain or shortness of breath. Some have likened coronary plaque to a pus-filled pimple that grows within the walls of arteries. If one of the pimples (plaques) pops open (plaque rupture), a blood clot forms over the spot to seal it, and the clot blocks the artery. The result: a heart attack.

There are a variety of diagnostic tests to detect the earliest stages of atherosclerosis. Pulse wave velocity studies measure stiffness of arteries using a finger tip sensor. Another test, carotid artery intimal thickness, uses harmless ultrasound on the neck to assess the thickness of the middle layer of the carotid artery, which is an early sign of disease. A third test, a specialized computed tomographic scan, using low dose X-ray, can detect calcium deposits in coronary arteries, confirming the presence of atherosclerosis.

Although cholesterol is a major component of atherosclerotic process, not all cholesterol is bad. In fact, cholesterol is needed by the body to synthesize important hormones such as estrogen and testosterone, manufacture vitamin D and maintain the health of nervous system cell function. About 80 percent

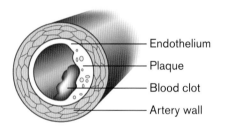

- Endothelium
- Plaque
- Blood clot
- Artery wall

Diseased Artery

of cholesterol is made by the liver and 20 percent is acquired by diet. Popular drugs called statins reduce high cholesterol levels (in particular "bad" LDL cholesterol levels) by blocking a liver enzyme involved in its production. Numerous studies have shown that statins decrease the incidence of stroke and heart attack as well as the need for bypass surgery and angioplasty. These drugs are relatively safe and have minimal side effects.

Atherosclerosis can be accelerated by genetics, especially cholesterol abnormalities, certain illnesses, risk factors and unhealthy lifestyle behaviors. Illnesses include inflammatory diseases such as lupus or arthritis, thyroid abnormalities and kidney failure. Traditional risk factors include diabetes, high blood pressure and obesity.

Behaviors that adversely affect coronary artery disease include cigarette smoking and a sedentary lifestyle. Collectively, these factors may directly trigger changes in cell metabolism and/or accelerate the atherosclerotic process by elevating cholesterol levels and intensifying inflammation.

Several interventions can help you reduce the risk of developing coronary artery disease. For example, lifestyle modification may be as effective as medication. Weight loss improves the good to bad cholesterol ratio, facilitates control of diabetes and significantly reduces blood pressure. Regular exercise complements weight loss to further reduce the factors that are known to accelerate coronary artery disease; it also provides a heightened sense of well being, improved functional capacity, increased strength and reduced fatigue. Avoiding excess alcohol intake, tobacco and dietary fat as well as compliance with prescribed medications are also proven interventions.

It takes decades for damage to occur within the arteries of your heart and body; thus, it's important to understand that it will take a major personal commitment, compliance and perseverance to successfully reduce your risk of future cardiac problems. Unfortunately, you're not cured by the coronary stent that we just implanted. Now the real work begins.

Lifestyle modification:
The '10' most powerful two-letter words?
If it is to be, it is up to me.
(Note: There's no pill or procedure that can take charge of your health the way you can.)

Heart Disease in Women— Is It Really Different?

Kavitha M. Chinnaiyan, M.D.

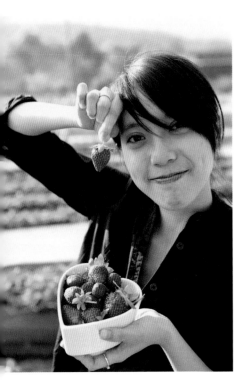

Over the last decade, heart disease, specifically, coronary artery disease (CAD), has resulted in a steady rise in deaths in women aged 35-54 years. Since 1989, more women than men have died annually from CAD. CAD and stroke result in three times more deaths in women than all cancers combined. One reason for this is that in women, the diagnosis of CAD can be challenging. Women often present with symptoms such as fatigue, shortness of breath, upper abdominal discomfort and back, jaw or neck pain, rather than crushing chest pain, which is more common in men. Also, compared to men, women with CAD have more adverse outcomes such as delays in getting care by emergency medical services, increased rates of pre-hospital cardiac arrest and a greater likelihood of dying when hospitalized for major heart attacks.

Risk assessment for CAD is recommended as the first step in diagnosis and treatment of this deadly disease. However, the most commonly used risk stratification model, the Framingham Risk Score (FRS), has several limitations in identifying women who are at risk for heart attacks and death. Based on new clinical trials since the development of the FRS in 1998, risk stratification guidelines in women were updated in 2007. These updated guidelines are designed to reduce the long-term risk of CAD and include a new risk assessment model based on risk factors and family history. Therefore, when being evaluated for the risk of heart disease, it is imperative for the treating physician to know the patient's risk factors and family history of heart disease.

CAD risk: What can you do to decrease it?

- Know your numbers and goals for cholesterol, fasting blood sugar, blood pressure, body mass index and waist circumference.
- Increase physical activity (at least 30 minutes of moderate exercise [brisk walking] daily).
- Make the right food choices: A diet low in saturated fat, cholesterol and sugar with an emphasis on fresh fruits, vegetables, low-fat dairy products and oily fish at least twice a week is recommended. Women with CAD or high triglycerides may consider taking a capsule supplement of omega-3 fatty acids.
- Quit smoking; avoid secondhand smoke.
- Know the current guidelines about hormone replacement therapy (HRT): HRT is not recommended to prevent heart disease in women.
- Know your supplements: Antioxidant supplements (such as vitamin E, C and beta-carotene) are not recommended for prevention of CAD or stroke.
- Consider aspirin therapy: Low dose aspirin may be considered in selected women with a low risk of bleeding complications.

Other diagnostic tests?

Several studies have examined newer ways of identifying heart disease in women at an early stage, using imaging tools that can directly "look" at blood vessels and the heart. One such tool is calcium scoring cardiac computed tomography. This rapid, noninvasive test can identify early stages of atherosclerosis, the process that leads to CAD and heart attacks. It provides powerful information on not just the presence of CAD but also long-term risks of having heart attacks and dying from heart disease.

In summary, heart disease should no longer be considered a "man's disease" since cardiovascular mortality is higher in women than men. The first step in changing this trend is to recognize one's risk factors and take steps to reduce them. The good news is that the above-referenced lifestyle changes are also beneficial in preventing and/or alleviating other chronic debilitating illnesses such as cancer. Risk stratification can include new imaging tools that detect early coronary heart disease.

VALUE OF CORONARY ARTERY CALCIUM SCORING

A few years ago, researchers reported on more than 44,000 consecutive asymptomatic individuals who were followed for an average of five years. Subjects without traditional risk factors but elevated coronary artery calcium (CAC) scores had significantly higher all-cause mortality (death rate) than individuals with multiple risk factors but no CAC. Conversely, the absence of CAC was associated with a favorable prognosis even among those with multiple risk factors. These findings challenge the use of risk factor assessments alone for determining the aggressiveness of primary prevention therapies and suggest that some patients without risk factors may benefit from further risk assessment (e.g., CAC scoring) and preventive therapies.

(*Circulation Cardiovascular Imaging*, July 2012)

Management of Coronary Disease: Which Way to Go?

Aaron Berman, M.D.

The management of coronary artery disease has significantly improved over the last 40 years. It has also become more complicated, as new devices, procedures and medications compete for the attention of health care providers and patients. This article clarifies the rationale for recommendations you may receive from your cardiologist, and potentially provides some questions for you to ask. The basis for any therapy is that it should be safe and effective, relieve symptoms, and/or potentially prevent acute cardiovascular events.

When you are diagnosed with atherosclerotic heart disease (i.e., clogged coronary arteries), your cardiologist will regularly recommend medications such as aspirin, cholesterol-lowering statins, beta blockers and nitrates. You'll receive advice regarding diet and lifestyle modification. If you have severe coronary blockages, with or without debilitating symptoms, you may also be advised to undergo coronary artery bypass graft surgery (CABG) or catheter-based revascularization such as angioplasty or coronary stenting, referred to collectively as percutaneous coronary interventions or PCI.

Cardiovascular medications have improved significantly over the last four decades. We now have powerful cholesterol lowering statins, which have been unequivocally shown to decrease the risk of heart attack in patients with coronary disease. Aspirin has become universally recommended for patients with coronary disease; beta-blockers and angiotensin converting enzyme inhibitors may also improve long term outcomes, especially in some patient subsets. But is this enough? When should CABG or PCI be added as complementary additions to lifestyle modification and medications?

The first studies comparing CABG to medical therapy were conducted in the 1970s. The Coronary Artery Surgery Study, European Coronary Surgery Study and the Veteran's Administration Surgery Study all compared survival and heart attack risk in cardiac patients randomized to medications alone or CABG (PCI was not performed until 1977).

Although these studies differed somewhat in their conclusions, patients with three vessel disease, especially if the major artery feeding the front wall of the heart was involved, and patients with significant heart muscle weakening from previous heart attacks, seemed to benefit the most in survival and symptom relief from surgery. Both medications and surgical technique have improved substantially since these early studies.

The next group of studies was conducted in the late 1980s and compared PCI with CABG in patients with multivessel disease. In these studies, short-term survival was equivalent in both groups, although PCI patients had a higher risk of having to return to the hospital for repeat procedures, and also had a lower likelihood of complete relief of anginal chest pain. With the advent of drug-eluting stents, this difference became less prominent, as drug eluting stents cause less renarrowing than the older bare metal stents, and it seemed that PCI was as good as surgery.

More recent studies have attempted to identify subgroups of coronary patients that may especially benefit from CABG. Diabetics, who often have a higher burden of diffuse atherosclerosis than non-diabetics, have received considerable attention and have been extensively studied over the past decade. One recent trial, the FREEDOM study, enrolled 1,900 patients with multivessel disease and diabetes and randomized them to PCI or CABG. The surgery group did significantly better, both with respect to fewer heart attacks as well as overall survival. On the other hand, they also had a higher risk of stroke.

Another aid to deciding whether to recommend CABG or PCI is the SYNTAX score, derived from the SYNTAX study, which compared these revascularization techniques, based on the severity of disease. Factors such as lesion length, the presence of chronic occlusions, and complex lesions are considered. If the SYNTAX score is less than 22, PCI may be appropriate; for scores of 22 to 33, either intervention may be used; and, for scores over 33, reflecting more atherosclerotic burden and a higher level of complexity of PCI, CABG may be preferable.

So where does that leave you? When appropriate, here are some good questions to ask your cardiologist:

- Does my diabetes make me a better candidate for CABG rather than PCI?
- If my heart function is impaired, will CABG improve my prognosis more than PCI?
- Are my arteries anatomically suited better for PCI or CABG?
- Am I more likely to get full symptom relief from CABG or PCI?
- Do I have risk factors that make CABG less attractive (more risky)?
- Can I achieve similar outcomes by combining aggressive lifestyle modification and prescribed medications, without undergoing PCI and/or CABG?

There are many approaches to a given patient's coronary anatomy, and many questions to answer. Do interventions besides medication and lifestyle change need to be done? If so, will PCI or CABG improve my lifestyle (symptom relief) and/or increase my survival? At what risk? Using the above questions, a frank and complete discussion with your cardiologist will give you a better understanding of which therapies will serve you best.

Coronary Artery Disease: The Fork in the Road

Nicholas Tepe, M.D.

The treatment of coronary artery disease (CAD) has markedly improved over the last 25 years. Contemporary cholesterol medications and blood lubricants are now common. Coronary angioplasty has become far more effective with the routine use of drug-eluting stents, reducing the likelihood that the blood vessel will clog or narrow again, a condition known as restenosis. We are now able to offer coronary artery bypass grafting (CABG) to virtually any patient. Many CABG patients are well into their 80s and today, operating on patients with renal failure on hemodialysis is routine.

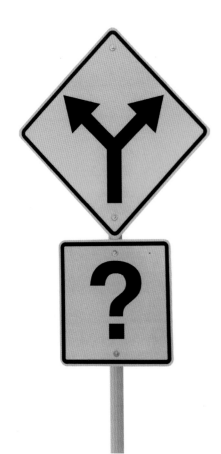

At one extreme are patients with limited CAD requiring only one or two stents. At the other extreme are patients with severe or advanced CAD requiring CABG and complex operations. Between these two black and white examples is a vast gray area of patients with CAD in multiple vessels and sites that technically could have either multivessel angioplasty or CABG. Often the choice is made on the basis of the complexity of the CAD. Patients with easily accessible lesions may opt for staged angioplasty with procedures done over two or more visits. Patients with complex blockages such as at a branch point or right at the beginning of a vessel or who have completely occluded vessels are usually sent for CABG.

For 17 years, the controversy has raged about staged angioplasty or CABG for the treatment of multivessel CAD. Which fork in the road should patients take? Studies have shown that in selected patient groups with multivessel CAD, angioplasty works just as well as CABG over the long term. However, most patients do not fall into this subset.

In a landmark study, the comparative effectiveness of these revascularization techniques was reported in patients with advanced CAD and diabetes mellitus. Investigators published the results of the FREEDOM trial (*New England Journal of Medicine,* Nov. 2012), which was a large randomized trial comparing multivessel angioplasty to CABG in coronary patients with diabetes. When followed for five years, the CABG group demonstrated a 30 percent greater reduction in death and heart attack, when compared with the angioplasty group. CABG showed a clear advantage over angioplasty in this large patient subset; however, stroke was more frequent in the CABG group. The accompanying editorial suggested that cardiologists discuss these findings with their coronary patients with diabetes before performing a diagnostic and interventional cardiac catheterization.

So, which fork? CAD is a chronic disease. Angioplasty and CABG are not mutually exclusive. You may need both over the long course of treatment for CAD. Early on, your treatment may be medications alone. Later, as blockages appear, one or more angioplasties may be done. If the disease progresses, CABG may be your best choice. If you are diabetic, the option for CABG should be offered earlier. In any event, talk to your cardiologist. Heed warning signs or symptoms suggesting progression of your heart disease, and keep your options open.

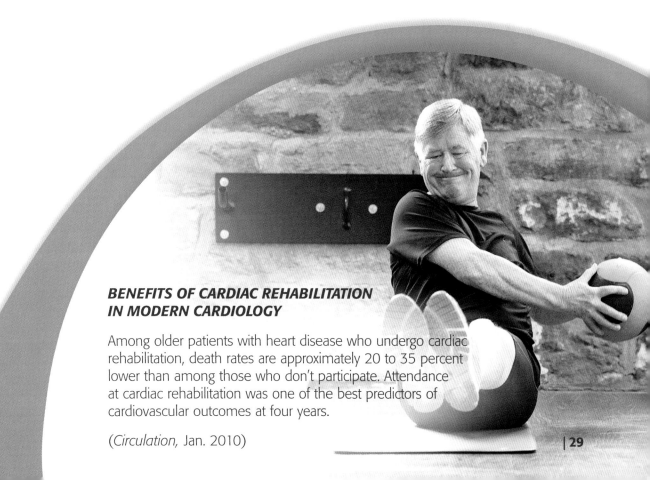

BENEFITS OF CARDIAC REHABILITATION IN MODERN CARDIOLOGY

Among older patients with heart disease who undergo cardiac rehabilitation, death rates are approximately 20 to 35 percent lower than among those who don't participate. Attendance at cardiac rehabilitation was one of the best predictors of cardiovascular outcomes at four years.

(*Circulation,* Jan. 2010)

Getting the Most Value From a Cardiovascular Appointment

David H. Forst, M.D.

In our expensive health care environment and with many people still uninsured, it is increasingly important for patients not only to maximize the quality of their medical visit, but also to minimize cost. Too often, the entire process is left in the hands of the cardiologist or cardiac surgeon, but every patient can play an important role in ensuring that the best possible outcome from a doctor's visit.

Communication

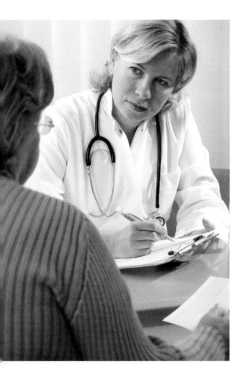

It is amazing how many tests are generated and how many prescriptions are written because of a lack of information. To minimize this, every patient should bring an accurate list of medications and appropriate test results when available. It's also important to ask the doctor to sit down; this creates an environment for more comfortable communication, which is necessary for a successful visit. Don't leave the office until you feel certain that you fully understand the test or treatment being prescribed. Taking a few extra minutes can prevent future problems. Also, don't hesitate to ask for handout materials or written directions; and always ask the doctor to clarify or repeat something if you still have questions.

Cost

Ask about different diagnostic and therapeutic options. A stress echocardiogram may cost less than a nuclear stress study, but oftentimes similar information can be obtained from either study. In many instances, generic drugs may be equally effective, but much less expensive. The cost of different pacemaker devices or coronary stents may also vary substantially with similar results as many other procedures. Do your homework before coming into the office and don't be afraid to ask about the financial implications of your proposed treatment.

Treatment options

Be sure to ask your doctor about the expected results of treatment. Many times a surgical or medical intervention may have similar outcomes, but very different recovery times and costs. This is also true of drug prescriptions. Always ask about side effects, drug interactions and therapeutic options. An allergic reaction is not only uncomfortable; but it also increases the cost of treatment and puts your overall health at risk. For those who are employed, valways ask about recovery time from a procedure and when you can reasonably return to work. This may make the difference when selecting a therapeutic option with similar risks and outcomes.

Insurance coverage

Always bring your insurance card with you. The last thing you want to happen is to get stuck with a large bill, especially if a different approach was possible had the insurance information been known. It is perfectly reasonable to ask the staff to explain deductibles and co-pays for different services. Also, note what insurance is accepted in a physician's office. You may wish to go elsewhere if an insurance plan is not accepted.

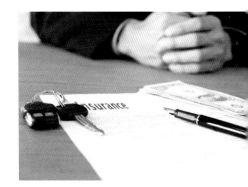

Clinical information

Always bring a list of diagnoses, past procedures, allergies and medications. This can save time and reduce errors. Likewise, know which hospital or clinic provided your service. The year or date may also be helpful. Today, even though electronic medical records are readily available, they may not be compatible among different hospitals or clinics. Hunting for records can waste time and delay decision-making and failing to note a past procedure or a medication may result in a medical error.

Summary

Providing appropriate information in your doctor's office can pay big dividends. Health care is collaboration between a doctor and a patient. Often, the better the information exchange, the better the outcome. Don't be afraid to ask about or even challenge a proposed diagnostic or treatment option. Communicating effectively increases the likelihood that you will receive the best possible care at the lowest possible cost, the outcome for which we all strive.

WHAT TO DO IF COSTLY MEDICINE ISN'T COVERED BY INSURANCE?

There are three approaches you can take. *First*, have the doctor who prescribed the medication write a letter of appeal to your insurance company. *Second*, contact the drug manufacturer to find out whether it has a special reduced-cost program for which you might qualify. *Third*, contact your state health department to find out if they have special programs to subsidize the cost of prescribed medications that residents cannot afford.

(Bottom Line's Outsmart the Health-Care Maze, 2013)

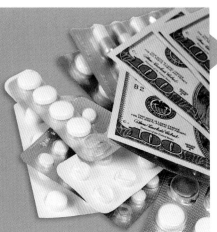

Maximizing Your Next Doctor's Visit: Five Strategies for Success

Andrew Hauser, M.D.

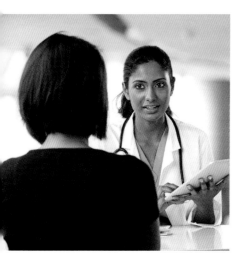

In a busy office practice where face-to-face time with your physician may be limited to 15 minutes or less, it's easy to become frustrated. How can you maximize the relatively brief opportunity you have to discuss your ailments and concerns and receive practical, understandable advice?

Over the last 30 years in practice, I've discovered five helpful strategies to optimize the time spent with your doctor. These include:

❏ *Do your homework.* This includes making accurate lists of all your current medications (drug name, dosages and frequency of use) and allergies (especially to drugs or x-ray dye). Bring the name and addresses of your primary care physician or specialists you wish to be contacted regarding your upcoming exam. If you have copies of previous test results, x-rays, consultation reports or hospital summaries, then bring these too. If the physician's office has mailed you a pre-visit questionnaire, complete it in advance of your visit and bring it with you. Bring a copy of all information items for the physician to keep in your chart. It is especially important to bring your medication list with you each time you see any physician and keep it updated (or bring all your medications in a bag). Wear loose, easily removed clothing to your appointment. Bring a book, knitting or other diversion in case of an extended wait.

❏ *Bring a spouse, knowledgeable relative or close friend with you.* This is especially important if you have trouble recalling past events, hearing, or remembering instructions that may be given.

❏ *Turn off your cell phone or pager while seeing your physician to avoid unnecessary interruptions.* (It may be unavoidable for the physician to do the same.)

❏ *Prioritize your concerns.* Tell the doctor at the beginning of your visit what concerns you most. If there is more than one concern, then bring a written list. When seeing a specialist, try to limit your initial concerns to his or her specialty. If other symptoms are important for a diagnosis, a skilled physician will lead you through a series of questions exploring other possible disease states or medical conditions.

❑ *Listen carefully to the doctor's questions and answer them as directly and succinctly as possible.* Don't ramble or go into excessive detail. If additional detail is required, the physician will usually ask for more explanation.

If strategies 1 through 5 are followed, this will allow more time to discuss the physician's impressions and recommendations. Before you leave the office, be sure you have a clear understanding of the significant findings and working diagnoses. You should also understand what additional testing or procedures have been advised and what risks might be associated with them. Understand clearly what medications are prescribed and what side effects might occur. Ask if you have any activity limitations, and whether exercise is advised. Request written material or pamphlets if they are available so that you may learn more about your health concerns. A full understanding of your evaluation will provide your first step to staying well … and staying out of doctors' offices.

RIGHT THINKING ABOUT CARDIOVASCULAR HEALTH

The current health care model in the U.S. supports a reactive, visit-based approach in which patients are seen when they become ill, typically during hospitalizations and at outpatient visits. This model falls short not just because it is expensive and often fails to proactively improve health, but also because health outcomes are primarily explained by individual behaviors. In fact, health care accounts for just 10 percent of the factors that determine premature mortality. Although patients with chronic illness may spend only a few hours a year with a doctor or nurse, they spend more than 5,000 waking hours each year making lifestyle choices (physical activity, diet, cigarette smoking, prescribed medications) that can profoundly affect their health. In the future, health care models must increasingly focus on initiatives to favorably modify the choices being made during these 5,000+ hours.

(*New England Journal of Medicine,* July 2012).

Helping Your Doctor Help You!

William H. Devlin, M.D.

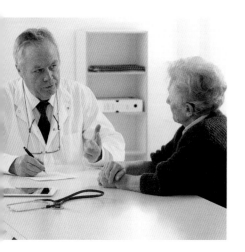

The relationship between patients and their physicians is unique to every individual situation. Oftentimes, little things can be done to optimize your care to help your physician help you. The following suggestions may be helpful to you, regardless of your physician network.

As a healthcare provider, it is essential to have details of a patient's prior history. We don't expect patients to remember every detail of every procedure they've had, so having prior hospital or physician records is especially helpful. Don't assume that the physician who refers you to a specialist or to another doctor will automatically send records. Generally, this is the responsibility of the patient to sign releases to allow records to be sent either by mail, hand delivered or faxed to another physician. Most offices will ask for the patient to obtain records, but as a general rule, it is also reasonable for the patient to have important aspects of their medical records immediately available. Some patients keep a brief summary on their computer and provide a copy to their doctor. I encourage all patients when visiting a new physician to make efforts to not only have records sent in advance, but to call one or two days prior to the appointment to verify that the records have been received. As many offices are using computers for their medical records, don't assume that all of these computers can instantaneously transfer patient records with the click of a button.

Another area that often causes confusion is obtaining test results. While some offices will simply say "we will call you if something is out of the ordinary," I prefer to make sure patients know the results of their tests, whether they are "good" or "bad." If you do not hear from your doctor's office within a couple of weeks of having had a test, you should contact the office and ask for the results. Having patients know what their cholesterol is and what it should be, or their latest blood pressure reading, makes them more likely to be compliant with medications or treatment. In our busy schedules, regardless of the system we have set up for "call backs," it is difficult to achieve 100 percent in tracking down every result, especially if tests are done outside of our usual network.

Oftentimes during a busy office visit, it is common for patients to forget questions that they wanted to ask the doctor or nursing staff. Accordingly, I encourage patients to write down their questions and have them available. Generally, these questions will be answered during the routine visit, but this simple suggestion will maximize communication and minimize follow up phone calls. No doctor wants to complete a scheduled office appointment and have to answer numerous questions the next day. Most physicians would prefer to take several minutes to answer questions in person, rather than having to return phone calls or have a patient uncertain about their medical condition.

The most common source of complications from medical care deals with medications. I encourage all patients to keep an updated list of medications with them at all times. You are taking medications not only when you see the doctor, but any time you are driving or out in public. Having your medication list on your person could save your life in an emergency. Despite modern technology, medical records are not readily available from one location to another. In our office, we ask for an updated medication list with every visit. It never ceases to amaze me how often prescriptions change, independent of visits to our office, as many patients have several physicians.

Sometimes, patients need to change physicians. This can occur on account of health coverage restrictions, because of loss of confidence in a physician, or due to a geographic move. Regardless of the cause, physicians will seldom get upset if you decide to switch to another doctor. It is your right to have access to your medical records, and to have them transferred to another physician without having to explain the reasons to your physician. Nevertheless, all patients should feel comfortable speaking with their physician if they are upset or concerned about a particular issue. Just as in any relationship, if communication cannot be kept open, then changes need to be made. By following some of these simple suggestions, you can help your doctor help you.

AMERICAN HEART ASSOCIATION (AHA): LIFE'S SIMPLE SEVEN

Cardiovascular health encompasses two basic components: ideal health behaviors and ideal health factors. The behaviors include not smoking, maintaining a healthy weight, and meeting or exceeding AHA recommendations for physical activity and eating a healthy diet. The health factors include blood pressure, fasting blood glucose and total cholesterol levels that are within AHA's recommended range— preferably without needing medication to keep them there. To receive your personal cardiovascular health assessment based on Life's Simple Seven and learn the steps you may need to take to improve heart health, visit: www.heart.org/MyLifeCheck.

My Life Check™
Live Better With Life's Simple 7™

 Get Active   Control Cholesterol   Eat Better   Manage Blood Pressure   Lose Weight   Reduce Blood Sugar   Stop Smoking

Take an Active Role in Your Heart Health: Be Your Own Advocate

Amy Fowler, B.S.

The most crucial role you have is as a "self-advocate," accepting the fact that achieving good health is primarily *your* responsibility according to the U.S. Department of Health and Human Services and the American Heart Association. Patient outcomes improve in those who take an active role in their medical care by communicating more thoroughly with their physicians, seeking information about their condition and following through with recommendations. By asking questions and fully understanding your plan of care, you become empowered to make well-informed choices. Indeed, some studies suggest that behavioral choices are the number one factor contributing to premature death and disability, exceeding genetic predisposition, social circumstances, environmental exposure and access to health care (*New England Journal of Medicine,* Sept. 2007).

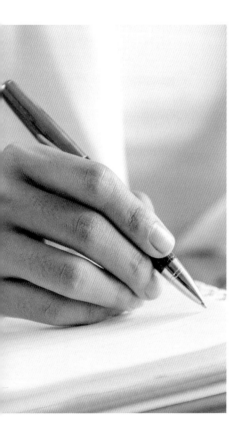

Becoming a self-advocate begins with advance preparation for medical appointments. Many physicians and other allied health professionals suggest patients bring a notebook or folder to each appointment that contains:
- current medications, including dosage and frequency
- concerns, such as symptoms you have experienced since the last visit
- questions, such as possible side effects to a new medication or treatment

Having this information on hand allows for focused discussions, efficient use of the limited time with a physician or other health care team member; it also results in the best treatment outcomes. Ideally, as you leave an appointment with any health care team member, you should feel satisfied and have a full understanding of your discussion, instructions, new medications, or upcoming procedures or tests. Also, most patients recall only a fraction of the information presented to them during an office visit; the presence of a friend or family member during appointments can enhance the likelihood of retaining important information.

Education is paramount to your success as a self-advocate. A physician or other health care team member is best for providing you with references to select educational sources. Valid information can be gathered online but caution should be employed; personal story-based sites may vary considerably in the accuracy of the information provided. The American Heart Association (www.americanheart.org) offers credible, research-based guidelines and information for the patient with cardiovascular disease.

The final component of becoming an empowered patient is to adopt healthy lifestyle behavior changes. Simply knowing that your cholesterol or blood pressure levels are abnormal will not prevent a heart attack. Taking your prescribed medications coupled with healthy eating habits and an appropriate exercise regimen can favorably modify numerous coronary risk factors.

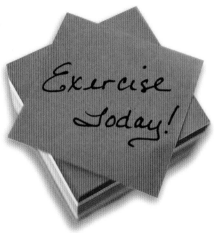

Changing longstanding behaviors can be challenging for many patients. The following are suggestions for identifying target risk factors, goal setting and maintaining new, healthy behaviors to reduce your risk:

- Discuss your risk factors like high blood pressure with your physician
- Know where you stand in relation to recommended values for each risk factor (e.g., your high-density lipoprotein, or HDL is 35 mg/dL; the recommended value is 40 mg/dL or higher in men and 50 mg/dL or higher in women)
- Understand which behaviors impact each risk factor. For example, regular exercise may modestly increase HDL
- Set measurable, reasonable goals. For example, aim for one to two-pound weight loss per week as opposed to a 30 pound loss for the year
- Anticipate obstacles to your behavior change and plan a course of action when you encounter them, such as listing "appointments" to exercise on your calendar on a busy week
- Get support from family and friends. Tell them about the behavior changes you are making so they can assist you in your goals
- Write your plan of action and post it in an area where you will see it often during the day
- Rebound from temporary lapses. For example, get back on track when you've neglected to exercise for a few days or weeks, instead of letting it become months.

The perfect health care storm originates when patients are afraid or unable to ask questions, relay concerns, answer questions inaccurately or neglect to follow through with physician recommendations. Moreover, many patients are ill prepared for the relatively brief period of time physicians and other health care team members have for each visit, which can lead to miscommunication. You can make an immeasurable impact on your future health and well-being when you:

- prepare for visits with your health care team.
- assume responsibility for your health education.
- take prescribed medications and make healthy lifestyle behavior changes.

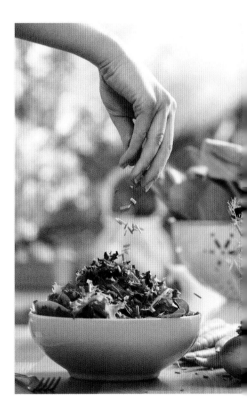

Achieving a Healthier Lifestyle: The Ultimate Secret of Success?

Barry A. Franklin, Ph.D.

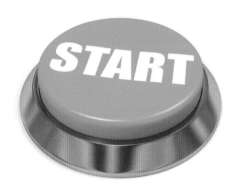

So you want to lose weight, improve your fitness, be healthier and live longer. What's the ultimate secret of success: In two words: *TAKE ACTION!* When you act, you set wishes in motion. When you set wishes in motion, you are rewarded with results.

Years ago, when I was in college, I decided I wanted to become a better writer—and maybe even write a book someday. How was I going to get myself to write? Then I remembered something I learned in my high school physics class: the law of inertia. A body at rest tends to remain at rest; a body in motion tends to remain in motion. What if inertia applied to human behavior and all I had to do was turn myself from the former (i.e., a body at rest) to the latter (i.e., a body in motion)?

I decided to find out by starting to work on a paper that was due at the end of the semester. I made a commitment—to write something every day, being persistent, even if a sentence or two was all that I could muster. I promised myself I'd do this for the next month and see what happened. During the first few attempts, my progress was agonizingly slow. Nevertheless, with each new day, I became more and more productive. I completed the paper, and learned one of the great lessons of my life: the moment you take action—any action—you will conquer inertia. And, once you transform yourself from a body at rest to a body in motion, you gain momentum (i.e., like a rock rolling down a hill).

According to Keith Ellis, author of *The Magic Lamp* (Three Rivers Press, 1998), "inertia is the single greatest barrier to success. It's also the easiest to overcome. All you have to do is act. Any action you take, no matter how trivial, will do the trick. The easier you make it on yourself to act, the easier it is to overcome inertia."

What are the implications for counseling patients? Let's take exercise, for example. When prescribing exercise to sedentary patients, I ignore conventional exercise guidelines (e.g., 30, 60, or 90 minutes per day), and give them something easily achievable to do. "Can you walk 5 or 10 minutes, just three or four times per week," I often ask. Similar to the physics principles of motion, a body at rest tends to remain at rest. The important thing is to get patients *moving* in the direction of their ultimate goals. Whether your goal is weight loss, starting an exercise program, or stopping smoking, a key principle of success is getting started. Try it!

CHAPTER
2

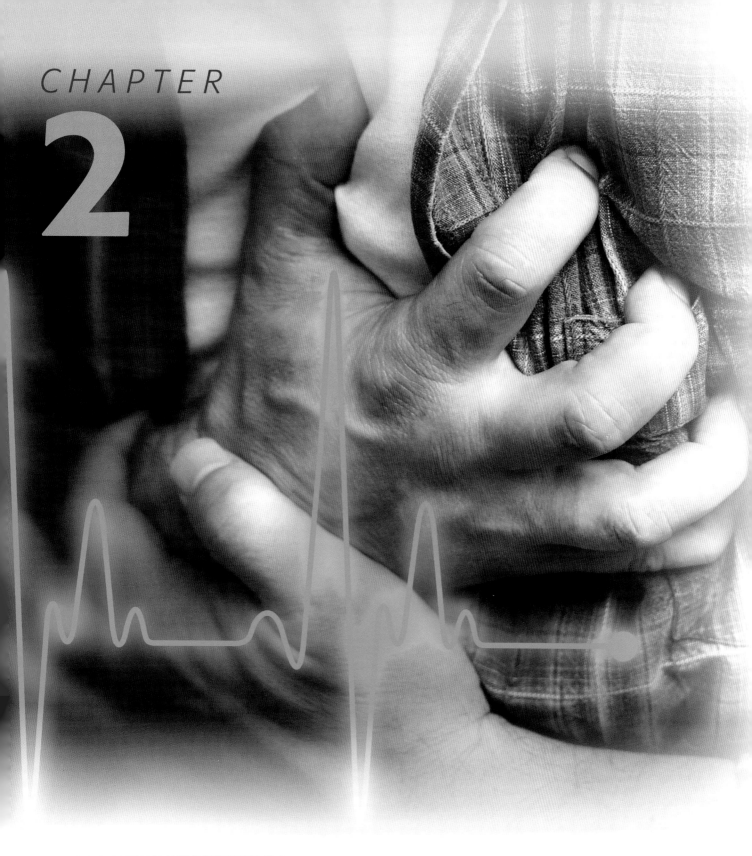

RISK FACTORS FOR CARDIOVASCULAR HEALTH

Preventing Your Next Heart Attack: Know Your Numbers!

Georges Ghafari, M.D.

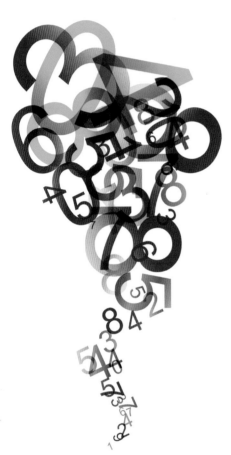

Most patients ask after surviving a heart attack, "What can I do to prevent the next one?" To begin the process of healing and recovery, one must understand the causes of heart disease and the risk factors that contribute to it.

A heart attack occurs when a coronary artery (about the size of a strand of cooked spaghetti) suddenly becomes blocked or obstructed. Oftentimes, this is a result of acute injury to the inner layer of these vessels due to inflammation and blood clotting. Over time, multiple risk factors contribute to the development of heart disease, and most of these risk factors are modifiable. This means a patient can favorably influence their long-term outcomes by aggressively modifying their lifestyle.

Unfortunately, many patients as well as the medical community continue to rely on costly heart bypass or angioplasty procedures and/or cardioprotective medications as a *first-line strategy* to stabilize or favorably modify established risk factors and the course of coronary disease. These therapies do not address the root of the problem, which are the underlying heart disease lifestyle factors such as poor dietary practices, physical inactivity and cigarette smoking.

Major modifiable risk factors and goals:
- **blood pressure** less than 140/90
- **cholesterol numbers:**
  - ✓ LDL less than 70
  - ✓ HDL greater than 40
- **obesity**—body mass index less than 25
- **sedentary lifestyle**—regular exercise, four to five days/week
- **diabetes mellitus**—hemoglobin A1c less than 6 (non-diabetics) or less than 7 (diabetics)
- **stress reduction**—positive attitude/outlook—respond rather than react to stressful situations
- **smoking cessation,** if appropriate

It's been said that, "It takes a village to raise a child." The same applies to heart disease—it takes a knowledgeable and committed team to prevent and treat heart disease. This includes internal medicine physicians and cardiologists, exercise physiologists, dietitians, pharmacists, spiritual counselors and nurses. However, you (the person you see in the mirror every day) probably have the single greatest influence on your destiny after a heart attack, bypass surgery or balloon angioplasty/stenting. In addition to medical management, favorably modifying your risk factors will help decrease your likelihood of having another cardiac event. It's also recommended that patients with cardiovascular disease have an annual influenza vaccination.

Don't be afraid to ask questions about the benefits and risks of varied treatment options with your team of caregivers. The key is to 'know your numbers' and to favorably modify your risk factors with aggressive lifestyle modification and cardioprotective medications (e.g., aspirin, cholesterol-lowering statins, beta-blockers), if necessary. The challenge is YOURS.

RESTING PULSE RATE INDICATES HEART ATTACK RISK

Postmenopausal women with a resting heart rate of more than 76 beats per minute are 26 percent more likely to suffer a heart attack in the next eight years compared with women whose resting heart rates are 62 beats or less per minute. Moreover, this relationship was independent of physical activity. A similar association between resting heart rate and heart attack risk has been reported in men.

(*British Medical Journal,* Feb. 2009).

Prediabetes: The First Road Sign "On Your Way to Diabetes"

Kathy Faitel, RN

According to the Centers for Disease Control and Prevention, more than 29 million Americans have diabetes. Moreover, it is estimated that there are an additional 86 million people that have pre-diabetes, that is, who are on the road to diabetes.

There are two types of diabetes. Type 1 diabetes is caused by an autoimmune destruction of the beta cells of the pancreas that produce insulin. People with type 1 diabetes are dependent upon giving themselves insulin to match the amount of carbohydrates that they consume. However, only a small percentage of people have this type of diabetes. Type 2 diabetes accounts for 95 percent of all people with diabetes. A precursor of type 2 diabetes is pre-diabetes, a road sign that reads "Diabetes Ahead," but the progression to diabetes is not necessarily inevitable. Diabetes does not occur overnight. But, like any road construction, ignoring the signs can have dire consequences. Because of the increased risk not only for developing diabetes, but cardiovascular disease and stroke as well, diagnosing pre-diabetes has taken on a greater urgency.

The hallmark of diabetes is high blood glucose levels that, over time, damage blood vessels, organs, and nerves. It is caused by insufficient insulin secretion from beta cells of the pancreas, or an inability of cells to utilize the insulin, called insulin resistance. Insulin is an important hormone that facilitates glucose transport into body cells to provide energy.

Type 2 diabetes is diagnosed by one of several blood tests. A normal fasting blood glucose (FBG), taken after an eight-hour fast, should be less than 100 milligrams per deciter (mg/dl). A FBG over 126 mg/dl is diagnosed as diabetes. It indicates that glucose is not being adequately cleared from the bloodstream following an overnight fast. Another blood test called an oral glucose tolerance test (OGT) can also be helpful. After fasting eight hours, a drink containing 75 gm of glucose is consumed and a blood glucose sample is taken after two hours. A blood glucose value of 200 mg/dl or higher signifies diabetes. A third test is called hemoglobin (Hgb) A1c. This test has become more widely used over the last 10 years. Because glucose attaches to the protein molecule of the red blood cell in proportion to the amount

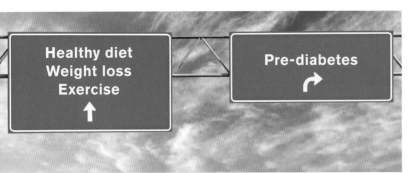

of glucose in the blood, this test gives a window into an "average" blood glucose over the previous three month period (because the life of a red blood cell is about three months). HgbA1c values over 6.5 percent indicate diabetes.

A FBG between 100 and 125 mg/dl, or an OGT between 140 and 199 mg/dl indicate "pre-diabetes"; blood glucose levels are elevated, but not yet high enough to be diagnosed as diabetes. HgbA1c values between 5.7 and 6.4 percent indicates pre-diabetes as well.

How do you know if you are at risk for diabetes or already on the road to diabetes? If you…

- are 45 years of age or older.
- are overweight or obese (body mass index greater than 25).
- are sedentary or not regularly physically active.
- have a member of your immediate family who already has diabetes.
- are of African-American, Hispanic, American Indian, Asian-American, or Pacific Islander decent.
- are a woman and delivered a baby weighing 9 pounds or more or developed gestational diabetes during pregnancy.
- have high blood pressure, low HDL (good cholesterol), or high triglyceride level (over 250 mg/dl).
- have been diagnosed with impaired fasting glucose or impaired glucose tolerance.

What can you do? The first step is to discuss your risk factors and blood glucose values with your doctor. Work with him/her to develop a plan of healthy eating, weight loss and regular exercise. A classic study called the "Diabetes Prevention Program," randomly assigned more than 3,000 overweight adults with pre-diabetes to one of three study groups. The first group (control group) was advised to simply lose weight and exercise. The second group (drug group) was placed on Glucophage (metformin, a common oral anti-diabetic medication) with diet and exercise recommendations. The third group (Lifestyle) got intensive counseling and follow-up to exercise at least 150 minutes a week and eat less (i.e., to achieve at least a 7 percent reduction in body weight). Results showed a 31 percent reduction in diabetes risk in the "drug" group, and a whopping 58 percent reduction in the "lifestyle" group, demonstrating the powerful effects of exercise and modest weight loss (*New England Journal of Medicine,* Feb. 2002).

The bottom line? The best way to prevent type 2 diabetes is a healthy diet, regular aerobic exercise, and weight loss—if appropriate.

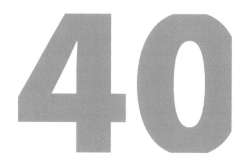

THE RULE OF "40"

Whatever your total cholesterol level is, reduction of that level by approximately 40 mg/dL reduces the relative risk of either an initial or subsequent cardiovascular event in half.

(*American Heart Journal,* Sept. 1995).

Diabetes And Heart Disease

Steven C. Ajluni, M.D.

Diabetes is a highly prevalent metabolic condition that has reached almost epidemic proportions in the United States. Today, more than 10 million diabetics are being treated, many of whom became diabetic at younger ages (even adolescents) due to the escalating prevalence of obesity and our increasingly sedentary lifestyle. Strictly speaking, diabetes is defined as fasting hyperglycemia (elevated blood sugar) that occurs due to either a relative lack or ineffectiveness of intrinsic insulin, a hormone secreted by the pancreas that is responsible for helping blood glucose transport into cells where it is used for energy.

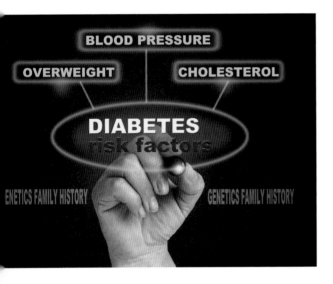

The predominant cause of type 2 diabetes (the most prevalent form) is a genetic or acquired resistance to the effects of secreted insulin. Accordingly, glucose transport does not occur effectively. Insulin resistance (aggravated by central obesity) leads to the systematic uptick in insulin secretion from the pancreas in an ultimately futile effort to restore normal blood glucose levels. In addition to its effect on blood glucose, insulin is known to behave as a growth hormone. As such, it aggravates and accelerates the growth of atherosclerotic plaques in our blood vessels and increases the formation of fibrous connective tissue in the heart. Ultimately, this results in a cascade of adverse clinical responses, including a more extensive burden of atherosclerosis, associated hypertension and renal vascular dysfunction (which results in protein leakage and worsening of kidney function). Over time, vascular consequences of diabetes include the progressive narrowing of coronary blood vessels and peripheral arteries as well as microscopic changes in small blood vessels in the kidneys, nerves, and retinae. This leads to clinical manifestations of diabetes with increased risks of heart attack, stroke, kidney failure, and vascular insufficiency of the lower extremities.

To combat the sobering consequences of diabetes, it is imperative to focus on the "at risk" patient (those with a family history of premature cardiovascular disease and associated conditions such as obesity, hypertension, hypercholesterolemia, and sleep apnea) which collectively increases end organ destruction by aggravating the underlying problem of insulin resistance. Treating obesity and sleep apnea, and optimizing cholesterol and blood pressure control have been shown to slow the progression of these devastating complications. Exercising regularly and maintaining a healthy low fat diet also play a major role in protecting one against the ravages of diabetes.

It is important for patients and doctors alike to optimally address the causes of diabetes and strive to adeptly play this lifelong poker game by minimizing vascular damage to reduce the risk of cardiovascular complications. Patients should become proactive in this process, attempting to achieve optimal weight control and treatment of sleep apnea, hypertension, and cholesterol abnormalities via lifestyle change and pharmacotherapies, if appropriate. Periodic physician-directed cardiovascular screening may be helpful in selected patients to identify the early signs of subclinical cardiovascular disease.

Perhaps the late General Normal Schwarzkopf summed it up best when asked how he would respond to an enemy attack. "Counterattack," he replied. When the enemy is heart disease, the strategy is no different.

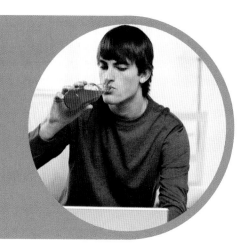

DIABETES EPIDEMIC?

According to the Centers for Disease Control and Prevention, one in three U.S. adults could have diabetes in 2050. Why? The predicted increase is due to aging of the population, obesity, our habitually sedentary lifestyle (e.g., too little exercise, excessive sitting time), and increases in the population of minority groups that are at higher risk for developing type 2 diabetes.

(www.cdc.gov)

Is Your Blood Pressure Low Enough?

Steven Almany, M.D.

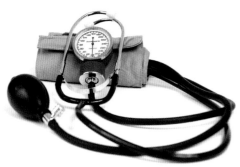

Approximately one out of three adults in the United Sates has high blood pressure (hypertension). Some people do not even know they have high blood pressure, as it is often without symptoms. Moreover, many have high blood pressure that is not adequately treated.

Current guidelines from the National Joint Committee suggest a systolic blood pressure of less than 140 mmHg for healthy people under 60 years of age and less than 150 mmHg for individuals aged 60 and older. For adults with kidney disease or diabetes, the recommendation is less than 130 mmHg. However, a new study may force us to reevaluate these recommendations.

A trial sponsored by the National Institute of Health called SPRINT, or the Systolic Blood Pressure Intervention Trial, in which approximately 9,300 men and women were involved, was stopped more than one year ahead of schedule in order to quickly disseminate the significant preliminary results. This investigation included patients that were 50 years and older who had kidney disease or were at increased risk for heart disease.

Patients were divided into two groups and treated with medications to lower their blood pressure. One group had a systolic blood pressure goal of 140 mmHg or less and, on average, took two different blood pressure medications. The other group, which was treated more aggressively, had an objective to achieve 120 mmHg or less and took an average of three medications. Both groups tolerated the medications without significant side effects. The results, which may surprise some physicians, showed a startling 25 percent reduction in mortality and a 33 percent reduction in cardiovascular morbidity in the group that was treated to the lower blood pressure goal.

The study was carried out at 100 medical centers throughout the United States and Puerto Rico. It began in 2009 and was scheduled to last nine years; however, it was prematurely halted because of the somewhat surprising results. The investigators used varied blood pressure lowering drugs, including diuretics, calcium channel blockers and angiotensin converting enzyme (ACE) inhibitors. These medications are typically available as low cost generics.

Although these preliminary results are intriguing, others suggest caution in recommending that all patients be treated to a systolic blood pressure goal of less than 120 mmHg, since the findings were based on a highly selected patient population. As a patient, your designated blood pressure goal should be discussed at length with your physician, especially if you have risk factors for cardiovascular disease. The results of the SPRINT trial, will likely affect future blood pressure guidelines.

Improving Cardiovascular Health: Combating the Metabolic Syndrome

Kirk D. Hendrickson, M.S.

In June 2008, Tim Russert, the beloved NBC correspondent and host of *Meet the Press,* died suddenly of a heart attack. He was only 58 years old. Apparently, a plaque ruptured in his coronary artery, triggering a clot and causing a fatal heart rhythm. Although Russert exercised regularly and received excellent medical care, he had high blood pressure, abdominal obesity, elevated triglycerides (blood fats) and low HDL "good" cholesterol—characteristics of the metabolic syndrome (MS).

MS is defined by a clustering of risk factors that appear to promote the development of atherosclerotic cardiovascular disease. These include: increased waist circumference (greater than or equal to 40 inches in men and greater than or equal to 35 inches in women); elevated triglycerides (greater than or equal to 150 mg/dl); reduced HDL or "good" cholesterol (less than 40 mg/dl in men and less than 50 mg/dl in women); elevated blood pressure (greater than or equal to 130 mm Hg systolic or greater than or equal to 85 mm Hg diastolic); and, elevated fasting blood sugar (greater than or equal to 100 mg/dl). Having at least three of these five characteristics indicates MS. MS is present in 24 percent of all adults in the United States and in more than 40 percent of men and women over age 65. This proportion is expected to grow to approximately two-thirds of the adult population. There is also a genetic predisposition to develop MS in patients of Hispanic and Asian Indian ethnicity.

The major underlying risk factors for MS are abdominal obesity and insulin resistance; other associated conditions include physical inactivity, aging and hormonal imbalance. Abdominal obesity, as signified by an increased waist circumference, predicts increased deposits of fat, known as visceral fat, surrounding the major organs such as the liver, kidneys and heart. The accumulation of visceral fat, and the excessive amounts of fat deposited under the skin in the abdominal region, give the patient a characteristic "apple" shape and are correlated with several cardiometabolic abnormalities. Conversely, individuals that have excess fat distributed in the lower extremities (legs and buttocks) do not appear to be at increased risk for MS.

The accumulation of visceral fat, and the excessive amounts of fat deposited under the skin in the abdominal region, give the patient a characteristic "apple" shape and are correlated with several cardiometabolic abnormalities.

The associated MS abnormalities include an increased production of triglycerides and small particle LDL-cholesterol, and decreased production of HDL or "good" cholesterol that, collectively, increase the risk of cholesterol plaque accumulation in the coronary arteries. Presumably, high blood pressure damages the walls of the arteries and increases the risk for clots, and the associated obesity is often accompanied by increased indices of inflammation (e.g., high sensitivity C-reactive protein) which can also heighten the risk of blood clots. Persons with MS have a fivefold risk of developing diabetes and a two to three fold increased risk of coronary disease or stroke. Insulin resistance diminishes the normal utilization of blood sugar for energy, increasing blood glucose concentrations, and resulting in overproduction of insulin by the pancreas. Ultimately, this may lead to the development of type 2 diabetes and/or increased cardiovascular risk.

The primary methods to prevent and treat those with MS include therapeutic lifestyle changes to reduce body weight and fat stores, structured exercise, increased lifestyle physical activity and the transition to a heart-healthy diet. Reduction of abdominal obesity, the prime underlying cause of MS, is the main therapeutic target. A reduced calorie diet that limits total fat to 25 to 35 percent of daily calories, decreasing saturated fat intake, with the majority of fat coming from polyunsaturated and monounsaturated fatty acids, such as fish, nuts, and vegetable oils, is recommended. Unsaturated fats can help reduce elevated triglycerides and raise the low HDL levels that are often found in individuals with MS. Sugar and starch (simple carbohydrates), including sugar sweetened beverages, should be severely limited or markedly reduced since they are major sources of excess calories and promote abnormally high insulin production. A modified Mediterranean-style diet high in fruits, vegetables, nuts, whole grains, and olive oil and lower in saturated fat (less than 10 percent), may have particular benefit for individuals with MS.

In summary, MS significantly increases the risk for coronary disease, stroke and type 2 diabetes. Adoption of a heart healthy, Mediterranean-style diet, and increasing physical activity/exercise aimed at reducing abdominal obesity and improving insulin resistance, can reduce the magnitude of all five risk factors associated with MS. Adjunctive resistance training also has beneficial effects. An increase in physical activity and aerobic fitness can improve insulin action and reduce visceral fat stores, even without an accompanying reduction in body weight, suggesting that physical activity is as effective in preventing insulin resistance as is losing body weight.

THERAPIES FOR TYPE 2 DIABETES AND HEART DISEASE

For the many patients with type 2 diabetes who have less extensive heart disease and for whom angioplasty is judged to be more appropriate than bypass surgery, prompt coronary intervention did not further reduce the risk of cardiovascular events, as compared with medical therapy alone.

(*New England Journal of Medicine*, June 2009).

Triggers of Acute Cardiac Events and Preventive Strategies

Barry A. Franklin, Ph.D.

Considerable evidence now suggests that heart attack or acute myocardial infarction (AMI) and sudden cardiac death (SCD, i.e., abrupt cessation of the normal heartbeat) can be triggered by physical, chemical and psychological stressors, including heavy physical exertion and situations that create heightened emotional stress (*Circulation,* July 2011). This review summarizes the evidence supporting the impact of selected triggers of acute cardiac events, as well as the potential role of various preventive strategies.

Physical stress

Although considerable evidence suggests that structured exercise, increased lifestyle physical activity, or both, may be cardioprotective, exertion-related cardiovascular complications have been reported in the medical literature and the lay press, suggesting that vigorous physical activity may actually trigger AMI or SCD in some persons. The increased risk appears to be largely limited to individuals with known or occult cardiovascular disease who were performing unaccustomed vigorous physical activity (*New England Journal of Medicine,* Dec. 1993). Thus, it is the combination of vigorous physical exertion and a diseased or susceptible heart, rather than the exercise per se, that seems to present the potential for exertion-related cardiovascular complications.

Strenuous physical activity, especially when sudden or involving unusually high levels of physical exertion, may transiently increase the risk for AMI and/ or SCD. These include high-intensity competitive and recreational activities (e.g., racquet sports). The excitement of competition can further augment sympathetic activity and epinephrine levels, increasing the likelihood of threatening heart rhythms. Other activities that are associated with increased cardiac demands and a greater incidence of cardiovascular events include deer hunting (*American Journal of Cardiology,* July 2007) and snow removal (*American Journal of Cardiology,* Oct. 2003), both of which involve superimposed isometric exertion in a cold environment.

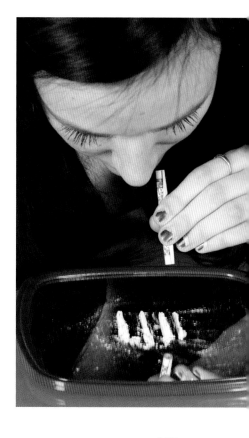

Chemical stress

There is considerable evidence to suggest that chemical stressors, including illicit drugs, can increase the risk of AMI in persons with and without underlying heart disease. For example, one study reported a 24-fold increase in the risk of AMI in the 60 minutes immediately following cocaine use (*Circulation,* June 1999). Similarly, the risk of AMI is elevated five times versus normal conditions in the hour after smoking marijuana (*Circulation,* June 2001).

In recent years, a growing body of research has reported consistent associations between active and passive cigarette smoking, short-term elevations in environmental air pollution, and increases in acute cardiovascular events, including AMI, threatening cardiac rhythms, and heart failure exacerbation. Even a very short period of passive or secondhand smoke has persistent vascular consequences. One analysis concluded that omnipresent air pollution exposure and the associated population risk may have considerable public health relevance, highlighting the potential cardioprotective benefits of lowering air pollution levels to current Environmental Protection Agency standards (*Lancet,* Feb. 2011). Moreover, city-wide smoking bans have unequivocally resulted in a reduced incidence of hospitalizations for acute cardiac events (*New England Journal of Medicine,* July 2008).

Psychological stress

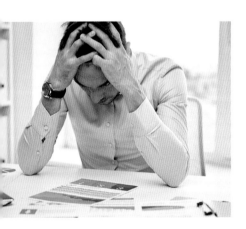

Psychological stressors that increase sympathetic activity also have the potential to trigger acute cardiovascular events. Emotional and stress-related psychological exposures that are associated with an acute, transient increase in the risk for cardiovascular events include earthquakes, sleep deprivation, sporting events, outbursts of anger, and distinct episodes of anxiety. More recently, natural disasters, such as Hurricane Katrina, and stock market crashes have been linked to a heightened risk of acute cardiovascular events (*Physician and Sportsmedicine,* Nov. 2011).

Perhaps the most widely-cited analysis involved the massive Northridge, California earthquake that occurred on January 17, 1994 (*New England Journal of Medicine,* Feb. 1996). Millions of people were awakened simultaneously at 4:41 a.m. by one of the strongest earthquakes ever recorded in a major North American city (Los Angeles County). A review of the county coroner's records suggested that the associated emotional stress likely triggered a disproportionate number of regional SCDs, from a daily average of 4.6 in the preceding week to 24 on the day of the earthquake! Most of the victims (96 percent) had either risk factors for or a history of heart disease. The researchers concluded that extreme emotional stress may precipitate fatal cardiac events in individuals with known or underlying heart disease.

Prophylactic interventions

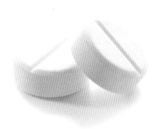

Is it possible to prophylactically reduce the adverse impact of potential triggers? Some clinicians suggest that high risk patients take cardioprotective medications (e.g., aspirin, short-acting beta-blockers) before engaging in activities that may impose excessive physical or psychological stress. Others suggest that such activities should be contraindicated. Additional preventive strategies include counseling inactive patients with known or suspected heart disease to avoid unaccustomed heavy physical exertion and high-risk activities (e.g., snow removal) and practices (e.g., illicit drug use), implementing anger management strategies, and strict enforcement of environmental regulations/public policy regarding air pollution. One of the most powerful interventions to prevent triggered acute cardiac events involves regular endurance exercise, which is associated with improvements in cardiovascular function that decrease the likelihood of coronary plaque rupture and thrombosis and/or threatening heart rhythms (*Physician and Sportsmedicine,* Nov. 2011).

In summary, SCD kills an estimated 850 Americans every day or 310,000 adults each year. Men with known or latent heart disease between the ages of 50 and 65 appear to be a particularly susceptible subset of the population. For example, consider the untimely deaths of the beloved newscaster, Tim Russert, and the fine actor, James Gandolfini, at 58 and 51 years, respectively. Unquestionably, some of these fatalities are triggered by physical, chemical, and psychological stressors, especially in combination. Understanding the potential triggers of acute cardiac events and avoiding them when possible, while embracing preventive strategies, will likely save lives.

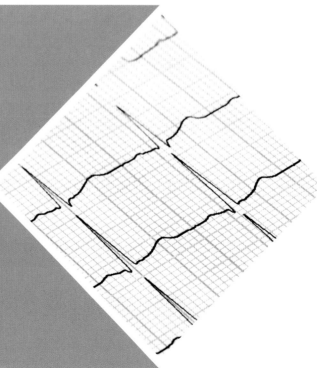

MANY HEART ATTACKS OCCUR WITHOUT DISCERNABLE SYMPTOMS

According to a just-published report of 9,498 participants who were free of cardiovascular disease at baseline and followed for an average of 8.9 years, new heart attacks were documented in 703 patients, and 45 percent of these had no discernible symptoms. These heart attacks were detected solely by accidental electrocardiographic findings during subsequent examinations. Nevertheless, both symptomatic and asymptomatic patients who experienced new heart attacks had a poorer prognosis. The investigators highlighted the importance of detecting "silent" heart attacks in clinical practice, using serial 12-lead electrocardiograms, and suggested that this patient cohort also warrants more aggressive prevention interventions in the future.

(*Circulation,* May 2016)

Air Pollution and Cardiovascular Disease

Barry A. Franklin, Ph.D.

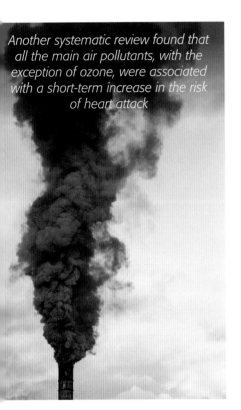

Another systematic review found that all the main air pollutants, with the exception of ozone, were associated with a short-term increase in the risk of heart attack

Increasing epidemiologic and clinical evidence has led to a heightened concern about the deleterious effects of air pollution and cigarette smoking on cardiovascular mortality. Of special interest are several environmental air pollutants, including carbon monoxide, oxides of nitrogen, sulfur dioxide, ozone, lead, secondhand smoke (the single largest contributor to indoor air pollution) and particulate matter. The latter are generally classified by size or diameter, as coarse, fine, or ultrafine. Fine particulate matter, which have been most commonly associated with increased hospitalization and cardiovascular mortality, can be generated from vehicle emissions, tire fragmentation and road dust, industrial combustion, metal processing, construction and demolition activities, residential wood burning and forest fires.

Relevant research

Compelling evidence that exposure to air pollution contributes to cardiovascular disease and death continues to grow, including three lines of epidemiologic research. First, population-based studies in 20 cities across the United States and in many cities abroad have found the death rate from cardiac causes to be elevated on the day following high levels of particulate air pollution. Second, several reports have shown that high levels of particulate air pollution are associated with increased hospital admissions for anginal chest pain and heart attacks. Third, an especially well-designed investigation strongly linked high levels of particulate air pollution in the greater Boston area with the triggering of acute cardiac events (*Circulation,* June 2001).

Additional reports have emerged to support the notion that these epidemiologic data truly reflect the adverse effects of particulate matter on the cardiovascular system. Another systematic review found that all the main air pollutants, with the exception of ozone, were associated with a short-term increase in the risk of heart attack (*Journal of the American Medical Association,* Feb. 2012). Other studies suggest that possible links between exposure to particulate matter and cardiovascular events may be related to abrupt increases in heart rate and blood pressure, blood coagulation, vascular inflammation, injury or dysfunction, and reduced variability in the heart rate response. These deleterious responses, alone or in combination, may serve to increase the likelihood of acute cardiac events.

Cardiovascular effects of secondhand smoke: Widely underestimated

Further support that the increased anginal symptoms and heart attacks attributed to air pollution comes from studies demonstrating that the cardiovascular system is highly sensitive to the toxins in secondhand smoke. According to one provocative report (*Circulation*, May 2005), the adverse cardiovascular effects of even brief periods of passive smoking are, on average, 80 to 90 percent as large as those from chronic smoking. Moreover, in the same report, non-smokers increased their risk of heart disease by approximately 30 percent if they lived with a smoker. Collectively, these studies and other reports (*Circulation*, Aug. 2013) suggest that workplace and community adoption of a smoke-free environment has the potential to rapidly improve the cardiovascular health status of its citizens while simultaneously reducing heart-related hospital admissions.

In closing, three important implications regarding the potential hazards of passive-smoking and maintaining smoke-free environments should be emphasized. First, physicians should counsel their patients, especially those with known or suspected heart disease, to avoid smoky environments (e.g., bars, casinos). Second, policy makers should ensure that all public environments are smoke-free. Finally, recognizing the insidious and pervasive nature of air pollution, and the fact that it is a widely underappreciated trigger of acute cardiac events, may serve to maximize the potential for cardiovascular risk reduction by addressing a portion of the incidence of coronary disease that is unexplained by traditional risk factors.

AIR POLLUTION AND HEART DISEASE

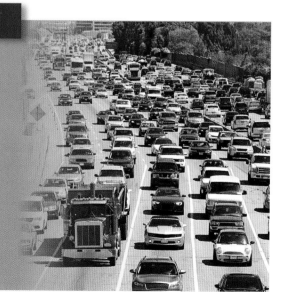

In a widely-cited report, researchers combined data from 36 separate studies and calculated the relative risk posed by varied known heart attack triggers, including the proportion of all heart attacks estimated to have been caused by each trigger. Although cocaine use was identified as the most likely to provoke a cardiovascular event in an individual, air pollution, particularly in heavy traffic, had the greatest negative population effect as more people are exposed to it. The investigators concluded that improvement of air quality is a very relevant target to reduce the incidence of cardiovascular disease in the general population.

(*The Lancet,* Feb. 2011)

Warning: Sleeplessness May Be Harmful to Your Heart

Steven Ajluni, M.D.

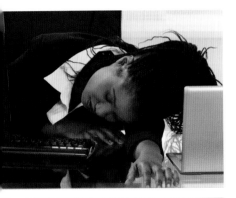

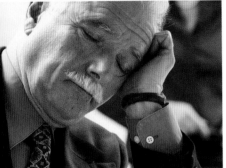

A common misconception among patients is that insomnia is primarily a social issue or simply an inconvenience, rather than a medical condition that can affect their health and well-being. Recently, however, we've begun to understand the important association between unhealthy sleep patterns and abnormal cardiac physiology. The basic reason for this connection concerns oxygenation, or the lack thereof, during the nighttime hours in patients who are afflicted with sleep apnea.

Sleep apnea occurs in two forms. The first involves obstructive sleep apnea (OSA). This is a mechanical obstruction to airflow that occurs primarily as the upper airway collapses when a patient is lying supine. This leads to a characteristic snore, associated hypoventilation and a reduced level of oxygen in the bloodstream. The other form is referred to as central sleep apnea (CSA), where breathing temporarily ceases due to a reduced respiratory drive. Whereas the typical patient with OSA tends to have a large body habitus and a thickened neck, a patient with CSA may actually be thin and more likely to be affected by impaired heart pump function (congestive heart failure and cardiomyopathy).

The common denominator between OSA and CSA is a lack of oxygenation during sleep. Oftentimes, this results in excessive stimulation of the sympathetic nervous system, producing a host of adverse vascular and physiologic effects, including hypertension and heart rhythm irregularities. It may also cause adverse structural changes in the heart's electrical conduction tissue, resulting in abnormal rhythms like atrial fibrillation and/or slow heart rates (bradycardia). In fact, when studying patients with a history of atrial fibrillation or those who may need a permanent pacemaker, we find coexistent sleep apnea in more than 60 percent of all cases.

Which patients should undergo evaluation for sleep apnea? Typically, these include individuals with a history of excessive daytime fatigue and hypersomnolence. Such persons may tend to nod off during the afternoon or require frequent naps. They tend to snore at night and frequently awaken. Others may experience gasping or nighttime periods where they actually cease to breathe as they struggle for ventilation. This can be frightening, to say the least. Once a history has been obtained, it is often recommended that a patient be seen by a sleep specialist, which may include an overnight study called a polysomnogram.

The treatment of sleep apnea involves confirming the diagnosis and improving oxygenation during the night. It may also involve simple maneuvers such as changing the position in which you sleep. Treatment may include a continuous positive airway pressure device using a CPAP mask. A structural assessment may also be performed by an ear, nose, and throat specialist who may recommend either surgical intervention or oral appliance therapy. Every patient is unique and an individualized approach will often lead to the most effective treatment options. Most patients will respond favorably to treatment if they persevere and attempt, in good faith, the interventions that their physician may suggest.

INSOMNIA RAISES HEART DISEASE RISK

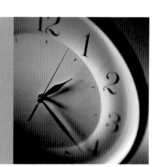

People who have trouble falling asleep or staying asleep have a higher risk of developing heart disease. Possible reason? Insomnia may be linked to increased stress hormones, blood pressure and inflammation, all of which increase the risk for heart disease.

(*Circulation*, Nov. 2011)

SLEEP DURATION PREDICTS CARDIOVASCULAR RISK

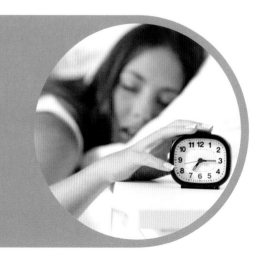

Currently, there is no evidence that sleeping between six and eight hours per day is associated with any long-term health consequences. On the other hand, people who report consistently sleeping five hours or less per night should be regarded as a higher risk group for nonfatal and fatal cardiovascular events. The mechanisms that underlie these associations are not fully understood.

(*European Heart Journal*, Jan. 2011)

Fainting: A Harbinger of Cardiovascular Disease?

David E. Haines, M.D.

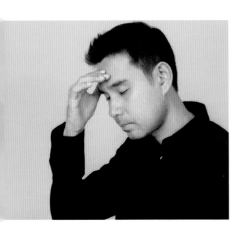

A simple swoon, a drop attack—these are symptoms that afflict as many as 50 percent of people during their lifetime. Clearly, the great majority of these fainting spells (syncope) are harmless, but occasionally, they represent a warning symptom of a dangerous, possibly life-threatening heart rhythm abnormality. It is the challenge of the physician to reassure the vast majority of patients with a benign form of fainting, and continue with an appropriate cardiac workup for patients at higher risk.

The common faint often occurs if patients stand too quickly, if they are fatigued, warm or nauseated, or are exposed to a fearful or unpleasant stimulus. Even the sight of blood may cause this response in some people. The physiology of the common faint is somewhat complex, and involves the autonomic or involuntary nervous system. The autonomic nervous system controls important bodily functions such as heart rate, blood vessel constriction, skin temperature, blood pressure, respiratory rate and the digestive movements of the gut. After a noxious stimulus or sudden positional change, the heart beats harder and faster. This stimulates sensory fibers in the heart muscle that send signals to the vasomotor center of the brain. Paradoxically, the brain sometimes responds with vagal nerve stimulation, dramatically slowing the heart, and withdrawal of stimulation of the alpha nerve receptors in the peripheral arteries, causing them to dilate and the blood pressure to fall. These responses may lead to diminished flow of blood and oxygen to the brain, and loss of consciousness. Because light sensors in the eyes are more sensitive to drops in oxygen and blood pressure than the rest of the brain, patients often experience a "black out" or "white out" before they actually lose consciousness. Loss of consciousness is very brief, with a return to normalcy within seconds or minutes. If the patient feels a fainting episode coming on, it can sometimes be aborted by performing a "squat and squeeze" maneuver. This involves assuming a squat position and tightly contracting all upper and lower body muscles in an isometric fashion, which temporarily raises blood pressure.

In most cases, a careful history, physical examination and electrocardiogram by a qualified health care provider is all that is needed to evaluate a patient with the common faint. Sometimes, additional testing is performed with more prolonged electrocardiographic monitoring, echocardiography, stress testing, and tilt table testing. The diagnoses that the doctor "can't afford to miss" include threatening slow or rapid heart rhythm irregularities, impending heart attack, or a neurological seizure disorder. Clinical factors that raise suspicion about more dangerous types of syncope include older age, history of prior heart attack, history of decreased heart function or heart failure, sudden drop attacks associated with physical injury, and slow recovery of normal wakefulness after the event. Syncope occurring post exercise is most often benign, but when an individual faints during physical activity or sport, this may be a sign of an underlying serious condition. In these cases, more extensive testing (and sometimes hospitalization) is warranted.

Some have suggested that fainting is an evolutionary-derived mechanism to protect us from predatory attack. However, it is difficult to view this as a positive adaptive behavior in modern times. Fortunately, most faints are non-sudden and are not associated with injury. If a patient is prone to more dramatic drops, then chronic medication to prevent these events may be prescribed. It may also be wise to have someone else climb the ladder to clean the gutters in the Spring.

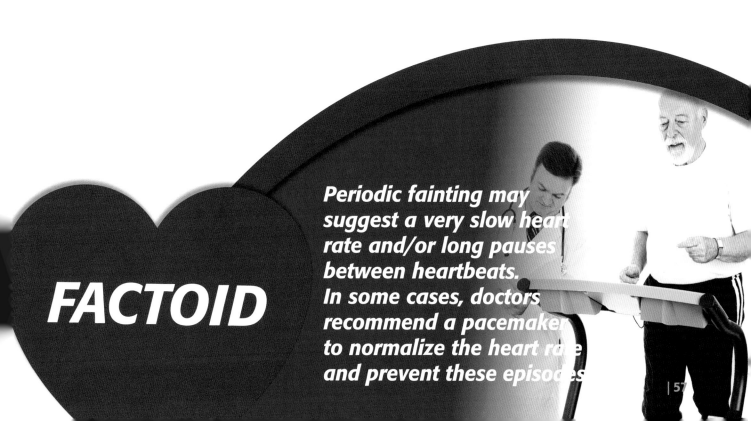

FACTOID

Periodic fainting may suggest a very slow heart rate and/or long pauses between heartbeats. In some cases, doctors recommend a pacemaker to normalize the heart rate and prevent these episodes

Prognostic Value of Coronary Artery Calcification

Harold Friedman, M.D.

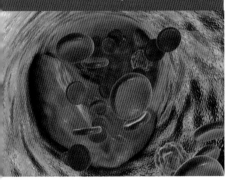

Research has shown that elevated CT calcium scores correlate with the risk of developing cardiovascular disease over periods ranging from three to 15 years.

Despite numerous studies involving thousands of patients with and without heart disease, the role of coronary artery calcium to assess a person's heart attack risk remains poorly understood and somewhat controversial.

The presence of calcium in the wall of an artery indicates the existence of atherosclerosis or "hardening of the arteries." This finding is part of the natural aging process but accelerates in bodily areas under stress due to chronic inflammation. Calcium appears within the coronary arteries over time due to inflammation caused by accumulation of cholesterol crystals, scar tissue and debris from dead cells. Once the calcium and cholesterol deposits form within the arterial wall, they never disappear. Autopsy studies have shown that in many cases the greater the amount of atherosclerosis or thickening of a blood vessel wall, the greater its calcium content.

A computed tomography (CT) scan, which uses X-rays, can accurately detect calcium deposits and calculates a score based on the total amount of the calcium that is present. The calcium score is highly reproducible and is typically adjusted based on a person's gender and age. The test takes approximately 10 minutes, requires no intravenous line and is relatively inexpensive. Modern-day CT scans produce pictures that use less X-ray exposure than a mammogram.

Research has shown that elevated CT calcium scores correlate with the risk of developing cardiovascular disease over periods ranging from 3 to 15 years. This means that a person with an abnormally high score is more likely to experience a heart attack, unstable angina (chest pain requiring hospital treatment), sudden cardiac death or stroke. The absence of calcium (score equals zero) signifies a very low risk with less than a 1 percent chance of a major cardiac event over the next five years. On the other hand, a high score (greater than 400) indicates a risk up to 12 times greater. This information can be extremely useful and alert a physician of a patient's heightened risk for heart attack or stroke, even in the absence of conventional risk factors.

Since the 1970s, risk factors used to evaluate the likelihood of a person developing heart disease have included age, diabetes, hypertension, cigarette smoking, elevated cholesterol, obesity and physical inactivity. However, the risk factor profile may be inaccurate and misleading in some population subsets. Thus, a coronary artery calcium score may be particularly useful when traditional risk factors indicate an intermediate risk for heart disease. In such cases, it may be difficult to decide whether cholesterol lowering therapy or further diagnostic testing should be recommended. One large European study reported that up to 50 percent of patients may be reclassified to either a higher or lower risk group based on the additional information provided by the calcium score (*Journal of the American College of Cardiology,* Oct. 2010).

Increasing evidence now suggests that the coronary artery calcium score may, in the future, become a routine component of a person's cardiovascular risk assessment. The American College of Cardiology has now endorsed limited use of calcium scoring in intermediate risk patients. The utility of the calcium score lies in its ability to identify persons without symptoms who may be at much higher risk for cardiovascular events than otherwise expected. An elevated coronary calcium score also serves to reinforce and stimulate patient counseling regarding the importance of diet, exercise and medications used for cholesterol and blood pressure control. It holds the promise of improving our ability to predict and possibly prevent the development of heart disease.

Do you know your coronary artery calcium score?

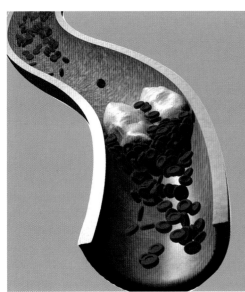

CONSIDER A CORONARY ARTERY CALCIUM TEST BEFORE TAKING STATINS

A coronary artery calcium test identifies signs of plaque in the heart's vasculature— a significant risk factor for heart attack. Persons with a 'zero' calcium score may safely choose to forgo statin therapy and instead control cardiac risk factors through a prudent diet, regular physical activity, and the avoidance or cessation of cigarette smoking. The absence of coronary artery calcium reclassifies approximately one-half of all candidates as not eligible for statin therapy.

(*Journal of the American College of Cardiology,* Oct. 2015)

Atrial Fibrillation, Risk of Stroke, and Long-Term Cognitive Function

David E. Haines, M.D.

The major focus of management of patients with AF has been two-fold; reduction of symptoms and reduction of the risk of blood clot and stroke.

Normal ECG rhythm

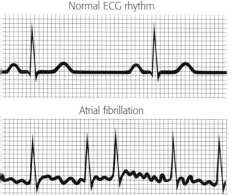

Atrial fibrillation

Atrial fibrillation (AF) is a common heart rhythm irregularity (arrhythmia), estimated to be present in more than 6 million Americans. While AF is more prevalent in older individuals, it can occur in patients of all ages. The major focus of management of patients with AF has been two-fold; reduction of symptoms and reduction of the risk of blood clot and stroke. Because the left atrium does not contract normally during AF, blood flow through the chamber is suboptimal. Eddies and stagnant pools of blood during AF can lead to clotting. If the blood clot remains adherent to the atrial wall, then there is no problem. But if the clot breaks off (embolizes), it flows downstream and lodges in an artery. If this artery is in the brain, part of the brain dies, leading to a clinical stroke.

The mainstay of stroke prevention in AF is the use of oral anticoagulation with warfarin (Coumadin), dabigatran (Pradaxa), rivaroxaban (Xarelto) or apixaban (Eliquis). All of these drugs have been demonstrated to substantially reduce the risk of stroke, and all have acceptably low risks of bleeding complications. An alternative to oral anticoagulants includes devices to occlude or obliterate the left atrial appendage (the source of more than 90 percent of clots). Although this approach is not necessarily better than medication, it is an important option for patients who cannot tolerate anticoagulant drugs. An alternative approach for reduction of blood clot risk is catheter ablation of AF. Catheters inserted into the heart are used to create ablation lesions that turn into lines of scar tissue that block the electrical transmission of AF impulses. Prevention of recurrent AF with catheter ablation should theoretically prevent stroke, but this is unproven at this time. Long term anticoagulation in high risk patients is still recommended even after successful catheter ablation.

Most physicians believe that we understand the exact link from AF to stroke—AF causes disrupted blood flow, clots form, then they embolize and cause a stroke. However, a recent report (*Circulation,* May 2014) challenged this simplistic view. In a trial of 2,580 patients with pacemakers, 51 suffered a stroke during follow up. Of those, 26 had some evidence of AF on the recordings from their implanted pacemakers. However, only five had AF episodes recorded within 30 days of their stroke. Thus, the presence of AF was strongly associated with the risk of stroke but the actual strokes were not linked to the AF episodes. What is clear is that appropriate anticoagulation in these patients with subclinical AF might have prevented some of these strokes from occurring.

In addition to stroke, a concerning association of AF to cognitive decline has been established. The risk of Alzheimer's dementia and vascular dementia is higher in AF patients as compared with those without this heart rhythm disturbance. Our hypothesis is that AF patients are at risk for "microembolism," that is, micro strokes that do not cause any direct symptoms but can result in progressive loss of brain function. Despite the strong association of AF to cognitive decline, a direct causal link has not been proven. Many medical conditions commonly found in AF patients (high blood pressure, diabetes, inflammation) may directly cause brain injury. So is AF the cause or just an innocent bystander? We and other researchers are trying to find the answer to this perplexing question.

While we are waiting for answers, what can we do? Optimal treatment of AF is a start. That includes appropriate blood pressure control, treatment of sleep apnea (if present), anticoagulation therapy in all patients with risk factors for stroke, and a heart-healthy lifestyle, including regular moderate intensity exercise (*Circulation,* Aug. 2008). The good news is that most patients with AF live long and normal lives.

LESSONS FOR LIVING LONGER

The average life expectancy in the United States is approximately 78 years, an age that is far less than our potential maximum life span. Yet according to studies of regions of the world where people commonly live active lives past the age of 100, the average American could live up to 14 more years by embracing most or all of the following habits: Regular, moderate intensity physical activity; eat less; limit meat; consider moderate alcohol consumption; cultivate a sense of purpose; de-stress; embrace your spiritual side; and put family first. (*Bottom Line Personal,* Oct. 2009).

HEARTFELT ADVICE

You (the person you see in the mirror each day) probably have the single greatest influence on your destiny after a heart attack, bypass surgery or coronary angioplasty/stenting. Perhaps the late General Norman Schwarzkopf summed it up best when asked how he would respond to an enemy attack. "Counterattack," he replied. When the enemy is heart disease, the strategy is no different. The best "counterattack?" Aggressive lifestyle modification and taking your prescribed cardioprotective medications as directed.

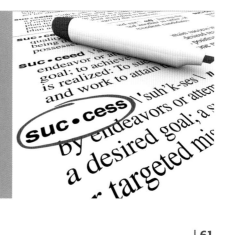

Do You Know Your CHA$_2$DS$_2$-VASc Score? If You Have Atrial Fibrillation, You Should

David R. Cragg, M.D.

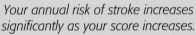

Your annual risk of stroke increases significantly as your score increases.

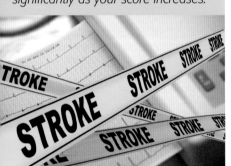

Atrial fibrillation (a-fib) is the most common heart rhythm abnormality that cardiologists treat. It affects 2 to 3 percent of the population and the percentage increases as you age. Four percent of people between 60 and 70 years are affected and more than 14 percent of people over 80 years of age have a-fib. One of the most feared complications of a-fib is stroke. Trying to predict who is at the greatest risk for a stroke can be challenging. Fortunately, there is a valuable clinical tool that cardiologists can use to stratify this risk called the CHADS$_2$ score. A few years ago, the CHADS$_2$ score was updated and became the CHA$_2$DS$_2$-VASc score (*Chest,* Feb. 2010). This new improved scoring scheme is an acronym that identifies risk factors for stroke. To calculate your score, review the eight conditions listed below, note those that apply to you (i.e., a "yes" response), and sum the total points.

CHA$_2$DS$_2$-VASc score	Stroke Risk %*
0	0
1	1.3
2	2.2
3	3.2
4	4.0
5	6.7
6	9.8
7	9.6
8	12.5
9	15.2
*Annual risk (i.e., risk per year)	

Your annual risk of stroke increases significantly as your score increases. The stroke risk is cumulative and for a patient with a score of 4, their annual risk would be 4 percent and 10 year risk of stroke would be 40 percent. The current guidelines recommend that if your score is above 2, anticoagulation with warfarin or one of the new oral non-warfarin anticoagulant drugs (called NOACs, e.g., dabigatran, rivaroxaban, edoxaban, or apixaban) is recommended.

	Condition	Points
C	Congestive heart failure (or left ventricular systolic dysfunction)	1
H	Hypertension: blood pressure consistently above 140/90 mmHg (or treated hypertension on medication)	1
A_2	Age, 75 years or older	2
D	Diabetes mellitus	1
S_2	Prior stroke or transient ischemic attack (TIA) or thromboembolism	2
V	Vascular disease (e.g., peripheral artery disease, myocardial infarction, aortic plaque)	1
A	Age 65 to 74 years	1
Sc	Sex category (female)*	1

*Female gender confers higher risk

Taking one of these drugs may lower stroke risk by as much as 75 percent. On the other hand, if your score is low (0 in men or 1 in women) no anticoagulant therapy is recommended. For men with a score of 1 or 2 or women with a score of 2, patient values and preferences need to be individually considered.

Recent studies have suggested that not only can the CHA_2DS_2-VASc score be used to predict who is at risk for a stroke, it can also predict who might develop a-fib in the first place (*American Journal of Cardiology,* Aug. 2015). The score even predicts those who may have a stroke in the absence of a-fib (*American Heart Journal,* Sept. 2011). Every patient with a-fib should know their own CHA_2DS_2-VASc score since it is such a good way to predict and potentially prevent serious medical problems. If you have a CHA_2DS_2-VASc score of 2 or higher, you should discuss anticoagulation therapy with your physician and seriously consider taking an anticoagulant such as warfarin or one of the newer NOAC agents.

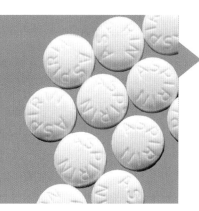

MINI-STROKE INCREASES RISK FOR HEART ATTACK

Patients who have suffered a mini-stroke are twice as likely to suffer a heart attack within the next five years. If you have had a mini-stroke: Reduce your risk for heart attack by achieving healthy blood pressure and cholesterol levels. Many men and women may also benefit from prophylactic aspirin therapy. Check with your physician.

(*Stroke,* April 2011)

HEART ATTACK: THE RISKIEST TIME OF DAY?

Numerous studies have now shown that the riskiest time of day for heart attacks is between 6 a.m. and noon. Why? Researchers now believe that cyclic morning increases in hormone levels, blood pressure and artery stiffness heighten the possibility of clot formation.

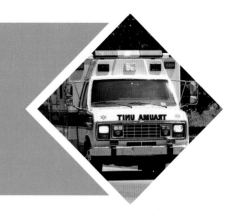

SHORT STATURE ASSOCIATED WITH HIGHER RISK OF HEART DISEASE

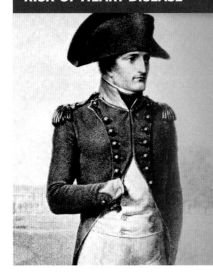

For many years now, clinicians have noted that shorter people are more likely to develop heart disease in a variety of populations and ethnic groups. A recent landmark study, including genetic data from nearly 200,000 men and women worldwide, found that each extra 2.5 inches of height was associated with a 13.5 percent reduction in heart disease risk. The investigators reported just one link between height and risk factors, and it was modest, to say the least: The genetic variants associated with shorter stature were linked to slightly higher levels of LDL-cholesterol and triglycerides, blood fats that are associated with the development of coronary atherosclerosis.

(*New England Journal of Medicine,* April 2015)

TOO MUCH SITTING AND CHRONIC DISEASE RISK

According to a sobering review and analysis of the existing scientific literature, prolonged sedentary time, independent of structured physical activity, is positively associated with various deleterious health outcomes, including a heightened cardiovascular and cancer mortality. Prolonged sedentary time was associated with a nearly twofold risk for developing type 2 diabetes.

(*Annuals of Internal Medicine,* Jan. 2015)

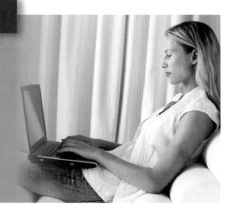

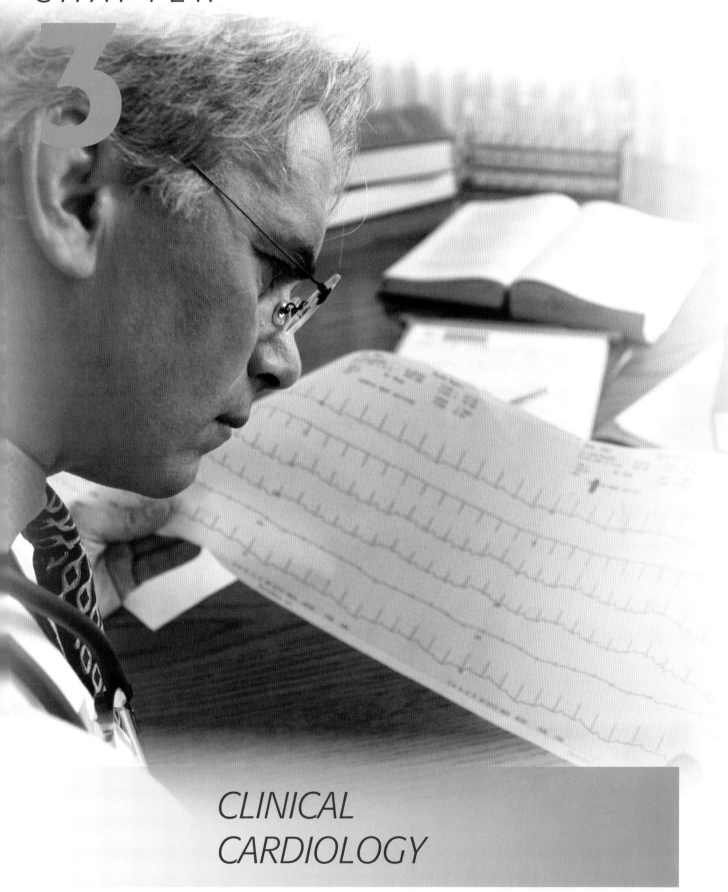

CLINICAL CARDIOLOGY

The Mystery of the Stethoscope Explained

Ivan Hanson, M.D.

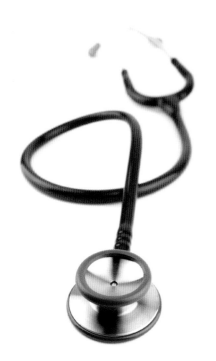

Have you ever wondered what a cardiologist hears when he or she listens to your heart? With the advent and refinement of non-invasive imaging tests, cardiac auscultation is becoming a lost art. However, the stethoscope remains one of the most useful clinical tools in the initial evaluation of many cardiovascular problems. The following is a brief synopsis of the link between heart sounds and cardiac function.

A normal heart beats regularly at a rate of 60 to 90 times per minute. If the rhythm is irregular, it could mean that extra heartbeats are periodically resetting the normal rhythm. It could also mean that an abnormal rhythm, such as atrial fibrillation, has completely overridden the normal rhythm.

The heart contains four valves that facilitate forward flow of blood from the low-pressure venous circulation to the high-pressure arterial circulation; aortic, pulmonic, mitral and tricuspid. Each normal heartbeat comprises two heart sounds, which are caused by valve closure. The first heart sound represents closure of the mitral and tricuspid valves, while the second heart sound represents closure of the aortic and pulmonic valves. Variations in the loudness of the first and second heart sounds may reveal medical conditions such as high blood pressure or pulmonary hypertension, as well as pathology of the valves themselves.

A murmur is a "whooshing" sound, which may signify that a valve is narrowed or leaky. The character, location and timing of the murmur help to identify the valve that is affected. The loudness of the murmur generally does not relate to severity. However, other physical examination findings are often useful in determining severity of the valve abnormality, which is usually confirmed by cardiac ultrasound (echocardiography). Severe valvular narrowing or leakiness may require surgical correction.

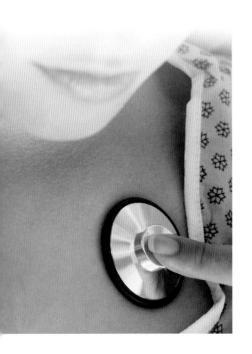

Other abnormal sounds may be present in the setting of volume, pressure overload or inflammation around the heart. These sounds may not be consistently present each time a patient is examined, and may disappear with medical therapy of the respective underlying condition.

The stethoscope is a gateway to cardiac function. Entirely normal cardiac auscultation is reassuring, though does not exclude the possibility that a cardiac structural abnormality is present. Auscultatory abnormalities, if properly appreciated and characterized, provide a starting point for confirmatory testing and management of cardiovascular disease.

The Electrocardiogram—Still a Treasure Trove After All These Years

James R. Stewart, M.D.

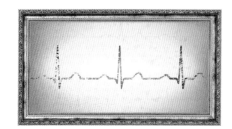

The original idea for the electrocardiogram (ECG) dates back to 1842 when Italian scientists demonstrated that each heartbeat generates an electrical current. The fact that these currents could be recorded from the body's surface allowed Willem Einthoven and others to develop the ECG, based on recording the electrical signal from 12 specifically placed leads (electrodes), a feat that earned him the Nobel Prize in 1924. The present day 12-lead ECG format was officially established in 1942.

Despite being the oldest of the cardiac noninvasive tests, the ECG remains an essential part of the present day cardiac evaluation and, in fact, is the most commonly used diagnostic test in all of medicine. The importance of the ECG relates to its versatility to diagnose a variety of cardiac abnormalities.

Heart rhythm abnormalities (arrhythmias) are among the most common problems seen by cardiologists and can only be diagnosed noninvasively by analysis of the ECG. Arrhythmias can originate from both the upper heart chambers (atria) or the lower chambers (ventricles) and range from benign to potentially life-threatening. Heart rhythm abnormalities generally increase in frequency as we age. For example, as many of 10 to 15 percent of the population over 80 years of age may experience an irregular heart rhythm called atrial fibrillation.

The ECG can also diagnose a delay in transmission of the electrical impulse through the heart's specialized conduction system, a condition that may lead to heart block and result in dangerously slow heart rhythms. Moreover, the ECG remains the most important test to diagnose a heart attack in patients presenting with chest pain. Specific ECG changes can often suggest which of the coronary arteries is occluded and help determine whether a patient will be treated emergently with cardiac catheterization and stent placement, or treated more conservatively with medication.

Changes in the ECG may also signify structural abnormalities of the heart such as enlargement or thickening of the cardiac chambers or may demonstrate previous heart attack or myocardial infarction (heart muscle damage).

Alterations in the electrical relaxation pattern of the ECG (repolarization) may suggest a genetic abnormality such as long QT syndrome or Brugada syndrome, which may indicate a high risk for dangerous cardiac rhythm disturbances. Changes in repolarization are also commonly seen with electrolyte anomalies such as abnormal potassium or calcium levels in the blood.

Finally, in patients that have implanted cardiac devices such as pacemakers or defibrillators, the ECG is essential to demonstrate whether these devices function normally.

The importance of the ECG is illustrated by the fact that a cardiology fellow in training is required to read 3,500 studies under supervision to satisfy minimum training requirements. At our institution, this is accomplished by spending three months during the first and second years of training specifically devoted to learning ECG interpretation.

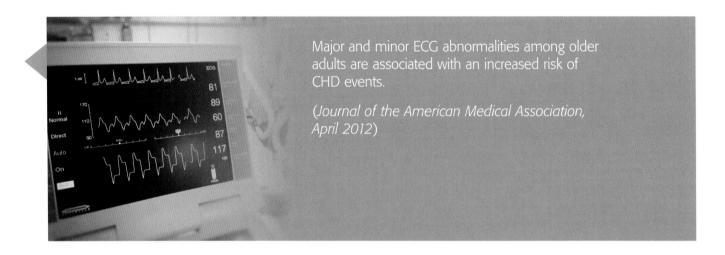

Major and minor ECG abnormalities among older adults are associated with an increased risk of CHD events.

(*Journal of the American Medical Association, April 2012*)

RESTING ELECTROCARDIOGRAM MAY PREDICT SUDDEN CARDIAC DEATH

Sudden cardiac death (SCD) accounts for one half of all deaths related to coronary heart disease (CHD) and presents as the first manifestation of CHD in approximately 25 percent of the deaths. One clinical study showed that a widened central spike on the resting electrocardiogram (ECG), referred to as a prolonged QRS duration, was an independent predictor of SCD over a 19-year follow-up. In fact, the added risk was comparable to that for established coronary risk factors such as cigarette smoking, elevated blood cholesterol, and type 2 diabetes mellitus. The investigators suggested that routine measurement of the QRS duration on the resting ECG may have clinical value in assessing the risk of SCD in the general population.

(*Circulation,* May 2012).

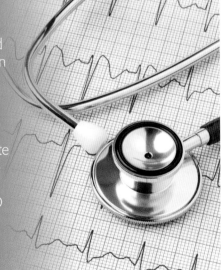

A Potentially Lifesaving "Walk Test"

Barry A. Franklin, Ph.D.

The 109 passengers and nine crewmen of a British Airways jet were not so fortunate at London's Heathrow Airport in June of 1972, when their plane crashed on takeoff, killing all aboard. A subsequent investigation established the accident's cause—a massive heart attack shortly after takeoff killed the plane's 51-year-old captain. His condition, said the report, "must have been developing for 30 years or more," yet the gradual narrowing of his coronary arteries had gone undetected in routine annual physical exams, including resting electrocardiograms, known as ECGs. The report went on to recommend exercise stress testing for all airline pilots.

What does an exercise stress test measure?

Exercise testing involves a medical evaluation of heart-lung fitness; heart rate and blood pressure responses to progressive exercise; abnormal clinical signs or symptoms (anginal chest pain); and associated changes in electrical functions of the heart, especially heart rhythm abnormalities and ECG signs of myocardial ischemia (inadequate blood flow to the heart).

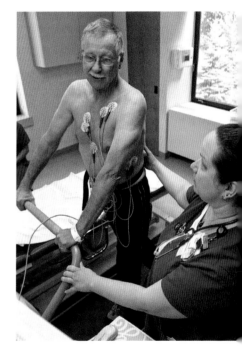

During incremental exercise, significant blockage of the coronary arteries (generally considered to be 75 percent or more) may cause anginal chest pain, a change in the ECG pattern (called ST-segment depression), or both. There is one limitation, however: Exercise stress tests are unable to detect mild-to-moderate coronary blockages, where most heart attacks occur. Consequently, an exercise stress test can be normal despite the presence of coronary plaque that may rupture.

Sometimes exercise tests suggest underlying heart disease when it does not exist; this is called a false-positive result and is associated with women in particular. Nevertheless, these tests provide enormously powerful prognostic information, especially when taking heart-lung fitness into account, expressed as metabolic equivalents or METs. A low exercise capacity of 4 METs or less indicates a higher mortality group. On the other hand, a MET capacity of 8 METs or higher designates a cohort with excellent long-term survival (*Journal of the American Medical Association*, May 2009).

What happens during an exercise stress test?

During an exercise stress test, an ECG is obtained during exercise, usually on a treadmill. The standard exercise stress test evaluates the heart when it's beating more rapidly than when it's at rest. The workload gradually increases as the test progresses (i.e., the treadmill speed and/or grade are increased every three minutes), and blood pressure readings are taken at intervals to assess the

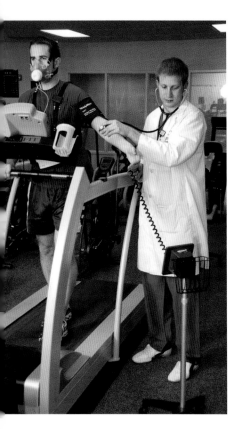

heart's pumping power. The test typically progresses to the point of volitional fatigue (the patient is too tired to continue) or to the point of adverse signs or symptoms, which suggest the test should be discontinued. These tests are often used to evaluate symptoms such as shortness of breath or chest pain, sometimes in conjunction with nuclear imaging or echocardiographic studies.

Are there any risks?

Several years ago we evaluated the complication rate of exercise testing in our laboratories. We reviewed more than 58,000 consecutive exercise stress tests and reported a mortality rate of 0.3 per 10,000 tests and a total complication rate of 2.4 per 10,000 tests. Thus, the test is associated with an extremely low risk of complications. Experts generally agree that the ability to maintain a high degree of safety depends on knowing when not to perform the test, when to terminate the test (i.e., recommended end points), and being prepared for adverse responses that may arise.

What does an abnormal result mean?

An abnormal result may suggest clogged coronary arteries, manifested as chest pain/pressure, ECG evidence of ischemia, or both. In some individuals, heart disease may be heralded by heart rhythm irregularities that develop during and immediately after exercise stress, or by a decreasing systolic blood pressure response to increasing workloads. The peak heart rate response to exercise or the decrement in heart rate after maximal exercise testing can also serve as important predictors of mortality.

By incorporating several exercise test responses into a mathematical formula or treadmill score, conventional exercise testing can often outperform the newer, more costly, noninvasive studies. According to Victor Froelicher, M.D., treadmill scores can help determine the type and advisability of further diagnostic testing. Low-risk patients could be spared from additional diagnostic studies, whereas high-risk patients would be referred for cardiac catheterization. Thus, for these patient subsets, treadmill scores would make additional noninvasive testing unnecessary.

If I get an abnormal result, what's next?

An abnormal result may suggest the likelihood of underlying heart disease, especially major blockage of one or more arteries. Depending on the abnormality, you may be directly referred for cardiac catheterization or coronary angiography, to obtain pictures of your heart's arteries and potential blockages. More likely, however, would be additional noninvasive tests (e.g., exercise echocardiography, exercise testing with cardiac imaging, computed tomography to detect calcium deposits in the coronary arteries, or cardiac CT angiography to visualize the coronary arteries). Patients who are limited in their ability to exercise may benefit from pharmacologic stress testing, which uses medications to increase heart rate or dilate coronary arteries. This form of testing is associated with an accuracy of up to 90 percent in detecting significant coronary blockages. If the results of these additional noninvasive tests are abnormal, cardiac catheterization may be recommended.

If heart disease is diagnosed, your doctor may recommend a number of options including medications (such as statin drugs to lower cholesterol or aspirin therapy), a low-fat diet, an exercise-based cardiac rehabilitation program, and smoking cessation. In addition, depending on your symptoms and/or the severity of the disease, you may be a candidate for an angioplasty procedure. For persons with multiple major blockages, typical in individuals suffering from severe heart disease, coronary artery bypass surgery may be recommended.

Epilogue

By ultimately identifying underlying, unrecognized coronary artery disease, an exercise stress test can change, or even save, your life—as it may have saved the lives of the unlucky 118 passengers and crew on the British Airways jet, who died because of someone else's heart attack.

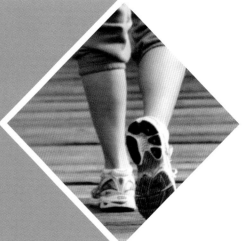

TIME FOR A SIX-MINUTE WALK?

Researchers found that cardiac patients who covered the shortest distance (bottom 25 percent) during a six-minute walk test, had four times the rate of new cardiovascular events over an eight-year follow-up period as compared with those who covered the most distance (top 25 percent). The ability of the walk test to predict cardiovascular events was similar to that of maximal treadmill exercise testing, highlighting the mantra 'survival of the fittest.'

(*Archives of Internal Medicine,* June 2010)

Exercise Stress Testing: Undervalued and Underappreciated?

Harold Friedman, M.D.

When performed by a trained exercise physiologist and carefully interpreted by a cardiologist, the exercise test provides a treasure trove of information that extends even beyond the diagnosis of heart disease.

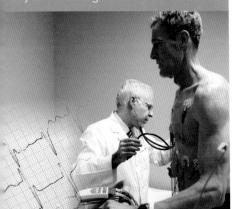

Exercise testing was one of the earliest studies doctors used to evaluate patients for heart disease. In the mid 1950s, the Masters Two-Step test was developed using patients with angina (heart pain) or a healed heart attack due to coronary artery blockage. The test results could confirm that a patient's symptoms were heart-related. It could also detect other patients who were symptom-free but had significant underlying coronary disease.

The test involved two 9-inch steps with a predetermined number of trips up and down. An electrocardiogram (EKG) with multiple wires attached to the patient's chest was obtained at baseline, during and after the test. Complaints of chest pain, changes in blood pressure, appearance of irregular heart rhythms and changes within specific areas of the EKG were found to be predictive of future cardiac problems. Stress testing soon became one of the earliest methods to establish a cardiac diagnosis.

Today, instead of stair steps, we use a treadmill, cycle ergometer, Air Dyne®, or arm crank as the exercise modality. The exercise is graded, indicating that the treadmill gradually speeds up and elevates or the resistance on the arm crank or cycle ergometer increases every three minutes. At every three-minute level or stage, after the vital signs have stabilized, blood pressure, heart rate, and perceived exertion are assessed and the supervising nurse or exercise physiologist records an EKG. Once exercise is stopped because of abnormal signs, symptoms or fatigue, patient monitoring is continued for at least six additional minutes of recovery. Testing is done in an environment where emergencies can be treated efficiently and expeditiously. Accordingly, emergency medications and a defibrillator are immediately available.

An exercise stress test may be administered for several reasons. Most commonly it is used to assess complaints of exertional shortness of breath and/or chest discomfort due to underlying heart disease. It can also be used to screen asymptomatic individuals who are at increased risk for developing heart disease as well as those with jobs involving public safety such as pilots or bus drivers. The test can assess the functional capacity or level of physical fitness to set exercise goals for those who are deconditioned or have heart and/or lung disease. Because physical exertion itself can provoke irregular heart rhythms that may require treatment, serial testing can be used to measure the response to prescribed medications.

When performed by a trained exercise physiologist and carefully interpreted by a cardiologist, the exercise test provides a treasure trove of information that extends even beyond the diagnosis of heart disease. Basic information such as blood pressure changes while lying, standing and during exercise can suggest heart valve disease, severely blocked arteries or conduction system abnormalities. The heart rate response to exercise and the rate of slowing immediately after peak exertion correlates with heart disease and prognosis. The origin of abnormal, irregular heart rhythms can be uncovered, classified and correlated with palpitations and dizziness complaints. Blood oxygen levels, continuously monitored by a finger sensor, can help sort out whether the patient's shortness of breath is primarily due to lung disease, heart disease or deconditioning.

Repeat stress testing, after treatment of heart artery blockage by either bypass surgery or angioplasty/stenting, can be used to demonstrate the successful restoration of blood flow to the heart, confirm the relief of symptoms and reassure the patient (and his or her doctor) that moderate-to-vigorous physical activity is safe. Annual stress tests comparing exercise time or peak energy expenditure level (termed METs or metabolic equivalents) are commonly used by physicians to assess prognosis and follow the natural progression of heart valve disease, which can help to determine the optimal timing of valve replacement. Treadmill testing can also unmask inadequate lower extremity circulation (referred to as peripheral arterial disease), as well as the severity of the problem.

Despite the widely publicized advances in diagnosing heart disease with computed tomography, cardiovascular magnetic resonance imaging and ultrasound, the fundamental value of an exercise stress test has withstood the test of time. It remains an inexpensive tool that is often the first step in assessing a patient with suspected heart disease as well as monitoring patients after coronary revascularization or other treatments.

A SIMPLE FUNCTIONAL TEST TO PREDICT MORTALITY?

Researchers in Brazil reported on the association between the ability to sit and rise from the floor and all-cause mortality in 2,002 adults aged 51 to 80. A standardized sitting-rising test (SRT) was objectively scored, using the minimum support that the subject felt was needed. Over a six-year follow-up, a low score on the SRT was associated with five-to-six-fold higher all-cause mortality in men and women. Take home message: Varied measures of poor functional status (i.e., beyond aerobic fitness) are associated with unfavorable health outcomes.

(European Journal of Preventive Cardiology, Dec. 2012)

Graded Exercise Testing: Diagnostic and Prognostic Implications?

Emily Balagna, B.S.

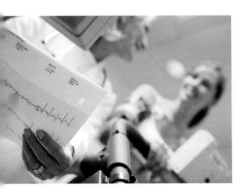

If you have ever had an exercise stress test, you may have wondered what is actually being evaluated. Is there more to it than all of the squiggly lines on the screen? Actually, yes, because no one specific response determines whether the findings are "normal," "abnormal" or "equivocal." Many different variables are simultaneously assessed, which help to build a snapshot of your overall cardiovascular health and fitness.

Two of the variables evaluated during the exercise test are your heart rate and blood pressure. Prior to exercise, resting values are taken to ensure that they are "within normal limits." During exercise, it is expected that both the heart rate and systolic blood pressure (top number) will rise. The normal response for diastolic blood pressure (bottom number) is to remain largely unchanged or slightly decrease. One of the objectives to ensure that we have a valid test is to achieve at least 85 percent of your age-predicted maximal heart rate, which is estimated by the formula (220 - age), and multiplying that number by 0.85. Certain medications that can cause a blunted heart rate and blood pressure response (e.g., beta-blockers) would be taken into consideration during test interpretation. In addition to the responses during exercise, heart rate recovery is also a telling indicator. The rate at which your heart rate drops at one minute after peak exercise is an index of both fitness and mortality. A delayed decrease in heart rate, defined as a reduction of 12 beats per minute or less from the heart rate at peak exercise, is associated with decreased long-term survival *(New England Journal of Medicine,* Oct. 1999).

Exercise capacity or cardiorespiratory fitness is another important variable evaluated during your exercise test. Treadmill tests are performed using standardized protocols which allow us to estimate your exercise capacity, expressed as peak metabolic equivalents (METs), based on the achieved grade and speed, as well as the number of minutes you are able to complete. A MET is the amount of oxygen or energy expended at rest, which generally approximates 3.5 mL O_2/kg/min. The longer that you can exercise on a progressive treadmill test, the greater your MET capacity or cardiorespiratory fitness. This is important because numerous research studies have shown that individuals with the lowest MET capacities (less than 5) have the highest risk of mortality, whereas those with the highest MET capacities (10 or greater) have a marked survival advantage (even those with underlying heart disease).

Another major component of the exercise test is the electrocardiogram (known as an ECG or EKG). Measurements are taken on 12 different leads or views of the heart at rest, during exercise and in recovery. This allows us to monitor the electrical activity of the heart. The exercise ECG can provide valuable information regarding the heart's rhythm as well as the likelihood of inadequate blood flow to the heart muscle, due to partially clogged coronary arteries.

In addition to all of the great technology that we have to evaluate cardiac health, we still rely heavily on the perception of overall effort, referred to as the rating of perceived exertion, and your conveying any symptoms that you may experience. One of the objectives of an exercise test is to gradually stress you to the point of volitional fatigue. Achieving this level of activity signifies a valid test. We also rely on you to report any adverse symptoms, for example, chest pain or pressure, shortness of breath or dizziness. Thus, your input provides an important contribution to the overall data being collected.

Once the exercise test is completed, the data can be used to estimate a patient's likelihood of heart disease and long-term prognosis. The Duke Score is a common method of risk stratifying patients. Variables considered include the duration of exercise, magnitude of abnormal ECG changes and the severity of chest pain, if any. This score can provide an estimate of future cardiac risk, as well as the need for additional diagnostic studies. Occasionally, your doctor may order complementary imaging studies during and immediately after your exercise test (myocardial perfusion imaging or stress echocardiography). These adjunctive studies may provide additional clinical information and/or increase the accuracy of the evaluation.

As you can see, there are many responses that are taken into consideration during an exercise test. Collectively, these provide us with important information regarding your heart health and exercise capacity.

WALKING VERSUS RUNNING FOR REDUCING CORONARY RISK

Using data from the National Runners' and Walkers' Health Study, investigators reported that equivalent energy expenditures by moderate-intensity exercise (walking) and vigorous exercise (running) produced similar risk reductions for the development of high blood pressure, elevated cholesterol and diabetes mellitus. These results should be used to encourage physical activity in general, regardless of its intensity. However, walkers would be required to devote more than twice the exercise duration (time) to achieve comparable risk factor reductions.

(*Arteriosclerosis, Thrombosis, and Vascular Biology,* April 2013)

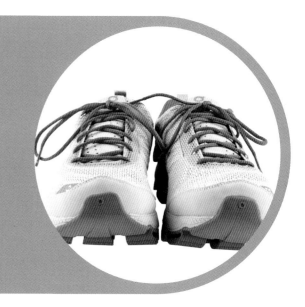

Why Exercise Stress Tests Don't Predict Heart Attacks

Simon R. Dixon, MBChB

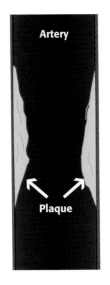

Artery

Plaque

The triggers for plaque rupture are not well understood

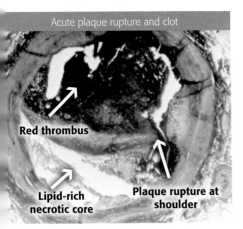

Acute plaque rupture and clot

Red thrombus

Lipid-rich necrotic core

Plaque rupture at shoulder

In February, I treated a 46-year-old man who came in to our Emergency Center with a heart attack. He had no prior history of heart disease or any other medical problems. In fact, he worked out daily and took pretty good care of himself apart from putting in long hours at work. He underwent emergency heart catheterization and we quickly opened a totally blocked artery with a stent, thus avoiding major heart damage.

Several months before this event my patient had an exercise stress test. The test was entirely normal with no findings to suggest lack of blood supply to the heart. Not surprisingly, one of the first questions that he asked me following the heart catheterization was "How did this happen? I just had a normal exercise stress test."

The answer to this somewhat puzzling question lies in what causes a heart attack. First, it is important to appreciate that exercise stress tests are often used to detect severe blockages in a coronary artery. During an exercise test we look for abnormal signs or symptoms, signifying that part of the muscle is receiving inadequate blood flow during stress, based on the ECG, nuclear or echo images, and anginal chest pain or discomfort. Typically a blockage needs to be greater than 75 percent to reveal these abnormalities. This might seem surprising, but most heart attacks occur at sites in the coronary artery where there is only mild plaque blockage (that would not be picked up on a stress test). For reasons we are still researching, the blockage suddenly becomes angry and ruptures like a shallow volcano, causing the contents (magma) to leak out and make the plaque sticky. A blood clot forms over the surface of the plaque resulting in sudden occlusion of the coronary artery (see figures). Once the artery is occluded the blood supply to that area of the heart is cut off, causing the muscle to die (heart attack) unless blood flow is rapidly restored.

These facts should not cause us to despair, nor lack confidence in the diagnostic and prognostic value of exercise stress testing. Rather it is important to appreciate that every cardiovascular test has some limitations, and exercise stress testing remains an excellent tool for evaluating patients with suspected or known coronary artery disease.

Accordingly, there is enormous interest in predicting which coronary artery plaques might cause a future heart attack. At present, this is about as easy as predicting when the next big volcanic eruption will occur; however, considerable progress has been made in the field with novel imaging techniques (e.g., coronary computed tomography angiography).

Until such time that newer tests are available, the best ways to reduce the risk of heart attack are to maintain a healthy lifestyle and body weight, exercise regularly (at least 30 minutes, five days a week), lower an elevated blood pressure or cholesterol level, if appropriate, stop cigarette smoking, and have regular check-ups with your primary care physician or cardiologist.

WHAT IS YOUR EJECTION FRACTION?

Ejection fraction or EF is the percentage of blood pumped out of the heart's main pumping chamber, the left ventricle, with each heartbeat. It is a key indicator in determining the health and function of your heart. Normal values range from 50-66 percent, which means over half of the blood that fills the left ventricle is pumped out to the body with each contraction. On the other hand, a major heart attack can reduce the EF to 15-35 percent.

A simple echocardiogram, among other tests, can determine this value. What's your EF?

Source: Anne Davis, R.N.
Cardiac Rehabilitation Center,
Beaumont Hospital, Royal Oak

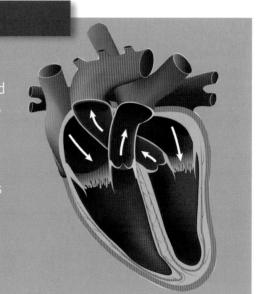

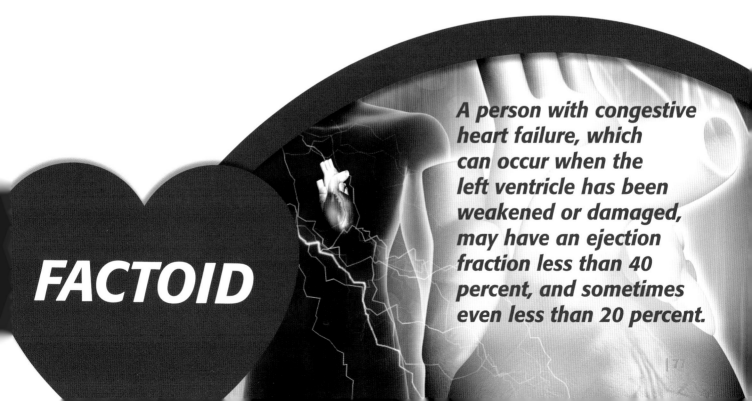

FACTOID

A person with congestive heart failure, which can occur when the left ventricle has been weakened or damaged, may have an ejection fraction less than 40 percent, and sometimes even less than 20 percent.

Cardiac Ultrasound: A Window Into the Heart

Nathan Kerner, M.D.

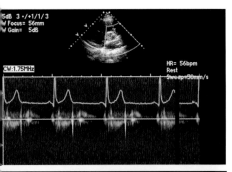

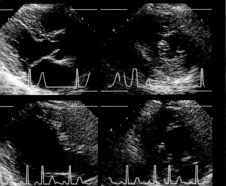

There are many imaging methods to assess heart function, although none used more than cardiac ultrasound. Ultrasound is an established, safe, and readily available modality that gives unparalleled data in terms of cardiac anatomy and function.

Cardiac ultrasound, or echocardiography, begins with two-dimensional imaging of heart structures. With 2-D imaging, we are able to visualize and measure abnormalities in the valves, pericardium surrounding the heart, and particularly the pumping function of the left ventricle, the main pumping chamber of the heart. This imaging modality is often coupled with treadmill stress testing to allow assessment of left ventricular function at rest and during exercise. Echocardiography is also helpful in detecting wall motion abnormalities, which may signify the presence of coronary artery disease (blocked arteries in the heart).

In addition to 2-D imaging, all current cardiac ultrasound equipment can also measure blood flow through the heart using Doppler ultrasound techniques. This allows the measurement of sound waves coming from red blood cells themselves as they travel through the heart. Being able to measure blood flow through the heart gives us the ability to identify abnormal pressures within the cardiac chambers and leaking or blocked valves in the heart.

A newer modality in echocardiography is three-dimensional imaging of the heart. Viewing the heart in this manner is performed using sophisticated computerized algorithms. Modern technology allows us to view cardiac structures from many different angles, which is extremely helpful to interventional cardiologists and surgeons performing valvular repair or replacement procedures, or correcting structural defects in the heart.

Cardiac ultrasound is an imaging modality that has been around for many years. It is proven as a safe and noninvasive means of imaging the heart. This relatively straightforward and constantly evolving tool yields a tremendous amount of information which can be of paramount importance in a physician's assessment and management of numerous and diverse cardiovascular conditions.

A New Window Into the Heart—Cardiac MRI

Michael Gallagher, M.D.

Over the past decade, advances in science, physics and medical technology have allowed doctors to examine the heart with a new camera. Cardiac magnetic resonance imaging (MRI) can actually take pictures of a beating heart. The pictures obtained through this new "lens" offer an alternative to the more common imaging tests such as heart ultrasound (echocardiography), nuclear imaging, and computed tomography scans. In fact, cardiac MRI has rapidly become a useful imaging test to diagnose many heart conditions.

What is a cardiac MRI?

Cardiac MRI is a safe, non-invasive medical test that creates detailed pictures of the heart using a specialized camera. MRI uses radio waves (radio frequency pulses), a powerful magnetic field, and a computer to make pictures. Doctors use cardiac MRI to assess the heart anatomy and function, as well as major blood vessels. Detailed MRI images help determine the presence of certain diseases that may not be identified with other imaging methods.

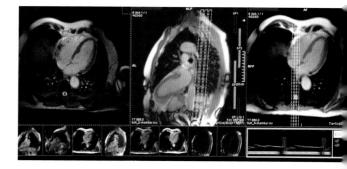

Why did my doctor choose an MRI of the heart?

MRI images of the heart are very clear, making the test invaluable for several conditions. Some common reasons to have the test include:

- To further investigate any abnormalities seen on other heart imaging tests
- To monitor heart muscle function, thickness and size (weak and dilated hearts called "cardiomyopathies" are accurately imaged with this test)
- To assess the amount of heart damage caused by a heart attack; and to determine if heart function has potential to improve after stent placement, bypass surgery or medical therapy. MRI is able to detect areas of heart tissue that have poor blood supply (due to coronary artery disease) or that has been damaged (from a heart attack)
- To evaluate structures in and around the heart, such as the pericardium (sack around the heart) and the aorta. MRI can also locate and characterize any rare tumors around the heart
- To better understand abnormalities of the heart the patient may have been born with (congenital heart defects)

The test: What should I expect; is it safe?

The test takes approximately one hour. It is an extremely safe test without any radiation exposure. The exam causes no pain. It is normal for the area of the body being imaged to feel slightly warm from the magnetic pulses. Although the strong magnetic field is not harmful, implanted medical devices that contain metal may malfunction or cause problems during an MRI (so tell your doctor if you have a pacemaker, defibrillator, or other implanted metallic devices).

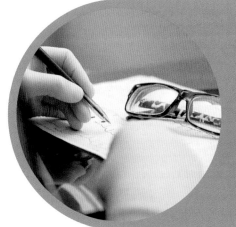

In a technical sense, state-of-the-art cardiac MRI approaches are mostly based on fast gradient-echo pulse sequence, which achieve synthetic "cine" representations of an average cardiac cycle, using retrospective electrocardiogram gating concepts.

(*Quantitative Imaging in Medicine and Surgery, October 2014*)

A heart MRI has minimal risks, as well as few, if any, side effects. On the other hand, a patient who is claustrophobic or who may feel besieged in enclosed spaces may not feel comfortable in the MRI machine.

FACTOID

What Should You Do About Leg Pain?

Robert Safian, M.D.

Some of the most common causes of leg pain include vascular disease (arterial and venous diseases), orthopedic problems, neurological conditions, infections, blood clots and trauma. So how can these common conditions be best diagnosed and treated?

Leg pain that occurs during walking or other types of physical exertion may be due to vascular causes. Patients with vascular pain often have a history of high blood pressure, high cholesterol, diabetes, and cigarette smoking.

Pain that occurs in the buttocks, back of the thigh, or back of the calf may be due to peripheral arterial disease (PAD), and may be caused by blockages in the arterial circulation to the legs. The pain is commonly described as a cramping sensation that occurs during walking or climbing steps, and the medical term for this type of discomfort is claudication. Claudication is usually quite predictable, which means that it occurs consistently while walking the same distance each day. Because blockages in the arteries can progress over time, patients with claudication may notice that their symptoms occur while walking shorter distances. PAD is easy to diagnose with special types of ultrasound (duplex ultrasound), computed tomography scans, and other vascular tests such as ankle-brachial index. Certain types of medications can be prescribed to alleviate the symptoms, and if symptoms do not respond, other potential treatments may include angioplasty, stents, and surgery.

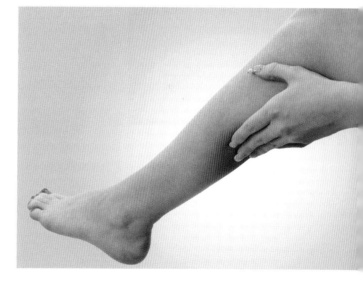

Another type of leg pain that may have a vascular cause is venous insufficiency. Patients with venous insufficiency may have a personal or family history of varicose veins, blood clots or phlebitis in the legs, or previous vein stripping. Venous insufficiency is caused by problems with the tiny valves in the veins in the legs (not blockages in the arteries), and common symptoms include heaviness in the lower legs and feet, swelling, purple or reddish-brown discoloration, dryness (eczema) and itching of the lower legs. Generally the swelling is worse during the day, once you are up and moving around, whereas it may diminish or disappear completely when the legs are elevated (such as after a night's sleep). Venous insufficiency is easy to diagnose with a careful physical examination and venous ultrasound. The mainstays of treatment include regular exercise (to activate the calf muscles), compression stockings (usually by prescription rather than over-the-counter), and venous ablation procedures if symptoms persist.

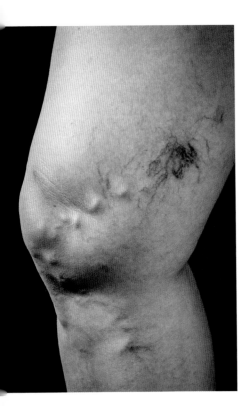

Many patients do not appreciate that leg pain can be due to lower back and spine problems, and such discomfort can be very disconcerting and disabling. Leg pain due to back and spine problems may be caused by narrowing of the spine canal (spinal stenosis) or compression of nerves as they exit the spine (due to disc or other back problems). Some patients develop severe shooting or burning sensations in their buttocks or legs. Others may complain of leg pain when they walk, which may be confused with claudication. Patients with back and spine problems can often be distinguished from patients with claudication since the former may have a history of back injury, chronic back pain, need for back injections, or previous chiropractic manipulations. They may experience leg pain while standing (such as cooking or waiting in long lines in stores), raising their legs overhead (such as while exercising at the gym), or during back extension. Leg pain due to back and spine problems can be readily diagnosed by a careful history and physical examination, and by special imaging studies (such as X-rays and magnetic resonance imaging). Treatment often includes physical therapy, anti-inflammatory medications, and other approaches, depending on the nature and extent of the problem.

Many patients are affected by pains in their legs and feet, particularly at night. These pains may be described as lightning bolts or searing pain, and may be especially troublesome in the soles of the feet and toes. These types of symptoms are almost always due to nerve injury (peripheral neuropathy), and the most common cause is diabetes. In contrast to the other causes of leg pain described above, which commonly involve one leg and sometimes two, peripheral neuropathy typically involves a "stocking and glove" distribution, and commonly involves both hands and feet. The diagnosis is established by careful history and physical examination, and may require special nerve tests (nerve conduction studies). Treatment is centered on the optimal management of diabetes and the use of special medications.

The causes of leg pain described above are usually chronic rather than acute medical conditions, and have been present for weeks, months or years. In contrast, there are a few causes of acute leg pain (over hours or a few days) that are important to know about, and usually require immediate medical evaluation. Obviously, traumatic injuries ranging from mild muscle strain to severe crush injuries are relatively easy to diagnose based on history and physical examination. Patients with acute pain, swelling and redness (usually of one leg) may have infections (called cellulitis) or blood clots (called phlebitis, or deep vein thrombosis); fever and chills are more characteristic of cellulitis. Patients with acute leg pain, associated with a cold limb and pale color, may have acute blockage of an artery to the leg. All of these types of leg pain should be considered medical emergencies, and patients should seek immediate medical attention.

The bottom line? Leg pain is fairly common, and almost all causes of leg pain can be readily evaluated and treated. See your physician for diagnosis and treatment.

Why Are My Legs Swollen?

Harold Friedman, M.D.

Edema refers to the build-up of fluid in tissues below the skin surface (peripheral edema), within the chest wall (pulmonary edema) or within the abdomen (ascites). By far, the most common presentation is the lower extremities. Edema of the legs can cause discomfort and, in some cases, may be an early sign of something more severe. The source of leg edema can most often be determined by obtaining a patient history, detailed physical examination, laboratory findings, an ECG and X-ray results.

Peripheral edema most commonly develops when the pressure in the smallest blood vessels, called capillaries, increases significantly or when the capillary walls dilate—permitting extra fluid to seep through into the surrounding tissue. This causes a painless puffiness, or swelling and stretching of the skin. It takes about 3 liters of fluid accumulation before leg edema begins to appear. Gravity increases fluid pressure into areas closest to the ground; thus, swelling typically appears in the feet and lower legs. Edema tends to increase gradually during a day of activity. Due to leg elevation overnight, the swelling is typically less in the morning. The degree of edema can be assessed by applying firm finger pressure producing a dimple (pitting) that persists for several minutes. Edema usually involves both legs unless it is caused by disease or injury to one leg.

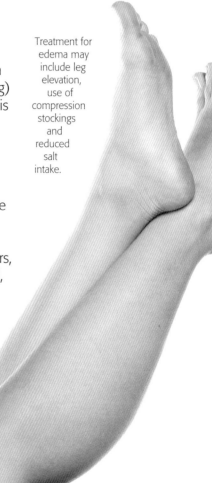

Treatment for edema may include leg elevation, use of compression stockings and reduced salt intake.

Benign causes of lower extremity edema include pregnancy and monthly periods due to the salt retaining effects of increased hormone levels. Also, specific medications for diabetes, cancer, pain control and hypertension can cause the kidney to retain excessive salt and water, creating increased pressure in the capillary system. Paradoxically, some antihypertensive medications indirectly raise capillary pressure as they lower the systemic blood pressure. A family of frequently used blood pressure medications, calcium channel blockers, dilate the blood vessels and increases fluid seepage. Although less recognized, the pain control medications for neuropathy, gabapentin and pregabalin, cause significant edema by a similar mechanism.

Chronic venous disease causes lower extremity swelling because the diseased veins progressively dilate. This may damage their one-way valves and impair venous return to the heart. Stagnation of flow increases the capillary pressure and creates the edema. Blood clots can obstruct blood returning to the heart, but more often affect one leg, causing pain with the edema.

Heart failure, caused by a weakened heart pumping action, can cause edema. Muscle damaged by either a heart attack, a leaking heart valve or a rapid heart rate can begin the process. The reduced cardiac output stimulates the kidney to retain extra sodium and water volume, which increases capillary pressure in the legs and lungs. Cirrhosis and low thyroid function are also medical conditions that can cause edema by similar mechanisms.

Treatment for edema may include leg elevation, use of compression stockings and reduced salt intake. Eliminating a culprit medication often will relieve the condition within several days. Diuretics, which cause the kidneys to release salt and water, can be cautiously prescribed, watching closely for lightheadedness and signs of decreased blood pressure.

Edema is a very common medical finding resulting from varied causes. The swelling itself, unless extremely severe, is harmless. If you experience signs or symptoms that suggest edema, contact your physician. The use of conservative measures, eliminating offending medications and treatment of the underlying disorder will often solve the problem.

Patients with congestive heart failure often experience sudden weight gain from fluid buildup, called edema. Fluid that backs up into the lungs can cause pulmonary edema—and extreme shortness of breath. A weight gain of 2-5 pounds or more over 1-4 days suggests edema and worsening of heart failure.

FACTOID

Congestive Heart Failure: Causes, Diagnosis and Therapy

James A. Goldstein M.D.

Congestive heart failure (CHF) is a common clinical diagnosis. Cardiac diseases leading to CHF include cardiomyopathies and pericardial disorders. The most prevalent manifestation of cardiomyopathy occurs when the heart is dilated (enlarged) and pumps poorly, resulting in reduced output of blood to the body, fatigue, and a buildup of fluid in the lungs and legs causing labored breathing and swelling of the lower extremities.

The CHF Epidemic. There are approximately six million Americans with CHF, representing nearly three percent of the adult U.S. population. It is the only form of heart disease that is increasing in prevalence. The lifetime risk of CHF at age 40 or 80 is one in five. There are 670,000 new cases diagnosed each year, contributing to 281,000 annual deaths and one million acute CHF hospitalizations. The associated mortality is 50 percent at five years, as dim a prognosis as many cancers. CHF is the number one reason for hospitalization of people greater than 65 years of age and is more costly than all forms of cancer combined, constituting the largest federal Medicare (37 cents/1 dollar) and Veteran's Administration ($39.2 billion) expenditures.

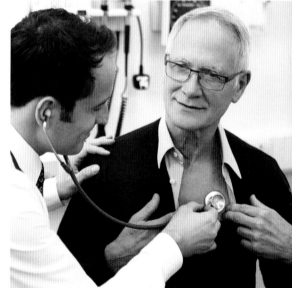

Causes of CHF. The most common causes of dilated cardiomyopathy include coronary artery disease (when severely blocked arteries cause heart attacks that damage the heart muscle), high blood pressure (hypertension) and valvular disease (blocked or leaky heart valves). CHF can also occur when the heart pumps well but is excessively "stiff," a condition that occurs when the heart muscle is abnormally thick (hypertrophied) due to hypertension or genetic causes. Diseases of the pericardium, the sac encompassing the heart, can also cause CHF; this can occur when the sac fills with fluid (effusion/tamponade) or becomes thickened and stiff (constriction). It should be emphasized that symptoms such as shortness of breath, fatigue and leg swelling are non-specific and may occur unrelated to cardiovascular disease; for example, breathing difficulty may reflect intrinsic lung diseases. Thus, the key to optimal CHF management is to characterize the underlying nature of the disorder to establish a precise diagnosis.

CHF: Diagnosis, therapy and outcomes. It is essential to identify diseases in which treatment of the primary underling problem may reverse CHF. For example, coronary artery disease and valvular heart disease may be

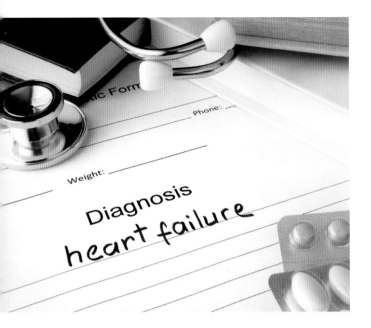

successfully treated in many cases by catheter procedures (for example, stents and heart valves) or by surgical interventions (coronary bypass and valve replacement). Coronary disease can be assessed by heart catheterization or, in some cases, non-invasively by computed tomography. Valvular disease is readily detected by non-invasive ultrasound (echocardiography). Other causes of CHF such as thick, stiff hypertrophic hearts can usually be identified non-invasively by echocardiography. Our cardiologists are experts in advanced diagnostic studies such as magnetic resonance imaging, which is helpful to exclude diseases that cause inflammation or infiltration of the heart muscle, as well as pericardial disorders. When such testing has excluded typical causes of CHF, the diagnosis is often inherited (familial) cardiomyopathy, which can be confirmed by diagnostic exclusion, followed by detailed genetic analysis.

CHF: Optimal therapy for best outcomes

- Precise diagnosis leads the practitioner to the preferred treatment and optimal outcome. Common therapeutic options include fixing blocked coronary arteries (stents or bypass surgery), valve interventions (catheter-based or surgery), medical therapies including vasodilators (drugs that relax arteries and improve the heart's output), diuretics (that stimulate the kidney to eliminate excess fluid build-up), beta-blockers (that improve heart function), or combinations thereof. Advanced therapies may include heart transplant and implantable ventricular assist devices.

- Appropriate drugs at dosages with proven efficacy are essential to achieving optimal outcomes. It is critical that CHF patients receive guideline-based prescriptions (optimal drugs adjusted to guideline-mandated dosages).

- Patients with severely depressed heart function are at increased risk for life-threatening heart rhythms. Accordingly, they should be evaluated for treatment with implantable defibrillators and sophisticated pacemakers that restore synchronized beating of the heart.

- Cardiac transplantation is an advanced, transformative therapy that can improve quality of life in patients with end-stage debilitating CHF. Patients less than 70 years of age with refractory CHF should be evaluated for this surgical intervention. Recognizing that the number of patients with CHF far exceeds available organs for transplantation, the last 15 years have seen the advent of surgically implantable ventricular assist devices, artificial heart pumps that can be both life-saving and improve the quality of life for patients with end-stage CHF. These devices are now widely available and can serve as a bridge to transplantation in those who are candidates and are awaiting a donor organ, but also can be employed as destination therapy in those with debilitating CHF who are not candidates for cardiac transplantation.

Heart Failure: Can You Get a Passing Grade?

A. Neil Bilolikar M.D.

There's a lot of confusion about what heart failure (HF) is among patients and even among some doctors who don't treat it often. Heart failure is commonly defined as the inability to pump sufficient blood to meet the body's needs. Experts agree that this definition is inadequate, largely because it does not encompass the full spectrum of disease. If you have hardening of the arteries, have ever had a heart attack, have diabetes or have high blood pressure, the likelihood that you will develop HF is five to 10 times that of a healthy person. Even if you don't have these risk factors, the chances of you developing HF in your lifetime are one in five.

There are two main types of HF. Either the problem involves poor pump function from the heart's main chamber (systolic HF) or the inability of the heart to relax properly to accept blood into that chamber, leading to backup of blood in the lungs (diastolic HF). Both of these conditions can cause shortness of breath and fatigue. A common test done to differentiate the two is called an echocardiogram, which is an ultrasound of the heart. This noninvasive test allows the physician to directly see the pumping function of the heart, as well as indirectly assess its ability to relax.

If you have systolic HF, your doctors may treat you with medications such as beta blockers (generics that end in –olol), ACE inhibitors (generics that end in –pril), diuretics such as hydrochlorothiazide or Lasix (furosemide), digoxin, or combinations thereof. Diuretics help to remove excess fluid from the body so that it does not remain in the lungs where it can cause shortness of breath. Many other medications work directly on the heart to improve its function. Depending on the cause of the systolic HF, sometimes your heart will strengthen over time; this is why it's very important to take all the medications your doctor prescribes.

If you have diastolic HF, therapy is directed at the cause of the disease. In this case, it is most often due to high blood pressure which can be treated with medications such as diuretics, beta blockers, ACE inhibitors and calcium channel blockers. If your HF is due to other factors, such as hardening of the arteries or a malfunctioning heart valve, then the therapy will target those conditions as well. Today, numerous studies are evaluating promising treatments for diastolic HF, which may make the heart less 'stiff' and better able to relax.

What other treatments may help with HF? Oftentimes, the best treatments aren't medications, but things that you can do to modify your lifestyle. For example, eating foods with less sodium (which cause you to retain water) and not consuming too much water can do wonders for your heart. A recent

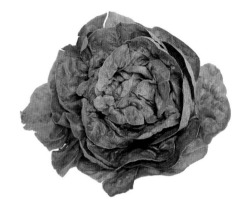

Newer studies show that a healthy diet that is largely plant-based will lengthen your life over food choices that are primarily meat-based.

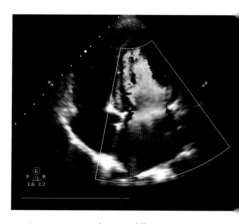

A common test done to differentiate the two forms of HF is called an echocardiogram, which is an ultrasound of the heart.

statement from the American Heart Association indicates that foods which have become a "staple" in most people's diets—soup, cold-cut sandwiches, pizza, and breads—have far more salt than is recommended for the patient with HF. This generally requires a complete shift in the types of foods you normally eat to remain healthy with HF. Newer studies show that a healthy diet that is largely plant-based will lengthen your life over food choices that are primarily meat-based. Lastly: moderate exercise! Physical activity may be difficult at first, but brisk walking 15 to 30 minutes a day for five to seven days a week can do wonders for your heart and cardiovascular system and improve your quality of life. If this amount of exercise is too taxing for you, it can be broken into shorter periods of activity (e.g., three five to 10 minute exercise bouts), repeated throughout the day. Discuss regular exercise and healthier eating practices with your doctor at your next visit, as these are your ticket to a passing grade in HF.

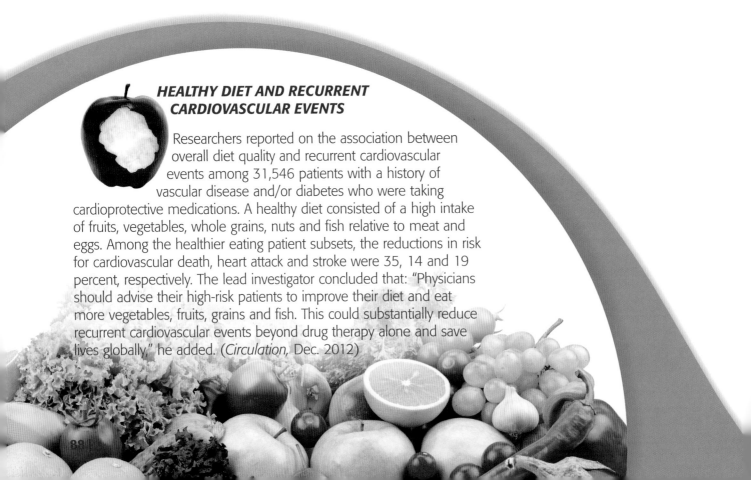

HEALTHY DIET AND RECURRENT CARDIOVASCULAR EVENTS

Researchers reported on the association between overall diet quality and recurrent cardiovascular events among 31,546 patients with a history of vascular disease and/or diabetes who were taking cardioprotective medications. A healthy diet consisted of a high intake of fruits, vegetables, whole grains, nuts and fish relative to meat and eggs. Among the healthier eating patient subsets, the reductions in risk for cardiovascular death, heart attack and stroke were 35, 14 and 19 percent, respectively. The lead investigator concluded that: "Physicians should advise their high-risk patients to improve their diet and eat more vegetables, fruits, grains and fish. This could substantially reduce recurrent cardiovascular events beyond drug therapy alone and save lives globally," he added. (*Circulation*, Dec. 2012)

Sex After a Cardiac Event: New Insights

Alan J. Silverman, D.O.

Is sexual activity strenuous enough to cause a heart attack or even sudden cardiac death? What happened to my sexual drive or desire? These questions are common among middle-aged and older patients with a history of heart problems; so here's what we know.

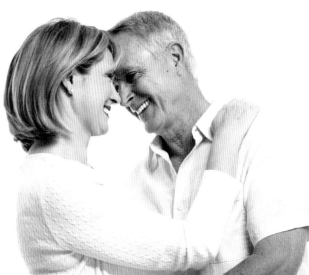

Sexual activity in a young married man with his usual partner is comparable to mild-to-moderate physical activity, approximating 3 to 4 metabolic equivalents (METs), which corresponds to walking on a level treadmill at 3 mph or at 2 mph up a 3.5 percent grade. Sexual activity is a probable contributor to heart attacks in fewer than 1 percent of patients. The absolute rate of events is very low because exposure to sexual activity is of short duration and the associated cardiac demands are modest.

Men and women with stable coronary disease who have no or minimal symptoms during routine activities can generally engage in sexual activity. This includes patients able to achieve at least 4 METs during peak or symptom-limited exercise testing without anginal symptoms, abnormal ECG changes, a decreasing blood pressure response, serious heart rhythm irregularities or excessive shortness of breath. In patients with unstable or decompensated heart disease (i.e., unstable angina, decompensated heart failure, uncontrolled heart rhythms or severe valvular disease), sexual activity should be deferred until the patient is stabilized.

Contemporary guidelines (*Circulation,* Feb. 2012) have been published addressing sexual counseling for patients with cardiovascular disease and their partners. This American Heart Association scientific statement included a review of medications and their potential effects on sexual function, cardiac risks related to sexual activity, the role of regular exercise in reducing the risk of acute cardiac events and supporting intimacy, and the importance of reporting warning signs or symptoms experienced during sexual activity.

Since the approval by the Food and Drug Administration for the treatment of erectile dysfunction, millions of prescriptions for sildenafil citrate (Viagra), vardenafil (Levitra) and tadalafil (Cialis) have been filled. Reported adverse complications associated with the use of these drugs include infrequent heart attacks, threatening heart rhythm irregularities, plummeting blood pressure, and in rare instances, death, especially in patients with heart disease who were simultaneously taking nitrates. If you're considering drug therapy to treat erectile dysfunction, check with your physician.

It is reasonable for patients with cardiovascular disease wishing to initiate or resume sexual activity after a cardiac event to be evaluated by their physician. Cardiac rehab and regular exercise can be useful to increase functional capacity and reduce the small risk of cardiovascular events during sexual activity. Patient and spouse/partner counseling by health care providers may be advised to assist in resumption of sexual activity after an acute cardiac event or revascularization procedure.

If heart trouble has cast a cloud over your sex life, talk to your doctor. With counseling and reassurance, many patients with heart disease can lead full, satisfying lives—sex included.

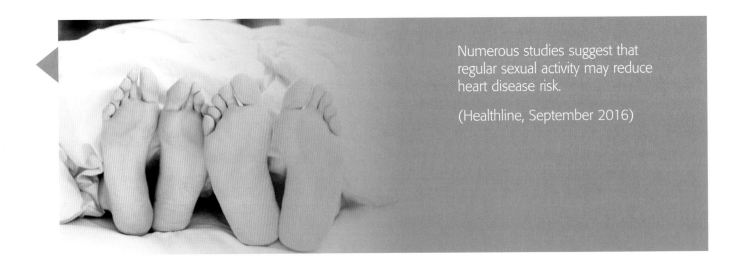

Numerous studies suggest that regular sexual activity may reduce heart disease risk.

(Healthline, September 2016)

SEXUAL ACTIVITY IS SAFE FOR MOST HEART PATIENTS

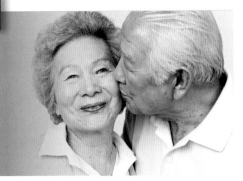

If a heart patient can achieve two minutes or more during a conventional treadmill test (1.7 miles per hour, 10 percent grade), without experiencing adverse signs or symptoms, the risk of cardiac events during sexual activity with one's spouse or regular partner is extremely low.

(*Circulation*, Jan. 2012)

Resuming Sexual Activity After a Heart Attack

Barry A. Franklin, Ph.D.

Is sexual activity strenuous enough to cause another heart attack? That question is commonly asked by middle-aged and older heart patients who have reason to be concerned about their cardiovascular health. Fortunately, numerous studies now provide reassurance to those who have such fears.

Sexual activity is associated with a very light-to-moderate energy expenditure, two to four metabolic equivalents (METs), and modest increases in heart rate. One MET approximates the amount of oxygen your body uses at rest. Consequently, if patients can exercise at four METs workloads (e.g., 3 mph, 2.5 percent grade; 2 mph, 7.0 percent grade) or higher, without adverse signs or symptoms (e.g., chest pain, excessive shortness of breath, electrocardiographic abnormalities), sexual activity should not impose excessive demands on the heart.

Other reports have now shown that sexual activity is a probable contributor to heart attacks in less than 1 percent of all cases. In the two hours after sexual activity, the relative risk of a heart attack increased two to three fold, but rapidly returned to baseline thereafter. An intriguing finding from these studies was that regular physical activity reduced the risk of a heart attack being precipitated by sex. In fact, individuals who exercised regularly did not have an increased risk of having a heart attack triggered by sexual intercourse.

Extramarital sex may be more demanding from a cardiovascular perspective for men with known or suspected coronary disease. According to one widely cited study, 80 percent of deaths associated with sexual intercourse occur in hotel rooms "in relations with lovers" rather than wives. It was suggested that alcohol, cigarette smoking and other changes in the environment may further increase arousal and the associated demands on the heart.

The bottom line? The next time you're out for a brisk walk and your neighbor asks you "Why your sudden interest in fitness walking?"... Just smile, and tell him you're training to safely resume your normal activities of "daily" living.

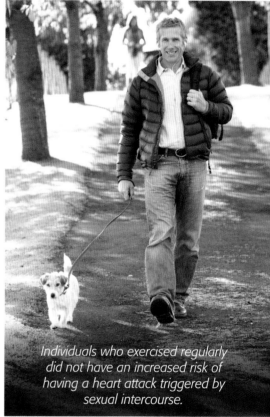

Individuals who exercised regularly did not have an increased risk of having a heart attack triggered by sexual intercourse.

No Bones About Erectile Dysfunction: ED Is Common, Especially in Heart Patients, and Is Nearly Always Treatable

Steven B.H. Timmis, M.D.

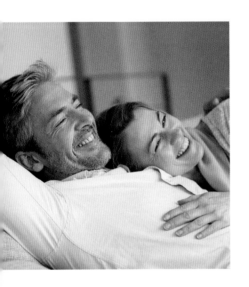

It is easy to talk to your doctor about your blood pressure, diabetes and heart disease. Heck, it's not all that difficult to discuss poor health habits, like cigarette smoking and excessive alcohol use. However, most patients are reluctant and embarrassed to bring up erectile dysfunction, or ED. When it is discussed, patients will often brush it off with statements like "what do you expect, I'm not a kid anymore." When it comes to my patient's health, I expect a lot! ED is not an insignificant personal problem; it is a common and serious medical issue.

Erectile dysfunction occurs in approximately 20 percent of men above the age of 40. Its prevalence increases with age. However, it is not a problem of getting older. Rather, ED is caused by the medical problems we commonly develop as we progress in life. Often it is the first sign of certain medical conditions. That is why it is crucial to tell your doctor if you have ED.

Hypertension, diabetes, cardiovascular disease and tobacco use directly contribute to ED. Certain medications, hormonal imbalances, prostate, bladder and rectal surgery also affect normal erectile function. Patients with spinal injuries and nerve problems (neuropathies) often suffer from ED. The more of these medical conditions that a person has, the more likely he will experience erectile dysfunction. Although many patients think that their sexual dysfunction is "in their heads," psychological causes account for only a minority of ED cases.

Each of these medical problems adversely affects erectile function by decreasing the vascular blood flow into the penis. An erection normally occurs when the penis is flooded with blood. As the shaft of the penis becomes engorged with blood it gets thicker, harder and erect. If the blood vessels are unable to permit normal blood flow into the penis during stimulation, it will remain flaccid. In short, ED is caused by vascular disease, just like angina, heart attacks and strokes. In turn, these lift-threatening problems are significantly more common in patients with ED. That is why patients need to tell their doctors about ED.

Fortunately, there are treatments. Almost everyone is familiar with Viagra, Levitra and Cialis. Today, it's virtually impossible to watch a ball game without seeing advertisements for these medications. These drugs are very effective in most early cases of ED. For more advanced cases, there are a variety of other remedies available under the care of a urologist. These treatments include vacuum devices, urethral suppositories, and penile injections. For cases that don't respond to these therapies, patients can consider surgical implantation of either an inflatable or non-inflatable penile implant. While such an approach may seem drastic, patients who have undergone an implant express a high level of satisfaction and often recommend it to others. Partners of those who have received an implant also express similar sentiments.

Erectile dysfunction is not a fact of life that must be endured. ED is a condition that often makes one feel incomplete. It is an important medical issue that should be discussed in a frank manner with your doctor. It can be successfully treated in up to 95 percent of cases. Furthermore, it may prompt your doctor to look for underlying medical problems that are responsible for the ED. Discussing ED with your doctor will lead to treatments that can restore your sexual health and may, along the way, save your life!

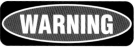

WARNING: ERECTILE DYSFUNCTION DRUGS AND NITROGLYCERIN MAY BE HAZARDOUS TO YOUR HEALTH

Drugs used for the treatment of erectile dysfunction (such as Viagra or Cialis) taken along with nitroglycerin (spray or tablet) can lead to extreme relaxation of blood vessels and, in some patients, a dangerous drop in blood pressure. Thus, nitroglycerin use in conjunction with these medications is strictly prohibited. (*Circulation,* June 2013)

New Cholesterol Guidelines: What Do They Really Mean?

Alan J. Silverman, D.O.

In November 2013, the American College of Cardiology and American Heart Association expert panel updated the national cholesterol guidelines. The purpose of these guidelines is to provide research-based recommendations to physicians in the treatment of elevated blood cholesterol. The panel addressed three critical questions:

1. What evidence is there for LDL-cholesterol (bad cholesterol) goals for the secondary prevention of heart disease (those patients who have had a heart attack, documented coronary disease, stroke or peripheral vascular disease)?
2. What is the evidence for LDL-cholesterol goals for the primary prevention of coronary disease (those patients who have no known cardiovascular disease)?
3. What is the impact of current cholesterol-modifying drugs on lipid levels, with specific reference to their safety and effectiveness?

The guidelines focused primarily on the treatment of blood cholesterol to reduce cardiovascular risk in adults. As always, emphasis continued to be placed on a heart healthy lifestyle including regular exercise, sensible dietary practices, and the avoidance of cigarette smoking as the foundation to reduce risk.

As always, emphasis continued to be placed on a heart healthy lifestyle including regular exercise, sensible dietary practices, and the avoidance of cigarette smoking as the foundation to reduce risk.

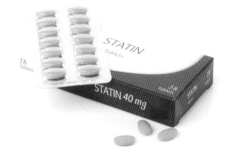

Four groups of patients were identified that appear to benefit most from treatment with cholesterol-lowering medications (e.g., statins such as Lipitor, Zocor, Crestor, etc.).

- *Group 1* Individuals with clinical cardiovascular disease (heart attack, documented coronary disease, stroke or peripheral vascular disease).
- *Group 2* Individuals with LDL-cholesterol greater than 190.
- *Group 3* Individuals 40 to 75 years of age with diabetes and LDL-cholesterol levels between 70 and 189 without known heart disease.
- *Group 4* Individuals without known heart disease or diabetes, aged 40 to 75 years, with LDL-cholesterol between 70 and 189 and an estimated 10 year risk of 7.5 percent or higher. This risk is estimated using a risk factor calculator.

Statin treatments are divided into high intensity, moderate intensity and low intensity therapy based on dosage and effectiveness.

In those patients who are not in one of the four groups, additional factors that may be considered in the treatment decision may include a family history of coronary disease, LDL-cholesterol greater than 160, or an abnormal coronary calcium score or ankle/brachial systolic pressure index. Such patients should discuss the benefits versus the risks of cholesterol-lowering therapy with their physician. These guidelines differ from those written previously, as for the first time, they focused on four major objectives:

1. The recommendations no longer list specific LDL-cholesterol levels as treatment goals (previously, patients were told their LDL-cholesterol levels should be less than 100 or less than 70 based on their risk). LDL-cholesterol levels are now used only to monitor that patients are taking their medications.
2. Only medications with proven effectiveness to reduce cardiovascular risk (e.g., statins) are advocated.
3. In the absence of contraindications or adverse effects, this guideline used the intensity of statin therapy (i.e., high dosage) as the goal of treatment.
4. Drug treatment is more strongly advocated for primary prevention (to prevent the development of cardiovascular disease in those without disease, based on those at the highest risk who would most likely benefit from cholesterol-lowering medications).

Finally, with the recent encouraging data regarding Zetia, which is a non-statin, and the release of the two new proprotein convertase subtilisin kexin 9 (PCSK-9) inhibitors, these guidelines will likely be revised in the near future. For now, however, we will continue to aggressively treat those patients with statins who appear to derive the greatest benefit from these medications.

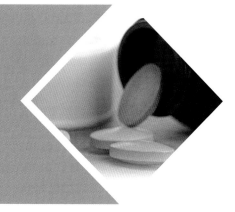

VALUE OF GENERIC CHOLESTEROL-LOWERING STATINS

Approximately 80 percent of patients can achieve the recommended levels of low-density lipoprotein cholesterol (LDL) by taking the cheaper generic statins, including atorvastatin or rosuvastatin.

(*Bottom Line Personal,* Nov. 2011)

How Low Can You Go? Studies on Reducing Cholesterol Levels

Harold Friedman, M.D.

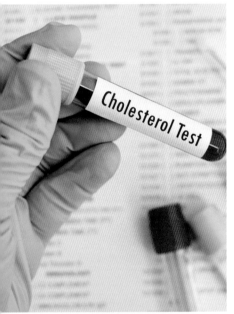

Numerous studies have shown that reducing LDL-cholesterol (the "bad" cholesterol) with drugs called statins decrease complications and recurrent cardiac events in patients with cardiovascular disease. It has been one of the major success stories over the past 30 years. The JUPITER trial demonstrated these benefits in apparently healthy middle-aged and older persons without known coronary disease. Additional data analysis from over 17,000 patients enrolled in the trial suggested enhanced benefits for "ultra responders," that is, those who demonstrated dramatic cholesterol reductions in response to statins. Patients who achieved LDL- cholesterol levels less than 50 mg/dL, far below the 'already aggressive' national goal of 70 mg/dL, had a 65 percent lower risk for new cardiovascular events as compared with their untreated counterparts. Equally important, there were no safety or side effect "red flags" within the group of over 4,000.

This provocative report may lead to a change in physician treatment practices. Instead of selecting an absolute number for the LDL goal, physicians may try to achieve a 50 percent relative reduction in LDL- cholesterol from baseline. Furthermore, studies from non-western nations with low rates of cardiovascular disease suggest that LDL-cholesterol levels in the range of 30 to 50 mg/dL may actually be normal.

Should we lower our goals? In all likelihood, we'll soon begin to see a trend toward treating the LDL to as low a level as reasonably achievable. This will be combined with greater use of more potent statins such as rosuvastatin and atorvastatin, which are now available as generics.

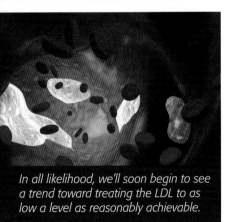

In all likelihood, we'll soon begin to see a trend toward treating the LDL to as low a level as reasonably achievable.

The niacin controversy

In the mid 1980s, a major Veteran's Administration study demonstrated that niacin increases HDL-cholesterol levels (the "good" cholesterol) and reduces cardiovascular events. Several subsequent studies came to similar conclusions. However, some suggested that the benefits may be due to other factors, since weight loss and smoking cessation also increase HDL levels and reduce risk.

Another large study to test the effects of slow release niacin added to a statin, the AIM-HIGH trial, was prematurely terminated by the National Institutes of Health, due to lack of clear benefit. This was a surprise, since it had long been accepted that adding niacin to statin therapy would offer the added benefit of increasing the HDL by 20 percent, while simultaneously lowering triglycerides and LDL-cholesterol levels. However, closer inspection of the study methodology (and several similar trials) led some authorities to question whether the conclusion leading to the study's premature termination may have been misleading. As part of the study, participants were strongly motivated to make substantive lifestyle changes and aggressively reduce their LDL-cholesterol levels. Thus, the study design markedly reduced the patients' cardiovascular risk, making it more difficult to detect the independent and additive benefit of niacin. The alternative interpretation? Niacin may, in fact, be beneficial for some patients. However, intensive lifestyle changes combined with aggressive statin therapy may make it harder to detect the benefits.

The new news may in fact be old news. Comprehensive risk factor modification including weight reduction, regular vigorous exercise and abstinence from tobacco products really works. These benefits also apply to apparently healthy people who may be at increased risk. Perhaps the study results may eventually lead to the reprioritization of lifestyle and dietary modification, combined with statins, as the first-line treatment approach, followed by the earlier identification of patients with a low HDL-cholesterol, since these individuals may have the most to gain from the addition of niacin.

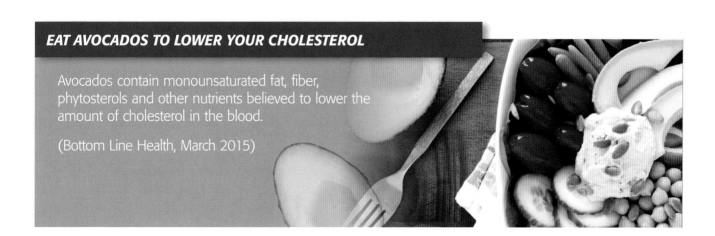

EAT AVOCADOS TO LOWER YOUR CHOLESTEROL

Avocados contain monounsaturated fat, fiber, phytosterols and other nutrients believed to lower the amount of cholesterol in the blood.

(Bottom Line Health, March 2015)

ESPECIALLY 'BAD' LDL-CHOLESTEROL SUBTYPES

Some LDL-cholesterol subtypes are more likely to cause heart disease than others. For example, a person with high levels of Lp(a), an extremely dense form of LDL-cholesterol, is up to 3 times more likely to develop heart disease than someone with lower levels, even when the total LDL is the same in both people. New cholesterol tests can measure individual types of LDL particles. Ask your doctor whether you should have one of the new cholesterol tests.

(*Bottom Line Health*, Aug. 2011)

A one-pound head of lettuce, which is about 95 percent water, contains just 60 calories.

FACTOID

CHAPTER 4

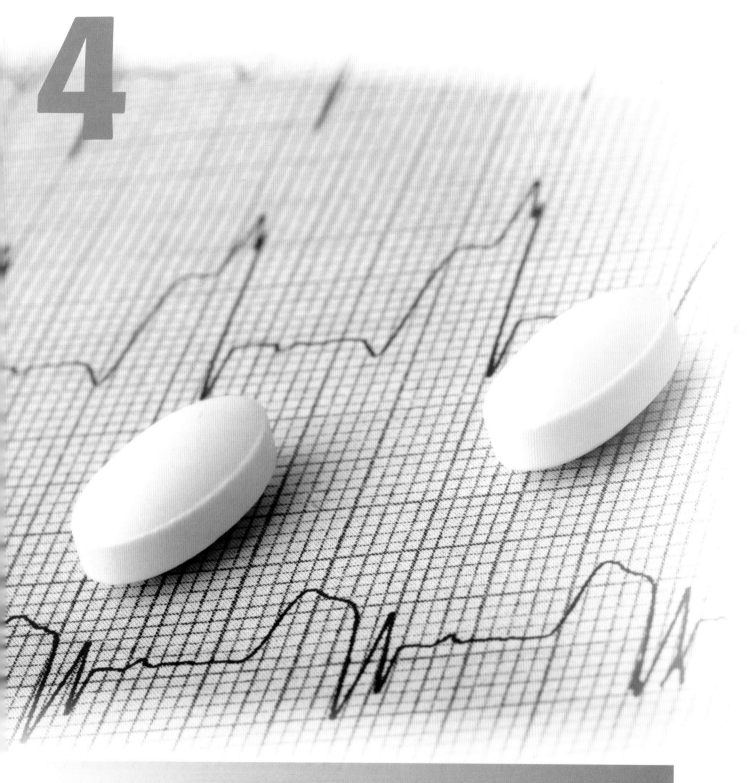

CARDIAC PHARMACOLOGY

Hit a Home Run for Your Heart

David H. Forst, M.D.

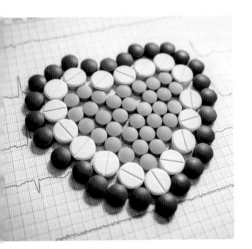

In an era where technologic advances dominate the medical scene, outstanding results can still be obtained by appropriately using cardioprotective medications. Understanding the four major classes of drugs used to prevent and treat a variety of cardiac disorders can save you money and a trip to the hospital.

Beta-blockers: These drugs slow the heart rate and lower blood pressure. Side effects are minimal. Many are generic with the drug name ending—olol. Beta-blockers are commonly used in the treatment of coronary artery disease, thickened or weak heart muscle, abnormal heart rhythms or high blood pressure. Examples are atenolol and metoprolol.

Angiotensin-converting enzyme (ACE) inhibitors/angiotensin-receptor blockers (ARBs): These drugs dilate your arteries, which can lower your blood pressure and the pressure in your heart. Consequently, the heart doesn't work as hard, decreasing the likelihood of irregular heart rhythms, promoting healing after heart attack and improving heart function in those with congestive heart failure. The most common side effect is a persistent dry cough, which disappears after stopping the drug. Many ACE inhibitors are generic with the drug name ending—pril. Examples are lisinopril and enalapril. ARBs are now available as generics and work similarly to ACE inhibitors. Examples are losartan or valsartan.

Platelet inhibitors (blood thinners): Aspirin remains a mainstay of therapy, decreasing inflammation in the arteries and preventing blood clot formation. Plavix® (clopidogrel) is a more powerful platelet inhibitor. These drugs are used for patients with coronary artery disease, including the prevention of clot formation in stents. Plavix must be used for at least one year after insertion of a stent. These drugs are also used in patients with peripheral vascular disease and to prevent strokes.

Statins: These cholesterol-lowering drugs have had a dramatic impact on preventing initial and recurrent heart attacks or strokes. They work not only by lowering cholesterol, but also by decreasing vascular inflammation. If one thinks of a coronary artery plaque as a pimple and a heart attack as a plaque that pops, these drugs decrease the likelihood of plaque rupture by decreasing inflammation, thickening the cap, and lowering cholesterol. This allows the plaque time to heal.

As we age, just like our joints, the heart and blood vessels become stiffer. By keeping our blood pressure and our HDL and LDL cholesterol levels in an acceptable range, and by decreasing the inflammation in our arteries, we can slow this process and prevent disease. These four classes of drugs, when used together, can decrease cardiovascular stress. Thus, it's not surprising that this combination is especially helpful in a wide variety of cardiovascular disorders including angina pectoris, atrial fibrillation or other rhythm abnormalities, congestive heart failure, heart attack, heart valve disorders and stroke. So the next time you see your doctor, ask about your prescribed medications and make sure you touch all the bases.

IMPLICATIONS OF THE JUPITER TRIAL?

The JUPITER trial was a landmark primary prevention trial that enrolled 17,802 apparently healthy men and women with a normal or near normal LDL-cholesterol level (less than 130 mg/dL), with an elevated level of C-reactive protein (greater than 1.9 mg/L), an inflammatory marker. Patients were randomly assigned to a statin drug (rosuvastatin) or a look-alike placebo, and followed for up to five years. The trial demonstrated that treatment with a statin was associated with a 44 percent reduction in cardiovascular events!

The investigators concluded that a high proportion of the cardiovascular events in adults worldwide could be prevented by treating populations that would not normally be prescribed a statin drug. (*New England Journal of Medicine,* Nov. 2008).

If you've stopped cigarette smoking and, in a weak moment, go back and have "just one cigarette," there is a 98 percent likelihood you'll start smoking again on a regular basis.

FACTOID

Aspirin to Prevent Heart Attack and Stroke: A Pound of Cure? Or Harm?

Steven B.H. Timmis, M.D.

It has often been said that an ounce of prevention is worth a pound of cure. For many years, aspirin has been touted to be that ounce of prevention and pound of cure for heart attack, stroke and cardiovascular death. Indeed, aspirin has been a lifesaver for patients in the midst of acute heart attack, lowering the risk of death by more than 25 percent.

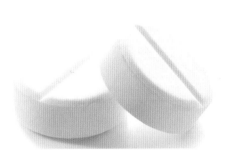

Aspirin has also been crucial for treating patients with documented coronary disease, such as those who have had a coronary stent or bypass surgery, as well as those who experience angina. Patients who have had a prior stroke have also proven to benefit from aspirin. The use of aspirin in these circumstances is known as secondary prevention, reducing the risk of heart attack, stroke and death in those who already have an established diagnosis of cardiovascular disease. A question of ongoing debate is whether aspirin has a role in the primary prevention for individuals who do not have a history of coronary disease or stroke.

In understanding the question of whether aspirin should be recommended to patients who have never been diagnosed with cardiovascular disease, it is important to understand how and where this drug works.

The blood vessels that supply the heart and brain can become narrowed by fatty plaque deposits, a process known as atherosclerosis. This plaque can become fragile and erupt, similar to a volcano. The blood vessel recognizes this ruptured plaque as a tear that "injures" the blood vessel, provoking a clot to be formed inside the artery in order to seal this "injury." However, this process of clotting is actually harmful, completely blocking the flow of blood feeding the heart or brain, resulting in a heart attack or stroke. Aspirin works as a blood thinner, preventing the clotting cells, known as platelets, from clumping together and forming a deadly blockage. By inhibiting clot formation, aspirin allows the blood vessel to maintain blood flow while it gradually heals.

Unfortunately, the many beneficial qualities of aspirin come at the cost of potential negative side effects. As a blood thinner, aspirin may cause bleeding. Patients often need to avoid aspirin if they have had a bleeding ulcer or have chronic stomach and esophageal problems such as reflux disease. Individuals who drink alcohol regularly also have a greater risk of bleeding. A patient may also be advised to avoid aspirin if they are scheduled to undergo certain surgical or dental procedures. Those that have suffered a bleed into their brain (a hemorrhagic stroke) may also be at risk for further injury with blood thinners such as aspirin. Lastly, patients may be unable to take aspirin due to allergic reaction. One should always check with their physician before starting an aspirin regimen.

Studies that have investigated whether aspirin helps to prevent heart attack, stroke and cardiovascular death in individuals without documented atherosclerosis have been mixed, showing either limited or no benefit. It seems that patients that are at low risk for cardiovascular disease do not experience any significant advantage by taking preventative aspirin. In these individuals, the bleeding risk of aspirin overshadows any potential benefit. On the other hand, individuals that have multiple risk factors for cardiovascular disease, especially a strong family history of coronary artery disease, elevated blood cholesterol, ongoing tobacco use, uncontrolled hypertension, diabetes mellitus, and peripheral arterial and aortic disease are more likely to have atherosclerosis affecting their heart and brain. As a result, they are more likely to benefit from the primary prevention of heart attack, stroke and death by taking aspirin (*Journal of the American College of Cardiology,* Jan. 2015).

However, even in high-risk patients, aspirin's benefit is controversial. The studies suggesting that aspirin lowers cardiovascular risk in high-risk individuals are getting old. Over the past two decades, other preventative measures such as better diet, smoking cessation and improved physical fitness may have mitigated, at least in part, the advantages of taking aspirin. The use of statin medications, such as Lipitor and Crestor, and better medical control of hypertension and diabetes in high-risk individuals might further attenuate the perceived benefits of aspirin for primary prevention. There are several ongoing studies that are readdressing the risks and benefits of aspirin in preventing heart attack, stroke and death in higher risk individuals who have not yet been diagnosed with cardiovascular disease.

In the meantime, consensus supports the use of low-dose aspirin in patients who seem to be at the highest risk. The optimal or preferred dosage has been suggested at 81-162 mg/day (*American Journal of Medicine,* Feb. 2010). Aspirin may, in high risk patients, represent a pound of cure. However, in lower risk patients with no history of cardiovascular disease, aspirin more likely represents a pound of harm.

Doctors now advise chewing and swallowing one regular uncoated aspirin (325 mg) in persons who think that they are having a heart attack (i.e., on the way to the hospital). It's estimated that this recommendation, if widely adopted, would save an additional 5,000 to 10,000 lives in the United States each year.

Dual Antiplatelet Therapy (DAPT) After Coronary Stenting: Do I Still Need Plavix?

Simon R. Dixon, MBChB

Recently, in our Cardiology Clinic, I was asked by a 72-year-old patient whether he still needed to take Plavix. He underwent cardiac catheterization 14 months ago for exertional chest pain (angina) and was treated with a drug-eluting stent in the left anterior descending coronary artery. He was doing well without chest pain and had no bleeding issues.

Aspirin and clopidogrel (Plavix) are extremely important after coronary stenting as these medications work together to prevent platelets forming a blood clot inside the new stent (this complication is called stent thrombosis). Some patients may be prescribed one of the newer anti-platelet medications in place of Plavix, such as prasugrel (Effient) or ticagrelor (Brilinta).

In general, dual anti-platelet therapy (DAPT) is taken for 12 months after the procedure until the metal struts of the stent are covered by a thin layer of scar tissue.

So, why might Plavix be helpful after 12 months? It is recognized that a very small number of patients may develop stent thrombosis several years after the stent is implanted. With current generation stents this complication is very uncommon; however, late stent thrombosis may result in heart attack or myocardial infarction (MI) and even sudden cardiac death. On the other hand, the downside of extended dual anti-platelet therapy is an increased risk of bleeding, as well as medication cost.

Several research trials have specifically addressed this important question. In the large DAPT trial, 9,961 patients were assigned to take DAPT for either 12 months or 30 months. Results showed that patients who took DAPT for 30 months had a lower risk of stent thrombosis and MI, but a higher risk of bleeding (figure) (*New England Journal of Medicine,* Dec. 2014).

Therefore, the decision whether to continue DAPT beyond 12 months must be customized to each patient, carefully weighing the pros and cons of extended therapy. For example, in a patient with a single stent who bruises easily or has a history of internal bleeding, I am inclined to stop the Plavix at 12 months. In a patient with multiple stents and no bleeding issues, I am likely to recommend staying on both aspirin and Plavix.

The decision whether to continue DAPT beyond 12 months must be customized to each patient, carefully weighing the pros and cons of extended therapy.

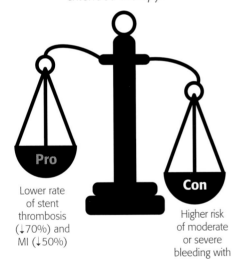

Pro
Lower rate of stent thrombosis (↓70%) and MI (↓50%)

Con
Higher risk of moderate or severe bleeding with DAPT

Drugs for Lowering Cholesterol: An Update

Heidi Pillen, PharmD

Heart disease is the leading cause of death in the United States. High blood cholesterol is a major risk factor for the development of heart disease. Indeed, according to Dr. William C. Roberts, editor of the American Journal of Cardiology, a strong case can be made for there being a single absolute risk factor for heart disease—that is, an elevated blood cholesterol level.

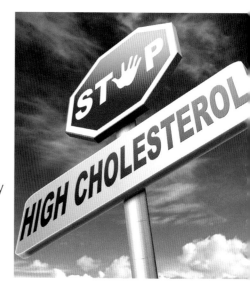

Cholesterol builds up on the insides of your arteries, making it harder for the blood to flow through them. It is important to know your cholesterol level. By lowering your cholesterol level, you can decrease the risk for the development of heart disease. Interestingly, research now suggests that whatever your total blood cholesterol is, reduction of that level by approximately 40 milligrams per deciliter (mg/dL) reduces the relative risk of a cardiac event (either a first one or a subsequent one) in half!

Many factors can affect cholesterol levels, including diet, weight, and exercise. Eating healthy food, losing weight, and increasing physical activity may all improve your cholesterol levels. Sometimes, however, these changes alone will not be enough, and you may require medications to favorably modify your levels. There are many different medications used to treat high cholesterol levels. Your doctor will decide which is right for you.

Statins: The statins (Mevacor, Zocor, Pravachol, Lescol, Lipitor, and Crestor) work mainly to lower your LDL cholesterol, but may also increase your "good" or cardioprotective HDL cholesterol and decrease triglycerides. Common side effects associated with statins include muscle aching, rash, insomnia and, less frequently, liver function changes. If you experience any unusual muscle soreness or weakness, you should contact your doctor immediately. Statins should be taken at bedtime to achieve optimal results.

Bile-acid sequestrants: This class of drugs includes Questran, Colestid and Welchol. These drugs also lower LDL cholesterol, but do not change HDL cholesterol and may even raise triglycerides. They are usually used in combination with other medications, and may cause gastrointestinal upset, including flatulence, bloating, and constipation. These medications may affect the absorption of other drugs, so ask your pharmacist if there are any interactions with the rest of your medications.

Niacin: Niacin, also known as nicotinamide, is effective at lowering LDL cholesterol, and can also raise HDL levels. Its use is limited by its side effects, however, as many patients experience flushing and itching within 2 hours after ingestion. Gastrointestinal upset and dizziness have also been reported.

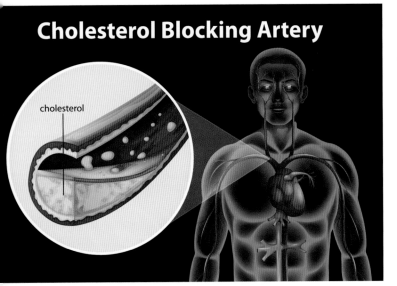

Cholesterol Blocking Artery

cholesterol

Fibrates: The fibrates (Lopid, Tricor, and Atromid) lower triglycerides and LDL cholesterol and increase HDL cholesterol. These agents are generally well-tolerated, with the most common side effects being rash. These drugs may interact with other medications you are taking, so be sure to ask your pharmacist if there are any interactions with the rest of your medications.

Zetia: Zetia reduces LDL cholesterol by preventing the cholesterol in food from being absorbed into the blood. It is often given with a statin. Vytorin contains both Zetia and Zocor in one pill. Common side effects include gastrointestinal complaints, body aches and back pain.

Knowing your cholesterol levels is a key step in preventing initial and recurrent cardiac events. Talk to your doctor about your need to decrease your levels and if taking medications to control your cholesterol is right for you.

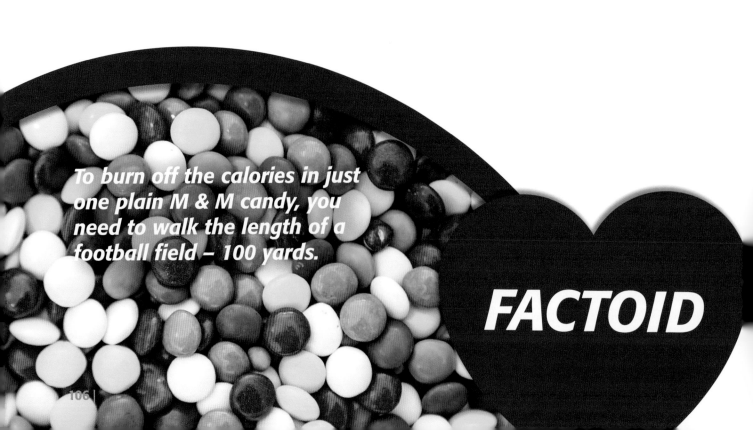

To burn off the calories in just one plain M & M candy, you need to walk the length of a football field – 100 yards.

FACTOID

Statin Drugs: Benefits Versus Risks?

Steven B.H. Timmis, M.D.

Over the past three decades, few medical developments have been as important as the emergence of statin therapy to both treat and prevent cardiovascular disease. Statin drugs are familiar to most patients, with names like Lipitor, Zocor and Crestor, all of which have been aggressively advertised on television. They derive their nickname "statin" from their generic names atorvastatin, simvastatin and rosuvastatin, respectively. Despite their tremendous benefit, few medications have been more difficult to convince patients to start taking. Patients are often fearful of potential side effects, whether real or perceived. Why does your cardiologist (and primary care doctor) prescribe these drugs? What are the concerns regarding these drugs? This article explores these questions and attempts to provide a 'fair and balanced" overview of their benefits and risks.

Benefits of statin therapy

Statin therapy has been studied in a broad range of patients in a wide variety of clinical situations. Patients with and without coronary artery disease who are taking these drugs have consistently demonstrated a significant reduction in adverse health outcomes, including death, heart attack and stroke.

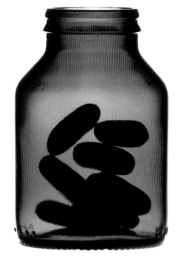

Statins are very effective in lowering bad cholesterol.

Patients at the greatest risk of these adverse events are those with known coronary artery disease, including individuals who have had a previous heart attack, angioplasty procedure, or heart bypass surgery, people who experience anginal chest pain or those who have had heart disease confirmed by cardiac catheterization or coronary computed tomographic scanning. People who have peripheral arterial disease, abdominal aortic aneurysms, carotid artery disease and previous stroke, diabetes mellitus or chronic kidney disease are also at substantial risk of similar outcomes. Those who have multiple risk factors including an elevated LDL cholesterol (bad cholesterol), a low HDL cholesterol (good cholesterol), hypertension, tobacco use and a family history of premature cardiovascular disease are at risk, as well. In each of these patient groups, statin drugs have resulted in a profound reduction in major adverse cardiovascular events, approximating 25 to 35 percent.

Statins produce these effects by lowering LDL cholesterol. Every study that has looked at lowering cholesterol levels has demonstrated a reduction in adverse cardiovascular outcomes that is proportionate to the degree of LDL cholesterol lowering. But statins don't just lower bad cholesterol. They have a favorable effect on good cholesterol and triglyceride levels (the other bad fat in the bloodstream). Statins also work on the blood vessels, where plaque develops and causes heart attack and stroke. Oxidation and inflammation aggravate plaque in the arteries, accelerating its development. Statins inhibit these processes, stabilizing the plaque. Long-term studies have shown that plaque progression slows and sometime even stops with statin therapy. One study showed that plaque regression, or shrinkage, actually occurred. These effects are not seen with other cholesterol lowering strategies.

The problem with statins

The answer is easy—side effects. While the concern for side effects is warranted, the likelihood of experiencing them is quite low. The most common side effect is muscle aches, which tend to be felt throughout the body. These muscle aches, also known as myalgias, can be uncomfortable, but are harmless. Further, they resolve quickly after stopping the medication. Often muscle and joint aches that occur from exercise, hard work, tendinitis or arthritis are mistakenly attributed to statin drugs. It may, therefore, be reasonable to restart statin therapy among patients who previously developed these symptoms while on treatment. In addition, a patient who is truly intolerant to one statin drug can often tolerate a different statin medication without side effects.

On rare occasion, patients taking a statin may develop inflammation of the muscle, a condition known as myositis or myopathy. Myositis is confirmed by a blood test that measures an enzyme called creatine kinase, or CK. If myositis occurs, the statin should be discontinued. The inflammation and muscle symptoms will gradually resolve. Again, like myalgias, myositis can be overdiagnosed. Patients can often have a brief increase in the CK that is unrelated to the medication. If symptoms are mild or absent when the CK is mildly increased, it is reasonable to wait and recheck the CK in about one week. If the CK returns to normal, statin therapy can continue. If, on the other hand, symptoms are more significant or weakness occurs, statin therapy should be immediately stopped. An extremely rare side effect is rhabdomyolysis, which is an intense inflammation of the muscle. When this occurs, the muscles are usually painful and weak, and CK levels are severely elevated. The kidneys can be injured or fail while trying to handle the protein released from the inflamed muscle. Early detection is crucial to prevent the most severe outcomes. Accordingly, for patients who are taking a newly prescribed statin drug, new muscle discomfort should be promptly reported to your physician. A CK can be drawn to exclude this condition. Fortunately, rhabdomyolysis occurs in less than one out of ten thousand people taking a statin drug.

Patients also worry about liver damage from statin therapy. Indeed, persistent minor elevations in liver enzymes can occur. However, this problem is seen in less than one percent of patients taking statins. These elevations are detected with a blood chemistry profile that measures the liver enzymes, aspartate aminotransferase (AST) and alanine aminotransferase (ALT). If a mild increase in liver enzymes is seen, it can safely be rechecked one to two weeks later. Usually the increases in AST and ALT occur without symptoms. Unless the increase in liver enzymes rises to more than three times the normal level, statin therapy can safely continue. Even when a significant statin-induced increase in liver enzymes occurs, it simply resolves when the medication is discontinued. As for liver failure, it is so rare that it is controversial whether statin-induced liver failure even exists. Nevertheless, it is appropriate that if unexplained abdominal discomfort or nausea occurs, an AST and ALT test should be done. Guidelines for cholesterol treatment also suggest these blood tests be routinely checked when monitoring cholesterol levels.

The 'take home' message

Statin drugs are tremendously important in preventing heart attacks, strokes and death. Further, they are incredibly safe. There is no class of medication that has been as thoroughly studied as statins. Although side effects can and do occur, they are uncommon and generally harmless. Serious side effects are exceedingly rare. Routine follow up and monitoring are an important part of any medical strategy, including statin therapy. In summary, the benefits of statin therapy in patients with known or suspected cardiovascular disease far outweigh the potential risk of these medications.

While various medications can lower blood cholesterol levels, statins are recommended for most patients because they are the only cholesterol-lowering drug class that has been directly associated with reduced risk for heart attack and stroke.

(www.heart.org; cholesterol medications; American Heart Association; 4/21/2014)

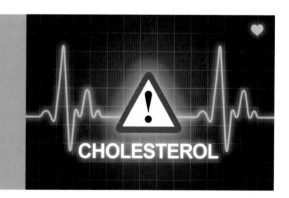

The net cardiovascular benefit for people at high cardiovascular risk strongly favors statin use.

(*New England Journal of Medicine*, May 2012)

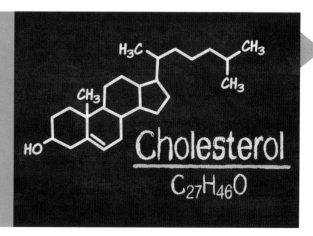

CoQ10: An Antidote to Statin-Related Muscle Aches and Pains?

A. Neil Bilolikar, M.D.

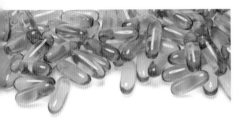

For the patient suffering from statin-related muscle aches and pains, the thinking has been that there is a deficiency in CoQ10 and supplementation might help

Are you taking a cholesterol-lowering statin drug and experiencing muscle aches? Is using Coenzyme Q10 (or CoQ10) right for you?

In order to protect you against future heart attacks, your cardiologist may have already prescribed a cholesterol-lowering medicine referred to as a statin. Ideal for lowering blood cholesterol, the generic drugs in this class, which generally end in 'in,' have been studied extensively in numerous randomized controlled trials. Unquestionably, these medications help lower blood cholesterol levels and prevent recurrent heart attacks. Numerous studies have also shown that statin medications are beneficial in preventing first heart attacks.

With these medications currently being prescribed to millions of patients, symptoms are reported to occur in 10 to 20 percent of all patients. The most common symptoms are muscle aches and pains, referred to as myalgias. Symptoms can range from mild to severe, and may ultimately lead to myositis, or muscle inflammation, which can be confirmed by a blood test. Lastly, a very rare complication from use of statins is rhabdomyolysis, which refers to actual muscle breakdown; this condition can also be verified by blood testing.

Other possible symptoms include foggy sensations and becoming more forgetful. Alert your physician if any of these symptoms arise, and he or she may prescribe a different statin. The rationale behind this is that each medicine is metabolized differently by the liver, and not every statin will cause the same symptoms in any given patient. However, even with changing statin medications, some patients continue to experience mild symptoms. What can be done about this?

Statins work by blocking an enzyme in the liver called HMG-CoA reductase. This enzyme is responsible for converting a cholesterol precursor into true cholesterol. A byproduct of this conversion of the cholesterol precursor to cholesterol is the formation of ubiquinone, a protein essential for cellular function and energy production. Once cholesterol synthesis is stopped, ubiquinone cannot be made and a deficiency in this substance results. Ubiquinone is also known as CoQ10, a substance similar to a vitamin, which also functions as an antioxidant that is used to help make energy in the mitochondria of all human cells. Specifically, it assists in the production of adenosine triphosphate, an energy currency used by the body to stimulate cellular reactions.

For the patient suffering from statin-related muscle aches and pains, the thinking has been that there is a deficiency in CoQ10 and supplementation might help. Use of CoQ10 has been studied in two small randomized controlled trials of 30 to 40 patients, and in those trials, CoQ10 reduced muscle aches in one study, but not in the other. Larger, non-randomized trials suggest that there is no difference in taking the drug versus placebo. Although the medical literature is controversial on this subject, it suggests that supplementation with CoQ10, while not harmful, may be of limited benefit for some patients with muscle aches and pains associated with statin usage.

Anecdotally, several of my own patients who have used this supplement have experienced a reduction in muscle soreness that began after starting a statin. Moreover, the impact of CoQ10 has been studied in several other disease states, and has been found to be useful among patients with breast cancer, and of modest benefit among patients with heart failure, diabetes, and high blood pressure.

Finally, recognize that CoQ10 is a supplement that is not Food and Drug Administration regulated; thus, the dose listed on the bottle may or may not be the actual dose of the medicine. The daily doses used in the above-referenced randomized controlled trials were 100 mg (worked) or 200 mg (didn't work). Moreover, CoQ10 has been shown to be relatively safe, with very few reported side effects. To be well absorbed, it should be taken with a fatty meal, or the capsule itself should be in a fat emulsion. If you are taking a dry pill of CoQ10, you are probably not absorbing it all.

If you have mild muscular symptoms while taking a statin medication, CoQ10 is certainly worth trying. After all, the benefits of taking statins and staying heart attack free are crystal clear, and this dietary supplement may help you to enjoy it pain free.

ONCE-A-DAY ANTI-STROKE, HEART PILL PROMISING

A single daily pill that combines aspirin and four blood pressure and cholesterol medicines may offer a cheap, simple way to prevent heart disease and stroke. The experimental "polypill" proved as effective as nearly all of its components taken alone, with no greater side effects, a major study found. Taking it could cut the risk of heart disease and stroke in half, the investigators concluded.

(*Lancet,* April 2009).

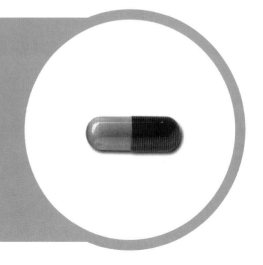

PCSK9 Inhibitors: A New Class of Medications for the Treatment of High Cholesterol

Jenna M. Holzhausen, PharmD, BCPS

Reduced levels of LDL result in decreased plaque build-up in the arteries, leading to fewer heart attacks, strokes, and other problems associated with cholesterol-clogged arteries.

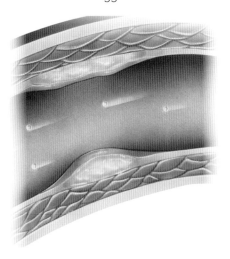

There has been considerable hype surrounding the recent Food and Drug Administration approval of a new class of medications for the treatment of high blood cholesterol, broadly classified as PCSK9 inhibitors. These new drugs, marketed as alirocumab (Praluent®) and evolocumab (Repatha®), are monoclonal antibodies that inhibit a protein called proprotein convertase subtilisin-kexin type 9 (PCSK9). The role of PCSK9 is to bind to low-density lipoprotein (LDL) receptors on the liver and promote their breakdown. By blocking the action of PCSK9, more LDL receptors remain on the liver surface to decrease the amount of harmful LDL cholesterol circulating in the bloodstream. Reduced levels of LDL result in decreased plaque build-up in the arteries, leading to fewer heart attacks, strokes, and other problems associated with cholesterol-clogged arteries.

Although the initial treatment of high cholesterol often relies upon modifications to diet and exercise, lifestyle modification alone may be insufficient to provide the desired protection for all patients. In these instances, medications are often relied upon to further reduce LDL levels. For several decades, the first-line option for reducing LDL cholesterol has been a class of medications known as the statins. Although statins have been shown to be effective for preventing cardiovascular events in a wide range of individuals, they don't always lower cholesterol to the desired degree, and may require a second cholesterol-lowering agent to be prescribed. Additionally, patients are occasionally unable to tolerate statins due to development of adverse side effects, such as muscle pain or liver damage.

The new PCSK9 inhibitors are administered as an injection beneath the skin in the thigh, abdomen, or upper arm every two or four weeks. These drugs have been studied both with and without concomitant statin therapy and have proven to be very powerful LDL reducers in short-term trials. Several longer-term (52 to 78 week) trials have recently been published (*New England Journal of Medicine,* May 2014; *New England Journal of Medicine,* April 2015; *European Heart Journal,* Sept. 2015), which reinforce the benefits seen with short-term use. In general, the PCSK9 inhibitors have been shown to reduce LDL levels by 50 to 60 percent compared to standard therapy alone. Additionally, preliminary data suggests the risk of cardiovascular events (including chest pain requiring hospitalization, heart attacks, stroke and death) may be reduced approximately 50 percent with the addition of a PCSK9 inhibitor. However, further research is required to confirm these initial findings.

As with all medications, PCSK9 inhibitors are not without their limitations. Due to the method of administration, the most common side effect is pain, tenderness, redness or itching associated with the injection site. Other side effects have also been reported, including muscle pain, headache, memory impairment and confusion. Additionally, the cost of these agents is anticipated to be thousands of dollars per year, which will limit access for many individuals.

Overall, the PCSK9 inhibitors are an exciting new class of medications that have demonstrated promise as an add-on to statin therapy in high-risk patients or as single-therapy in individuals unable to tolerate statins. However, their therapeutic role remains unclear and data regarding their long-term safety and effectiveness are currently lacking.

EXCESS SALT BLAMED FOR CARDIOVASCULAR DEATHS WORLDWIDE

Salt intake worldwide is at least twice what it should be, with a negative impact on global cardiovascular health, researchers reported. Daily sodium intake averaged 3,950 milligrams (mg) in 2010, according to an analysis covering all of the world's population. The recommended daily intake is 2,000 mg by World Health Organization standards and 1,500 mg by American Heart Association guidelines. The impact of the excess dietary sodium: an estimated 2.3 million deaths from cardiovascular disease in 2010 alone. These findings highlight both the tremendous disease burden caused by sodium as well as the need for food industry and policy makers to take rapid and decisive actions to reduce sodium in the food supply.

(American Heart Association Nutrition, Physical Activity and Metabolism and Cardiovascular Disease Epidemiology and Prevention meeting, March 2013)

The Problem With Abruptly Stopping Beta-Blocker Therapy

Harold Friedman, M.D.

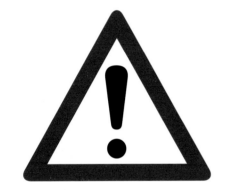

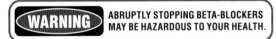

Beta-blockers are a class of drug used to treat a variety of cardiovascular conditions. Referred to by either their generic names, which commonly end in "ol" (atenolol, metoprolol, nadolol, propranolol, timolol), or their brand names (Tenormin, Lopressor or Toprol, Corgard, Inderal and Blockadren), they work by affecting the response to certain nerve impulses throughout the body. These drugs are commonly used to treat hypertension, irregular heartbeats, rapid heart rates, anginal chest pain, heart attacks and congestive heart failure. Because beta-blockers are widely prescribed, understanding their safe use is important.

Beta-blockers block adrenalin in the bloodstream from binding to beta-receptors on a variety of cells in the body. The receptors are part of the "flight or fight" stimulating mechanism. Beta-receptors are located in many cellular sites, including the heart and blood vessels. With prolonged exposure to beta-blocker drugs, the body begins to adapt by increasing the numbers of receptors on each cell. This serves as a counter response to heighten adrenalin sensitivity. This adaptive response, which occurs in everyone, results in a series of predictable and serious problems if the medication is abruptly stopped.

Abrupt drug discontinuation results in an upsurge in cellular adrenalin-like activity since more receptors have formed and many of these become unblocked. The response may include increased angina, accelerated heart rates, heart attack, stroke, and potentially dangerous spikes in blood pressure. Less serious symptoms include palpitations, increased perspiration and malaise. Such symptoms often occur in up to 50 percent of the patients with angina.

Beta-blockers are typically tapered over 10 to 14 days in elective situations. If "rebound" symptoms appear, the dose or frequency of the beta-blocker can be modified. If you suspect medication-related side effects, consult your physician immediately. There may be a different beta-blocker formulation that is better for you or a non-beta-blocker medication alternative.

Beta-blocker therapy can be useful for preventing recurrent heart attacks and potentially fatal rhythm disturbances in heart attack survivors. Patients who may also benefit from these medications include the elderly and individuals with heart failure. Nevertheless, abruptly stopping beta-blocker treatment can lead to a rebound effect, including adverse signs and symptoms. In some cases, these may be life-threatening.

As a reminder, I'd suggest making a copy of the above-referenced label and pasting it on your medicine tray.

New Drug Therapy for Heart Failure: Spotlight Entresto

Steven Ajluni, M.D.

Patients being treated for congestive heart failure (CHF) have enjoyed numerous treatment advances over the past three decades that have dramatically improved their prognosis and quality of life. These include: CHF-specific medications (Carvedilol, sold under the brand name Coreg among others, a nonselective beta-blocker/alpha-1 blocker, angiotensin converting enzyme [ACE] inhibitors, angiotensin receptor blockers [ARB] and aldosterone antagonists); implantable cardioverter defibrillator (ICD)/dual chamber pacing or cardiac resynchronization strategies; and, more recently, left ventricular assist devices or LVADs. Conservative interventions such as treatment of sleep apnea, weight loss, exercise, and salt restriction, or combinations thereof, have aided in the treatment of CHF as well.

Another agent has been recently added to the above-referenced arsenal, namely a combination pill of a new class of pharmacotherapy (neprilysin inhibition) combined with an ARB. The neprilysin inhibitor, Sacubritil, is an antihypertensive drug used in combination with Valsartan, an ARB. This drug, trade name Entresto, coupled with beta-blockers and other standard of care agents has been studied in a large randomized double-blinded study conducted worldwide (the Paradigm HF Trial) (*Journal of the American College of Cardiology,* Nov. 2015). In that study, selected CHF patients on stable standard of care medications including ACE inhibitors and beta blockers were randomized either to continuing the ACE inhibitor or substituting it with Entresto. The results demonstrated a clear superiority in using Entresto compared with ACE inhibitors (along with other standard of care CHF medications). There was a 16 percent reduction in mortality due to heart failure and nearly a 20 percent reduction in rehospitalization rates among patients treated by Entresto as compared with the ACE inhibitor group. These significant results became even greater in magnitude with more marked divergence in outcome curves over time. This highly significant result led to premature termination of the trial along with an expedited Food and Drug Administration approval.

Although the use of Entresto may offer significant treatment advantages in the future, certain precautions should be considered. Low blood pressures (hypotension), particularly in patients on aggressive diuretic plans, should be carefully monitored, as well as elevated potassium levels and an increased risk of angioedema (allergic swelling). The physiologic effects on chemical metabolism and drug interactions associated with Entresto are still being evaluated and its long-term health implications remain unclear.

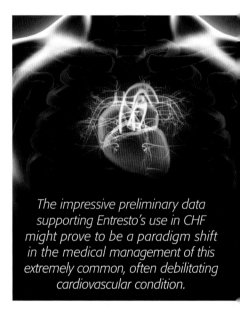

The impressive preliminary data supporting Entresto's use in CHF might prove to be a paradigm shift in the medical management of this extremely common, often debilitating cardiovascular condition.

Moreover, the impact of Entresto on amyloid deposition in selected tissues, including the brain, requires additional investigation. Still, the impressive preliminary data supporting its use in CHF might prove to be a paradigm shift in the medical management of this extremely common, often debilitating cardiovascular condition. Both patients and doctors alike should be aware of this promising new drug.

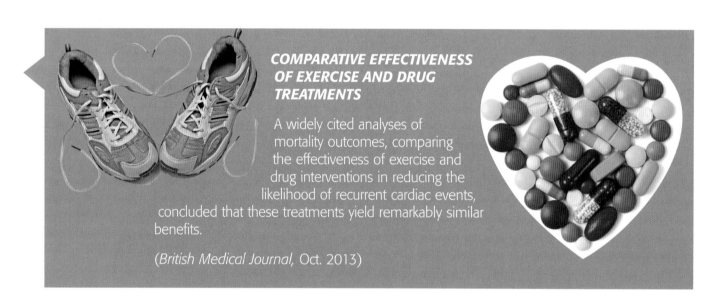

COMPARATIVE EFFECTIVENESS OF EXERCISE AND DRUG TREATMENTS

A widely cited analyses of mortality outcomes, comparing the effectiveness of exercise and drug interventions in reducing the likelihood of recurrent cardiac events, concluded that these treatments yield remarkably similar benefits.

(*British Medical Journal*, Oct. 2013)

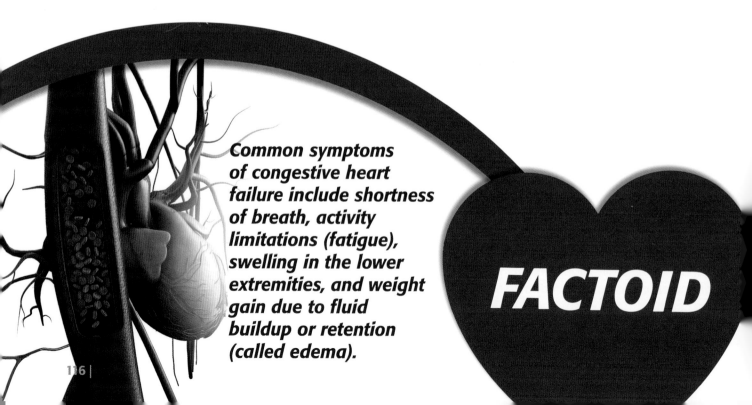

Common symptoms of congestive heart failure include shortness of breath, activity limitations (fatigue), swelling in the lower extremities, and weight gain due to fluid buildup or retention (called edema).

FACTOID

Optimizing Medication Dosing and Addressing Nonadherence

Susan Halley, RN

Most prescribed heart medications are designed to reduce the workload on the heart, improve the risk factor profile, and decrease the likelihood of future heart attacks or life-threatening heart rhythm irregularities. These drugs provide independent and additive cardioprotective benefits when combined with healthy dietary modifications, moderate exercise, weight loss and avoidance of cigarette smoking (*American Journal of Cardiology,* July 2004), resulting in improved artery dilation, ambulatory blood pressure, and lipid/lipoprotein profiles. Ultimately, the combined therapy results in a reduced risk of acute cardiac events.

In order to optimize overall cardiovascular health, medication dosing and adherence serve as an integral part of the treatment regimen. Although nearly 90 percent of patients are discharged from the hospital with appropriate cardiac medications after experiencing a heart attack, at 12-month follow-up visits, most patients receive doses of beta-blockers, statins, angiotensin converting enzyme inhibitors and angiotensin receptor blockers that are substantially below those with proven effectiveness (*Journal of the American College of Cardiology,* Nov. 2013). These findings highlight the need for increased education and awareness of the most appropriate doses and therapeutic levels of prescribed cardiac medications. Thus, patients need to be proactive in communications with their physician, regarding the medications and therapeutic doses needed to achieve optimal medical management.

Along with prescribed and up-titrated medication dosages, long-term adherence should be addressed. In one widely-cited study (*Circulation,* Jan. 2006), nearly 30 percent of cardiac patients were not consistently using aspirin, and fewer than half reported consistent long-term use of beta-blockers, cholesterol-lowering drugs, or combinations of these life-saving medications. High risk patient subsets such as the elderly, diabetics, and those with congestive heart failure were less likely to take their prescribed medications. Unfortunately, medication noncompliance is a significant factor associated with increased all-cause mortality, recurrent cardiac events, repeat hospitalizations and revascularization procedures (*American Heart Journal,* April 2008). In this report, over an average follow-up of 4.1 years, medication nonadherence was a common problem, with one in four patients being non-adherent to their prescribed beta-blockers, angiotensin-converting enzyme inhibitors or statins.

Although cardioprotective medications can unequivocally reduce the incidence of acute cardiac events, many of these drugs, especially when

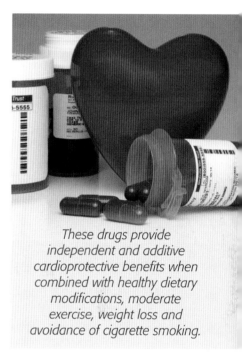

These drugs provide independent and additive cardioprotective benefits when combined with healthy dietary modifications, moderate exercise, weight loss and avoidance of cigarette smoking.

combined, can result in lightheadedness, marked reductions in heart rate and/or blood pressure, and orthostatic hypotension. Indeed, more than one in four hospitalizations among seniors are due to adverse drug reactions, and approximately 32,000 older adults suffer hip fractures each year due to falls attributed to the hemodynamic consequences of cardiovascular medications (*Healthcare Cost Utilization Project Statistical Briefs,* 2011).

In light of the above-referenced statistics, serious efforts are needed to improve the appropriateness of medication dosing and long-term compliance. Is nonadherence due to misunderstanding or underestimation of the negative impact on cardiovascular disease on the part of the patient and/or physician? Do patients stop taking medications due to associated symptoms and/or excessive costs? Are optimal prescriptive doses, titration and follow-up possible? Can we better educate and advocate? Are we targeting high risk populations that often need medications the most, but may be more likely to be non-adherent? These are intriguing questions to address to optimize cardiovascular health outcomes and decrease the likelihood of acute cardiac events. Collectively, these data suggest that optimization of cardiovascular medication dosing and addressing medication nonadherence should be high priority performance measures for patients and the physicians that care for them.

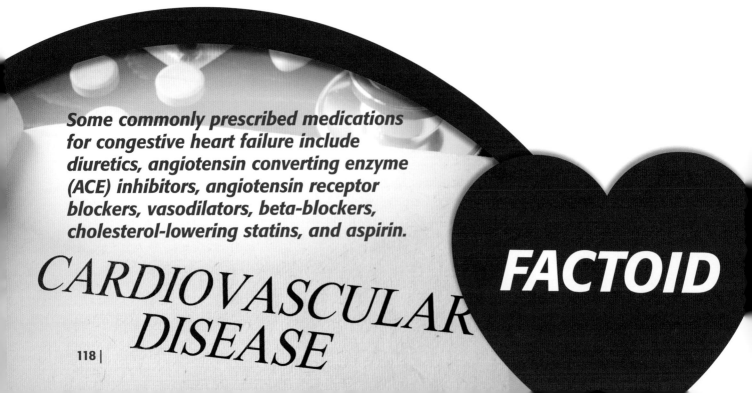

Some commonly prescribed medications for congestive heart failure include diuretics, angiotensin converting enzyme (ACE) inhibitors, angiotensin receptor blockers, vasodilators, beta-blockers, cholesterol-lowering statins, and aspirin.

CARDIOVASCULAR DISEASE

FACTOID

Medications: A Double-Edged Sword?

William Devlin, M.D.

Most people who see a physician, whether it is for a cardiac problem or for any other medical issue, generally take several medications. The science of pharmaceuticals is incredible, as these agents can help us prevent, control and even cure diseases. Although there is considerable evidence substantiating the safety and effectiveness of drug therapy, there is the potential for harm.

Each year, medication errors account for many patients being hospitalized and even deaths. Some medicines can counteract or enhance the effects of other medications. Depending on what medical problems one has, medications can have toxic or dangerous effects on certain body functions. Health care providers are constantly concerned about potential side effects of medications and medicine interactions. Accordingly, it is essential that we know what medicines a patient takes. It amazes me when we occasionally get resistance from patients to review medications. "It has not changed since the last time I was here" and "It is in the computer" are common responses we get.

When you come to the office or hospital, it is routine practice that your medications are reviewed. This is usually done by a medical assistant or nurse. Medications commonly change and patients often see more than one physician. We even see patients who make changes to their own medications. Sometimes this is appropriate, but often it is not. Medication errors can occur in three different ways; when the medication is prescribed, when the prescription is filled, and when and how the prescription is taken by you, the patient. Of course dealing with medication interactions are a vital part of practicing safe medicine.

To help you and your physician, every patient should keep an accurate and up-to-date list of their medications in their purse or wallet.

Most health care providers now use electronic devices to prescribe medications. The prescription can either be printed and taken to the pharmacy or sent electronically. Either way the issue of mistaken handwriting has virtually been eliminated from medical practice. Additionally, computer-based prescribing provides safety messages through alerts to us when we write the prescription. These systems have also helped pharmacists dispense medications with unparalleled accuracy and safety. Thus, prescribing medications is now safer than ever and mistakes have been dramatically reduced.

The medications listed in your medical record or at your local pharmacy don't really matter

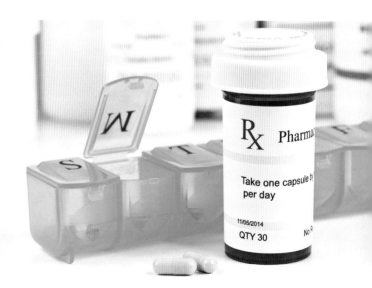

if you are not taking them. To help you and your physician, every patient should keep an accurate and up-to-date list of their medications in their purse or wallet. We cannot identify medications by shapes and sizes, though sometimes it is tempting. Generic medications can change colors, or even pill shapes depending on the manufacturer. Don't rely on your memory alone for something this important. As I say to patients on a regular basis: "Heaven forbid that you are in an accident and cannot talk. Having an accurate medication list on you could save your life."

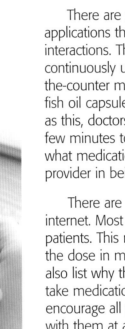

There are multiple sources online or even smartphone applications that can be used to help identify medications and their interactions. This is also why it's important for your physician to be continuously updated as to what medications you're taking. Over-the-counter medications and related supplements (e.g., omega-3 fish oil capsules) should also be listed. With something as important as this, doctors and patients cannot make assumptions. It takes a few minutes to review a list that could save your life. Not knowing what medications a patient takes essentially handicaps a health care provider in being able to deal with any medical problem.

There are numerous sample lists that are available on the internet. Most hospitals supply a medication card for discharged patients. This medication list simply provides the medication name, the dose in milligrams, and how frequently it is taken. Some patients also list why they take it, or even designate the time of day that they take medications. Regardless of how you want to format your list, I encourage all patients to have an accurate, updated medication list with them at all times.

Each year I give a lecture to the first year medical students at Oakland University, William Beaumont School of Medicine on Cardiovascular Disease in the Elderly. This is an enjoyable experience for me. I was once in their shoes and who knows, someday I might be treated by one of these students. One of the key points that I make is that as we get older, there is a trend to need and take more medications. There is also a tendency to have more medication errors and to have medication side effects due to the increasingly complex medical issues that elderly patients often have. This message is given to medical students, interns and residents as well as to our cardiology fellows. We try to educate future doctors that it essential to be aware of medications not just as a tool to treat diseases but also as a potential cause of medical issues. Remember, a cardinal tenet of medicine is, "first, do no harm."

Keeping an updated medication list is one way that you can help yourself. Please allow nurses or medical assistants who ask you about your medications to do their job. This is after all, in your best interest. If we can cut down on medication errors and adverse interactions, you will likely enhance your health and health care experience.

5

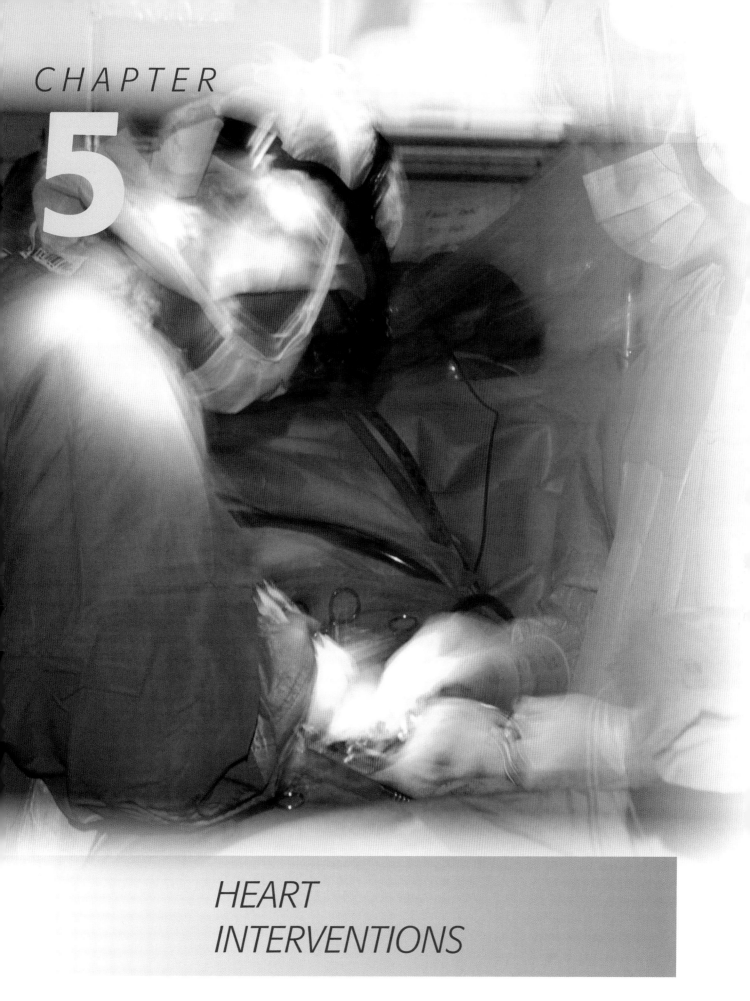

HEART INTERVENTIONS

Inside a Modern Cardiac Catheterization Room

Simon R. Dixon, MBChB

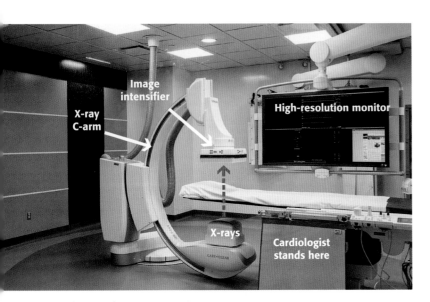

Image intensifier

X-ray C-arm

High-resolution monitor

X-rays

Cardiologist stands here

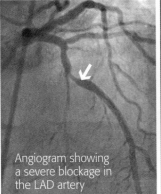

Angiogram showing a severe blockage in the LAD artery

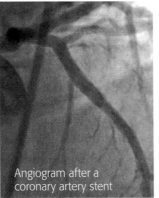

Angiogram after a coronary artery stent

A cardiac catheterization lab (cath lab) is a special room in the hospital where heart catheterization procedures are performed to diagnose and treat coronary artery disease and other heart conditions. Some cath labs are also configured to treat vascular disease such as carotid or leg blockages, or implant pacemakers and defibrillators.

At the "heart" of the modern cath lab is sophisticated X-ray imaging equipment which allows the physician to advance thin tubes called catheters in real-time from the wrist or groin into the heart. The X-rays pass through the patient from the bottom of the "C-arm" to the image intensifier where they are displayed on a high-resolution monitor in front of the cardiologist. The catheters are used to record pressure measurements inside the heart and also to inject contrast dye into the coronary arteries to identify blockages (called an 'angiogram'). With advances in X-ray technology, very detailed images of the blood vessels in the heart can now be obtained, including tiny collateral vessels (natural bypass channels). If a severe narrowing is identified, the cardiologist passes a balloon through the catheter into the coronary artery to stretch open the blockage and then place a stent. A modern cath lab costs about $2 million to build and needs to have the X-ray equipment replaced every seven to eight years.

These specialized procedures require an extremely well trained team of nurses, technicians and cardiologists. For example, a typical heart cath procedure requires three nurses and two doctors. One nurse monitors the patient and administers sedation to keep the patient comfortable, one nurse gets equipment for the physician during the procedure (for example different catheters or balloons), and the other documents every step of the case in the medical record. The room also has a lot of other equipment that is necessary for these procedures.

As a patient, entering a cath lab for the first time can be quite a scary experience. To help patients prepare for a heart cath we created a virtual tour of one of our cath labs. Not unlike visiting a realtor website, this allows you to do a "360" inside the room and familiarize yourself with a modern cath lab. View the tour at heart.beaumont.edu/cardiac-catheterization.

Stents or Bypass Surgery for Severe Coronary Artery Disease?

Simon R. Dixon, MBChB

Recently, I performed a heart catheterization on a patient who had been experiencing exercise-induced pain (angina) between her shoulder blades for about one year. She had diabetes and high cholesterol but had never smoked and kept herself in good physical condition. The heart catheterization revealed severe blockages in all three of the coronary arteries that supply the heart muscle (we call this multivessel disease). Significant blockages in the right coronary artery and left anterior descending (LAD) artery are shown in the adjacent figures. Because of the multiple severe occlusions, I did not think she could be treated with medicines alone; that is, she needed something done to fix her compromised blood supply. Those options included stents and coronary artery bypass surgery. In this patient's case, I recommended bypass surgery.

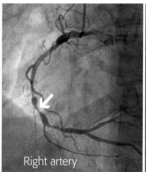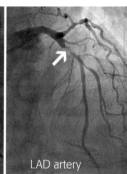

Right artery   LAD artery

The bottom line is that bypass surgery is generally better than stenting, especially in patients with diabetes, and those with complex, multivessel disease.

This common scenario raises the important question of how we determine whether a patient is best treated with stents or bypass surgery when multiple blockages are identified during the heart catheterization. Historically, this issue created friction between cardiologists and surgeons who often had opposing views on the optimal treatment course. Fortunately, those days are long gone, and decisions are now founded in excellent science, clinical guidelines and the adoption of team-based decision making.

The bottom line is that bypass surgery is generally better than stenting, especially in patients with diabetes, and those with complex, multivessel disease. This might seem like a bold statement for a physician who trained to put in stents, but the facts are the facts. There is no question that stents are an easier fix in the short term and have a faster recovery—the real issue at hand is which plumbing option is better over the long term.

Several recent landmark trials have compared stents versus bypass surgery for patients with multivessel disease or blockage involving the left main artery. In patients with more complex disease, bypass surgery was associated with a lower risk of heart attack and repeat procedures, more complete relief from angina, but a small increased risk of stroke. Cardiologists often grade the extent of disease on the heart catheterization films using a scoring system called the Syntax score. The higher the score the more likely the patient appears to do better with bypass than stents.

With that said, stents remain an excellent treatment option in those patients with less complex blockages, and many other factors must be taken into account when we decide whether to place stents or recommend bypass surgery. For example, patients with a weak heart, lung or kidney disease, advanced age, or prior stroke might be better to undergo stenting if it is felt that surgery is too risky. The quality of the blood vessels where the surgeon attaches the bypass graft is also an important consideration.

Because of these complex issues, it is very important for the cardiologist, surgeon and patient to come to consensus together on the optimal treatment course. What is right for one patient, might be totally different for another patient.

As a rule, it will take a patient about 4-to-6 weeks to start feeling better after undergoing cardiac bypass surgery.

FACTOID

Bypassing Blocked Arteries: The Road to Recovery

Marc Sakwa, M.D.

Learning that you need coronary artery bypass surgery can be a devastating experience. Besides the initial shock regarding your urgent medical condition, patients often begin to worry about their recovery and what their future quality of life will be like. Assuming that there are not serious complications, most patients are grateful that they had the procedure and recover very quickly.

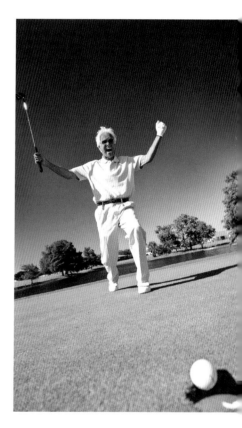

Regardless of the approach, any major surgical procedure is disruptive and debilitating. Your body needs time to heal and your mind needs time to cope. After cardiac surgery, it is not surprising that many patients are depressed. After all, most of us feel we are invincible. We go to work every day, we take care of our families and, for the most part, fulfill needs for many people. Because these people may depend on us, it can be extremely difficult to accept our own illness.

Initially after surgery most patients are not self-sufficient and may require special assistance from spouses or family members. Yes, this can be challenging; however, it is generally short-term. After 2 to 3 weeks, most patients begin to resume their normal lifestyle. The notion that patients require 2 to 3 months to get back to their full activity is antiquated. Patients are now encouraged to increase their activities almost immediately upon hospital discharge. Within 2 to 3 weeks, most patients begin to drive cars, increase their physical activity, and if desired, return to work. Once this increased activity occurs, the postoperative depression generally dissipates.

Many older patients are retired and worry about what their quality of life will be like after heart surgery. Fortunately, most patients rapidly return to their presurgical activities and are able to do them at a much higher level because they are now symptom-free. Being an avid golfer, I always relate to patients who are also golf enthusiasts. After surgery, we usually ask patients to wait 2 to 3 weeks before they begin to resume their chipping and putting. Full swings can be undertaken within 4 to 6 weeks, once the sternum has had a chance to heal. Although most patients will initially have a slight increase in their handicap, I've had patients who experienced their first "hole in one" after bypass surgery!

Cardiac surgery, although not without risk, can improve the quality of life of many people. After an initial recovery period, most patients perceive an improvement in lifestyle, not only resuming their former activities, but often having the energy to try new ones.

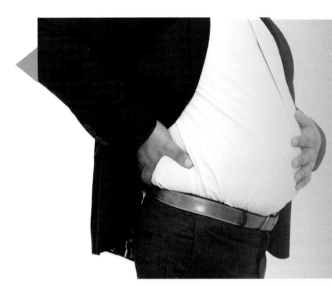

According to new research, compared to coronary artery bypass patients with normal weight, patients with severe obesity were three times more likely to develop an infection after bypass surgery.

(*Physician's Weekly,* June 2016)

Most patients who have a coronary stent inserted can resume normal activities within a few days.

FACTOID

New Frontiers: The Bioabsorbable Stent

Simon R. Dixon, MBChB

In 1994, the first coronary artery stent was approved for use in the United States. The concept of stenting arose in the early days of coronary angioplasty to overcome recoil of the artery after balloon dilation. Coronary stents are essentially a metal frame designed to prop open the narrowing like a scaffold, and maintain blood flow to the heart muscle. Over the past decade many new generations of stents have been developed to improve the ease of insertion and long term results for our patients. While we often take it for granted, modern stents are remarkable pieces of engineering technology, and have revolutionized the treatment of coronary artery blockages, enabling many patients to avoid open heart surgery.

Bioresorbable Stent

More recently, it has become apparent that the "scaffolding" effect of a coronary stent is really only needed for a few months after implantation, while the artery wall is healing. Accordingly, there has been escalating interest in developing stents that are fully absorbed by the body, rather than leaving behind a permanent implant. The goal is for the stent to be gradually resorbed by the body over six to 12 months. The idea of the "disappearing stent" has several theoretical benefits such as restoring the artery to its natural function, minimizing the need for long-term medications such as clopidogrel (Plavix), and improving the accuracy of subsequent diagnostic testing with techniques such as coronary computed tomographic angiography.

Several bioabsorbable stents are currently being studied. One type uses a biodegradable polymer; another is a made of a magnesium-alloy. The technology that is most promising is made by Abbott Vascular, and has two layers of a biodegradable polymer. One layer contains the drug everolimus to limit scar tissue formation, and the other layer provides the structural backbone. This stent, which was first tested in New Zealand and the Netherlands, was approved for use in the United States in 2016.

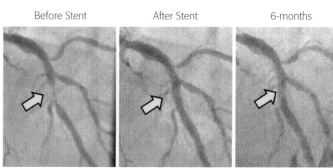

Before Stent   After Stent   6-months

Promising New Heart Attack Treatment: "Supersaturated Oxygen"

Simon R. Dixon, MBChB

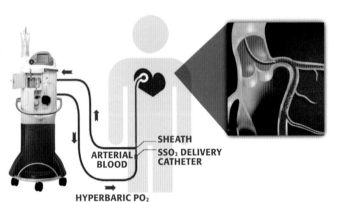

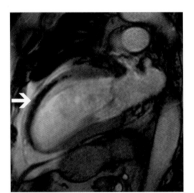

MRI of the heart after a large heart attack. There is extensive injury in the front wall of the heart (arrow)

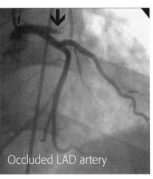

Occluded LAD artery

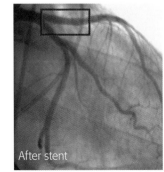

After stent

A heart attack is caused by sudden blockage in one of the coronary arteries that supply the heart muscle with oxygenated blood. Prolonged interruption in blood flow causes the muscle cells to die which may weaken the pumping ability of the heart and result in congestive heart failure or death. The most common cause for myocardial infarction (heart attack) is formation of a blood clot at the site of an inflamed atherosclerotic plaque inside the coronary artery tree.

Emergency coronary angioplasty and stenting is the most effective method for relieving the obstruction in the coronary artery and abating the course of the heart attack. The faster the occluded artery can be opened the better, since the longer the heart is starved of blood flow, the more extensive the muscle injury. The amount of muscle damage is the most important factor that will influence a patient's recovery and future well-being.

Over the past two decades, we have explored numerous additional treatments that might help prevent permanent damage after a heart attack. One promising new treatment is supersaturated oxygen (SSO_2). This therapy is based on the known beneficial effects of hyperbaric oxygen in patients with burns and wounds. The technology (which was developed in Detroit) provides the equivalent of a hyperbaric oxygen chamber, but just to the heart.

The treatment is delivered after the cardiologist has opened the occluded coronary artery with a stent. Using a small circuit, the patient's blood is supersaturated with oxygen, and then returned directly into the main coronary artery through a small catheter for 60 minutes. The high level of oxygen appears to improve healing, and has been shown to reduce the size of the heart attack by 25 percent!

Our health system has been one of the few centers in the U.S. pioneering SSO_2 therapy and is now leading a new clinical trial with this innovative technology. However, the therapy is not FDA-approved at this time and may not be suitable for all heart attack patients. Nevertheless, for those with large heart attacks, the treatment looks extremely promising.

What Is Coronary Brachytherapy?

Simon R. Dixon, MBChB

The introduction of coronary artery stents in the early 1990s revolutionized the treatment of coronary artery disease. The metallic frame of the stent scaffolds open the blockage in the artery to maintain blood flow to the heart muscle. After implantation, a thin layer of scar tissues grows over the metallic struts so the stent basically becomes part of the vessel wall. Modern stents, known as drug-eluting stents, also have a thin layer of drug on the outside surface of the stent to limit how much scar tissue forms.

Although relatively uncommon, some patients develop excessive scar tissue inside the stent that results in the artery re-narrowing. This process, which is called "restenosis," may cause the patient to experience chest pain or shortness of breath and therefore need another catheterization procedure to open the artery.

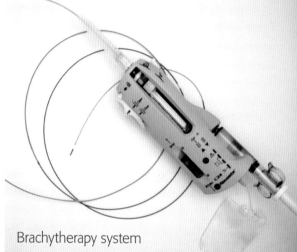

Brachytherapy system

The treatment of coronary restenosis varies depending on the extent of scar tissue inside the original stent. In cases of focal restenosis, balloon angioplasty alone may be used to stretch open the scar tissue. Sometimes a new drug-eluting stent is placed inside the old stent.

Another treatment option that is now available involves the use of radiation (brachytherapy) inside the old stent to prevent regrowth of the scar tissue. This is a very safe and effective option, especially for patients who have diffuse restenosis or multiple layers of stents.

How does this work? Brachytherapy is performed as part of the usual angioplasty procedure. First the interventional cardiologist opens the scar tissue with a balloon (angioplasty). Next, a thin radioactive ribbon is advanced inside the artery that delivers radiation to the wall of the artery. The radiation passes only into the wall of the artery and does not affect the rest of the body. After three to four minutes, the radioactive ribbon is withdrawn and the procedure is completed.

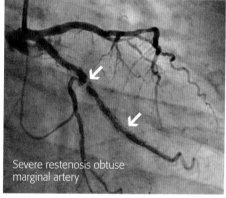

Severe restenosis obtuse marginal artery

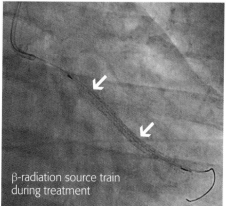

β-radiation source train during treatment

New Frontiers for Totally Blocked Coronary Arteries

Simon R. Dixon, MBChB

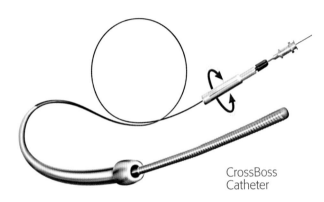

CrossBoss Catheter

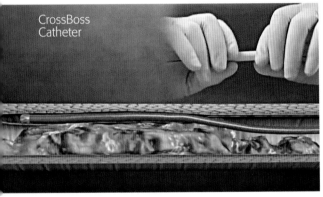

CrossBoss Catheter

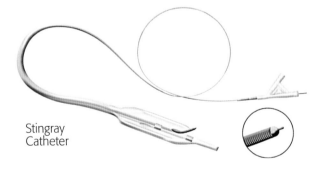

Stingray Catheter

About one in 10 patients undergoing heart catheterization for suspected angina are found to have total blockage (occlusion) of one of the major coronary arteries that provide blood to the heart muscle. This is known as a chronic total occlusion (CTO). It may be surprising, but in many cases an artery can become 100 percent occluded without causing a heart attack because the heart has time to adapt and build natural bypass channels (collaterals) to the affected area. Nevertheless, the blocked artery might cause symptoms such as chest pain, shortness of breath or fatigue during physical activity.

Until recently, totally blocked arteries have been extremely difficult to treat with traditional balloon angioplasty and stent techniques, with a success rate of about 50 percent. Imagine the coronary artery is like a tunnel with a total cave-in. During the procedure, the cardiologist must create a new channel through the cave-in with a small guidewire in order to use the balloon and stent. Sometimes the blockage is rock hard so the guidewire will not pass.

Fortunately, there are now several new techniques to treat these totally occluded arteries. One approach is to use a device called the CrossBoss catheter to open the artery through the front-door. This novel device is used to create a channel between the wall of the artery and plaque blockage. Subsequently, a Stingray catheter is used to access the true lumen of the artery beyond the blockage and a stent is then placed to scaffold the artery open.

Another novel approach is to treat the total blockage via the back-door (or retrograde approach). In these cases the cardiologist threads the guidewire down a good artery, through collateral channels and then backwards up the blocked artery to the site of occlusion (this side of the cave-in is often easier to get through compared with the front-door). After crossing the blockage the guidewire is pulled out, which then provides the rail for placing the stent.

While these new techniques have revolutionized the treatment of CTO, careful case selection and planning are critical to determine the best approach for each patient. Special training is also required for the cardiologist.

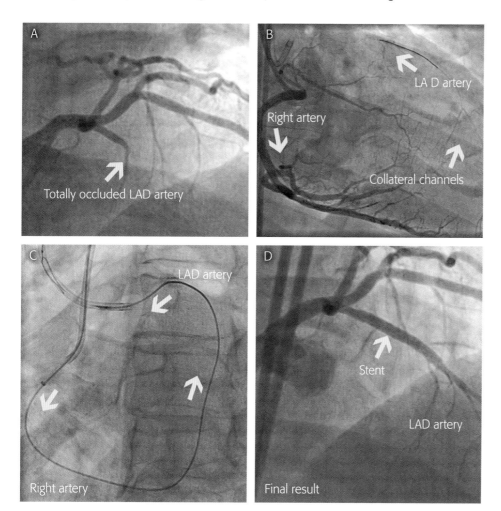

MitraClip for the Treatment of Mitral Regurgitation

George S. Hanzel, M.D.

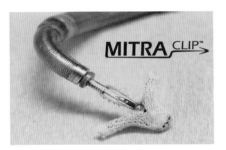

Mitral regurgitation is a common cardiac condition that affects up to 7 percent of people over the age of 75. It is estimated that 4 million Americans have mitral regurgitation with 250,000 new cases diagnosed annually and 50,000 mitral valve operations performed each year. With the aging baby boomers, the absolute number of patients with mitral regurgitation is expected to dramatically increase over the next 15 years.

Understanding the problem

The mitral valve is a one-way valve that separates the left atrium (the heart chamber that receives blood as it leaves the lungs) from the left ventricle (the heart chamber that pumps oxygen-rich blood to the body). When the left ventricle squeezes, the mitral valve closes to prevent blood from traveling backwards and reentering the left atrium and even the lungs. Mitral regurgitation is, in essence, an incompetent or "leaky" mitral valve.

The leakiness of the valve burdens the heart and causes it to work harder. Eventually, if the regurgitation is severe enough, the heart becomes weakened and enlarged. This leads to congestive heart failure, which is often manifested by fatigue, fluid retention and shortness of breath. It can also cause an irregular heart rhythm called atrial fibrillation. More severe degrees of mitral regurgitation can lead to worse outcomes, including fatal cardiovascular events. There are many causes of mitral regurgitation, but the two most common causes are mitral valve prolapse and heart muscle damage, frequently due to a heart attack, which may result in weakened, enlarged hearts (where the leaflets are pulled apart).

Catheter

MitraClip in position

Treatment options

Unfortunately, there are no medications that can directly treat or reduce mitral regurgitation. Milder degrees of mitral regurgitation do not require treatment and can be monitored over time. Symptoms caused by more severe degrees of mitral regurgitation can be treated with diuretics, or water pills, and blood pressure medications. Currently, the standard treatment for more severe degrees of mitral regurgitation is open-heart surgery to repair or replace the mitral valve. This is a proven and effective means of eliminating mitral regurgitation and improving symptoms of heart failure.

Unfortunately, many patients are too high risk to undergo conventional surgery. The MitraClip is a novel device that can be used to treat severe mitral regurgitation in high-risk patients. The device is based on a surgical procedure called the Edge-to-Edge Repair, or Alfieri technique, named after the surgeon who invented it. The MitraClip is placed through a vein in the groin and advanced into the heart via a catheter, or small tube. The clip then grasps and pulls together the two leaflets of the mitral valve in order to improve valve closure and reduce leakage.

In November 2013, the Food and Drug Administration approved the MitraClip for the treatment of patients with mitral valve prolapse and severe mitral regurgitation who are at high-risk for conventional surgery. Cardiologists and cardiac surgeons at our center and others are collaborating to investigate the MitraClip in patients who have severe mitral regurgitation due to weakened hearts (called functional mitral regurgitation). These patients who are too high-risk for conventional surgery are randomized to the MitraClip versus continued medical therapy. The results of this trial will determine whether treating severe mitral regurgitation in patients with a weakened heart will improve their heart failure symptoms.

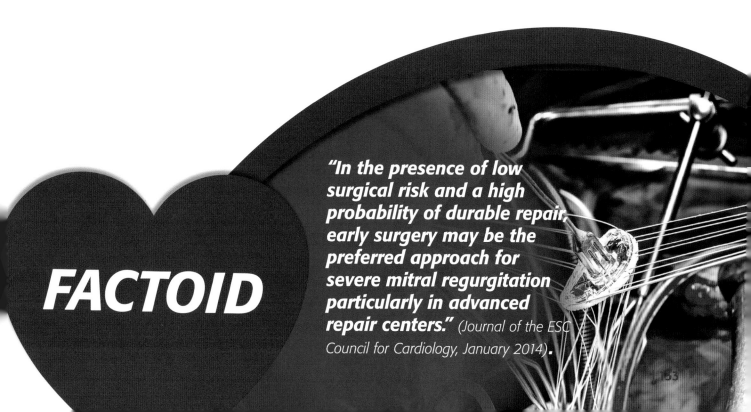

FACTOID

"In the presence of low surgical risk and a high probability of durable repair, early surgery may be the preferred approach for severe mitral regurgitation particularly in advanced repair centers." (Journal of the ESC Council for Cardiology, January 2014).

Transcatheter Aortic Valve Replacement

George S. Hanzel, M.D.

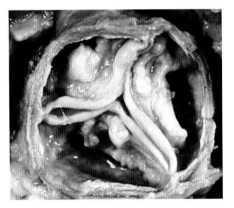

Aortic Stenosis

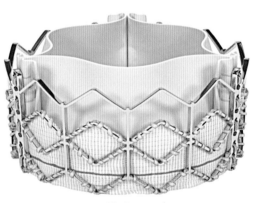

Stent with tissue valve

Aortic stenosis is a common cardiac condition that affects approximately 5 percent of people over the age of 75. Moreover, an estimated 80,000 aortic valve operations are performed each year in the United States. With the aging "baby boomers," the absolute number of patients with aortic stenosis is expected to dramatically increase over the next 15 years.

Understanding the problem

The aortic valve is a one-way valve that separates the left ventricle (the heart chamber that pumps oxygen-rich blood to the body) from the aorta (the main blood vessel of the body). When the left ventricle squeezes, the aortic valve opens and allows blood to flow from the heart to the body. Aortic stenosis is a narrowed aortic valve that prevents efficient and unimpeded flow of blood from the heart to the rest of the body.

The narrowing of the valve burdens the heart and causes it to work harder. Eventually, if the narrowing is severe enough it can lead to congestive heart failure, (which is manifested by fatigue, fluid retention and shortness of breath), angina (chest pain) or fainting. Severe aortic stenosis is associated with poor long-term outcomes, including fatal cardiovascular events. There are several causes of aortic stenosis, but the two most common are bicuspid aortic valves (a congenital defect in which a person is born with two instead of three aortic valve leaflets) and "senile" degeneration of a normal trileaflet valve.

Treatment options

Unfortunately, there are no medications that can treat or improve aortic stenosis. Milder degrees of aortic stenosis do not require treatment and can be monitored on a routine basis. Currently, the standard treatment for more severe degrees of aortic stenosis is open-heart surgery to replace the aortic valve. This is a proven and effective means of correcting the structural defect and improving symptoms and life expectancy. Cardiac surgeons at our medical center have helped pioneer new minimally invasive ways of performing traditional aortic valve replacement surgery. Unfortunately, approximately one-third of older symptomatic patients do not undergo this life saving surgery due to either age or the coexistence of additional medical problems.

Several years ago, Beaumont was the first site in the North America (and the second in the world) to perform transcatheter aortic valve replacement (TAVR). During this procedure, a tube (or catheter) is inserted into the artery in the groin and threaded to the heart. A stent with a tissue valve sutured inside it is advanced to the aortic valve and implanted, pushing aside the old narrowed valve and allowing the new valve inside it to open and close normally.

Clinical trials of TAVR have demonstrated significantly improved survival and quality of life in patients who are not candidates for traditional surgical aortic valve replacement. In high risk patients, TAVR has been shown to be equivalent to surgical aortic valve replacement in terms of survival and quality of life.

Based on these clinical trials the Food and Drug Administration approved transcatheter heart valves for the treatment of inoperable and high risk patients. Today, cardiologists and surgeons are routinely treating high risk and inoperable patients with TAVR, and evaluating its effectiveness in intermediate risk patients. Patients who are considered intermediate-risk for traditional aortic valve surgery are randomized ("a flip of the coin") to traditional surgery or to TAVR. Additionally, we are studying TAVR for the treatment of degenerated bioprosthetic heart valves.

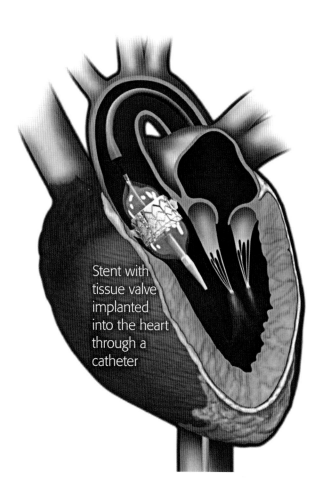

Stent with tissue valve implanted into the heart through a catheter

Atrial Fibrillation: Treatment Options

Phillip Robinson, M.D.

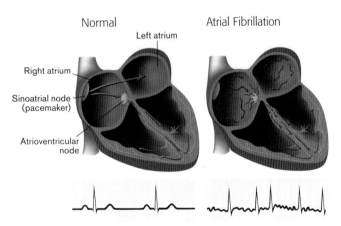

Normal

Atrial Fibrillation

Left atrium

Right atrium

Sinoatrial node
(pacemaker)

Atrioventricular
node

Atrial fibrillation (a-fib) is a heart rhythm irregularity affecting approximately 3 million people in the United States. It is usually recognized by patients who notice that their heartbeats are erratic at times or that they are skipping beats. The older you are, the greater the risk for developing this abnormal heart rhythm. About 3 percent of patients in their forties and up to 10 percent of those in their eighties experience this irregular heart rhythm.

There are three classifications or types of a-fib. These are based on the duration of time you spend in a-fib, and what makes your heart revert back into its normal rhythm, known as sinus rhythm. Many patients spend short periods of time in this rhythm and will spontaneously convert back to normal on their own. Others spend longer periods of time and may require electric shocking of the heart to return to a regular rhythm. For some patients, the heart may never resume its regular rhythm and the patient stays in a-fib permanently.

The basic problem with this electrical conduction disturbance is that the upper chambers of the heart (the atria) do not beat in the usual fashion. The atria lose their ability to produce forceful contractions which adequately fill the lower pumping chambers (the ventricles). The consequences of this rhythm can include feelings of tiredness; fast, irregular hearts beats called palpations; or even strokes. In fact, the risk of a stroke is seven times higher for a patient in a-fib than a patient in normal sinus rhythm. Twenty-five percent of all strokes in this country are from a-fib. These strokes are usually more debilitating than strokes from other reasons and often occur multiple times over a patients' lifetime if not treated.

The primary medical treatment for patients with a-fib uses medications to control the heart rate and lower the risk of strokes. Blood thinners such as Coumadin or newer medications reduce stroke risks, but can be associated with bleeding complications. Recently, newer medications have been introduced to help with some of the inconveniences associated with Coumadin like frequent blood testing. Those patients that are very symptomatic and have trouble coping with normal daily activities while in this heart rhythm may require more aggressive treatment plans. This may involve using medications which can convert a-fib to sinus rhythm. However, the side effects of these medications are significant and can lead to even more serious complications.

Highly symptomatic patients may require a procedure called ablation, which can also be used to treat a-fib. An ablation makes a precisely controlled scar on the inside or outside of the heart which isolates the diseased area of the heart where the a-fib starts from the healthy part of the heart which controls the normal rhythm. The scar is usually made by heating the heart tissue to a high temperature with lasers or other energy sources which produce the desired results. The scars are strategically placed around veins in the heart, which connect from the lungs, or other areas which are known to trigger the a-fib. These ablation lines can either be placed by specially trained cardiologists who perform the procedures through the groin like a heart catheterization, or for more difficult types of a-fib, by surgeons through very small incisions or robotically. The results have been very encouraging with a success rate ranging from 75 to 95 percent, depending on the type of a-fib.

Successfully treated a-fib allows patients to be weaned from their medications and stop the blood thinners. For the best long-term chance to remain free from a-fib, patients should be very diligent in watching their blood pressure, keeping it as close to normal as possible. For patients with obstructive sleep apnea, a mask that keeps the airway open during sleep may solve the problem. A healthy lifestyle of regular exercise and weight reduction, if appropriate, is also highly beneficial (see Chapter 7: Treatment of Atrial Fibrillation: Fitness and Fatness Matter).

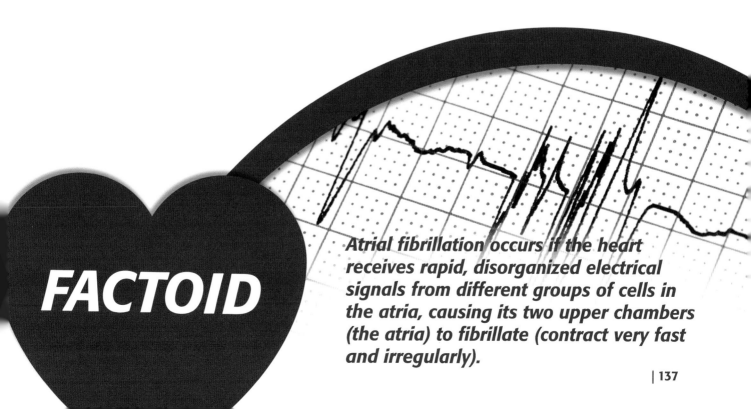

FACTOID

Atrial fibrillation occurs if the heart receives rapid, disorganized electrical signals from different groups of cells in the atria, causing its two upper chambers (the atria) to fibrillate (contract very fast and irregularly).

WATCHMAN Left Atrial Appendage Closure to Reduce Atrial Fibrillation-Related Stroke

George S. Hanzel, M.D.

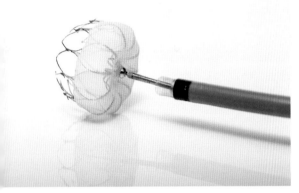

Atrial fibrillation, a common medical condition affecting more than 6 million adults in the United States, can cause palpitations, fatigue and shortness of breath. However, the greatest threat of atrial fibrillation is clot formation within the heart, ultimately leading to a stroke. On average, atrial fibrillation increases a person's risk of stroke five-fold, and 20 to 25 percent of all strokes are due to atrial fibrillation.

The standard strategy to reduce atrial fibrillation related stroke is anticoagulation therapy with warfarin (Coumadin), dabigatran (Pradaxa), rivaroxaban (Xarelto), apixaban (Eliquis), or edoxaban (Savaysa). However, nearly 50 percent of patients with atrial fibrillation are unable to tolerate anticoagulant therapy. There are many reasons for this, but the main one is risk of bleeding complications. For this reason there is great interest in reducing the dreadful complication of stroke without increasing the risk of major bleeding.

Interestingly, 90 percent of all clots in atrial fibrillation arise in an out-pouching of the left atrium called the left atrial appendage. Because of stagnation of blood flow within this structure, clots are prone to develop there. If this structure could be occluded or sealed off it is thought that atrial fibrillation related strokes could be reduced without the need for anticoagulation therapy. Accordingly, the risk of bleeding complications from long-term anticoagulation therapy could be eliminated.

Since 2005, our physicians have been investigators in four clinical trials of the WATCHMAN device to achieve left atrial appendage closure. This device is placed into the left atrial appendage to "plug" it. The procedure is performed via a small tube placed in the vein in the groin and takes approximately an hour to complete. The clinical trials demonstrate that the WATCHMAN device is similar to warfarin in terms of stroke reduction but carried a dramatically lower risk of bleeding complications. In March 2015, the WATCHMAN device was approved by the Food and Drug Administration as an alternative to anticoagulation therapy in selected patients with atrial fibrillation. Ideal patients include those who are not optimal candidates for anticoagulation but who can tolerate at least a short course of anticoagulation therapy since a six week course of warfarin is required after the procedure.

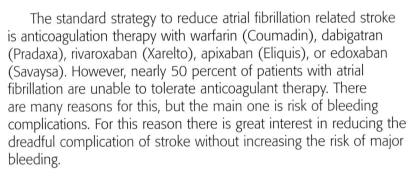

Traveling With Pacemakers and Defibrillators

Alan J. Silverman, D.O.

A common question for patients with defibrillators and pacemakers is, "what do I do when I travel"?

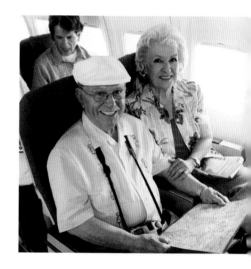

Most patients who have pacemakers and defibrillators are enrolled in a device clinic. This is usually run by a registered nurse, physician assistant or a specially trained pacemaker technologist under the supervision of a cardiologist. Every patient is given a device identification card. This is important to have with you at all times when you travel. Besides having all your device information, it is also proof to all airport screening personnel that you have a device.

Though many patients with implanted cardiac devices express concern about airport security systems, there really is no need to worry. When you arrive at security, walk through the metal detector at a normal pace. If the alarm sounds, it means the system has detected the metal in your pacemaker or defibrillator. Show airport security your identification card. Ask for a hand pat-down search. If they use a wand, it should be held over your device for no more than 30 seconds.

In addition, when traveling, it is helpful for patients to have with them a printout from their last pacemaker or defibrillator evaluation. This will include all of the current device settings. This information can be very helpful in the event of an emergency while traveling.

Finally, always have your device clinic and doctor's phone number with you. If you have any concerns about your device while traveling, we are only a phone call away. Have a great trip!

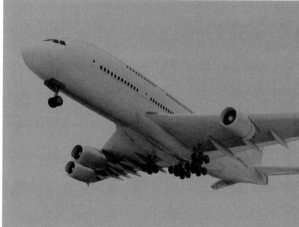

Sitting motionless for prolonged periods of time may put some travelers at increased risk for deep vein thrombosis, or DVT. A blood clot that develops in the lungs (pulmonary embolism) is especially dangerous and can be fatal. To reduce your risk of DVT during a long-distance flight, wear loose comfortable clothes, consider graduated compression stockings, walk around often during the flight, drink plenty of water, and avoid alcohol consumption. Sitting in an aisle seat may also be helpful in getting regular physical activity at 30,000 feet.

The COURAGE Trial: Lessons Learned …

Barry A. Franklin, Ph.D.

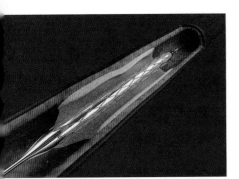

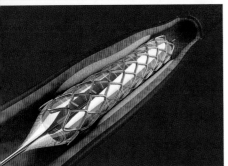

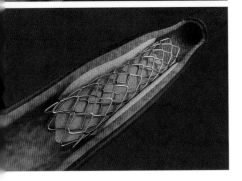

During an angioplasty procedure, a doctor inserts a catheter into an artery in a patient's arm or leg and advances it into the coronary arteries where a balloon is inflated to open the blockage. Usually, a tiny mesh-like tube (stent) is implanted into the artery to keep it open.

Angioplasty is a highly effective treatment to halt heart attacks in progress and improve anginal symptoms. Many patients also believe that if they undergo angioplasty and stenting, they'll be less likely to have a heart attack or they will live longer. Indeed, these procedures are performed more than 1 million times each year, and the vast majority are undertaken electively in patients with stable heart disease.

Although coronary angioplasty is known to improve survival when done to restore blood flow during a heart attack, no study has examined the ability of coronary angioplasty to improve survival over and above modern, optimal medical therapy in coronary patients with or without anginal symptoms. Several years ago, this question was addressed in an important study called the COURAGE trial.

Researchers enrolled 2287 patients with known heart disease at 50 hospitals in the U.S. and Canada, randomizing them to one of two treatment groups: angioplasty (to "fix" existing coronary blockages) plus optimal medical therapy (n = 1149) or optimal medical therapy alone (n = 1138). Thus, both groups received aggressive medical therapy, which included an array of antianginal and cardioprotective medications designed to reduce symptoms and achieve recommended cholesterol and blood pressure levels, as well as lifestyle programs such as smoking cessation, exercise, weight management, and nutritional counseling.

Enrolled patients had signs and/or symptom of insufficient coronary blood flow and at least a 70 percent blockage of one or more coronary arteries. A majority of the patients in the study were men (85 percent) and nearly 40 percent had suffered a previous heart attack. Most exhibited several risk factors for heart disease.

Over a follow-up period averaging 4.6 years, a total of 211 deaths or nonfatal heart attacks (the primary focus of COURAGE) occurred in the coronary angioplasty group (19 percent), compared with 202 in the medical therapy group (18.5 percent), a statistically nonsignificant difference. When stroke and hospitalizations for anginal symptoms were examined, again there were no differences seen between groups. On the other hand, the angioplasty group reported less anginal symptoms during the trial. Moreover, a greater number of the medically managed patients went on to have either angioplasty or bypass surgery (at their doctor's discretion) to relieve worsening symptoms.

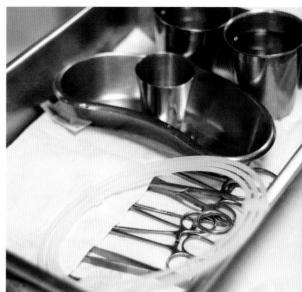

Do the COURAGE results apply to all coronary patients? Probably not. Were there limitations to the study design and potential confounding variables? Most definitely.

The investigators acknowledged that the preponderance of male patients limited the generalizability of their findings, as did the lack of ethnic diversity (only 14 percent of the patients were non-white). In addition, many of the sickest cardiac patients were excluded from participating in the study. Others emphasize that bare-metal, rather than drug-eluting stents were employed, and that during the study period, more aggressive anti-clotting drug regimens were adopted before and after angioplasty procedures. Finally, a greater number of the medically managed patients went on to receive angioplasty procedures or bypass surgery to relieve worsening anginal symptoms.

Collectively, what do the results of the COURAGE trial really signify? According to Dr. Steve Nissen, Director of Cardiology at the Cleveland Clinic: "… the results suggest that it's probably OK to defer angioplasty and give medical therapy a try—and, you're not going to compromise your health." Dr. James Stein, Director of the Preventive Cardiology Program at the University of Wisconsin, Hospital and Clinics, Madison, commented: "This study clearly shows something we all knew—but many did not want to believe—that angioplasties don't save lives, except in acutely ill patients, and don't prevent heart attacks."

According to an accompanying editorial, the COURAGE trial should lead to changes in the initial treatment of many patients with stable coronary artery disease, with expected substantial healthcare savings.

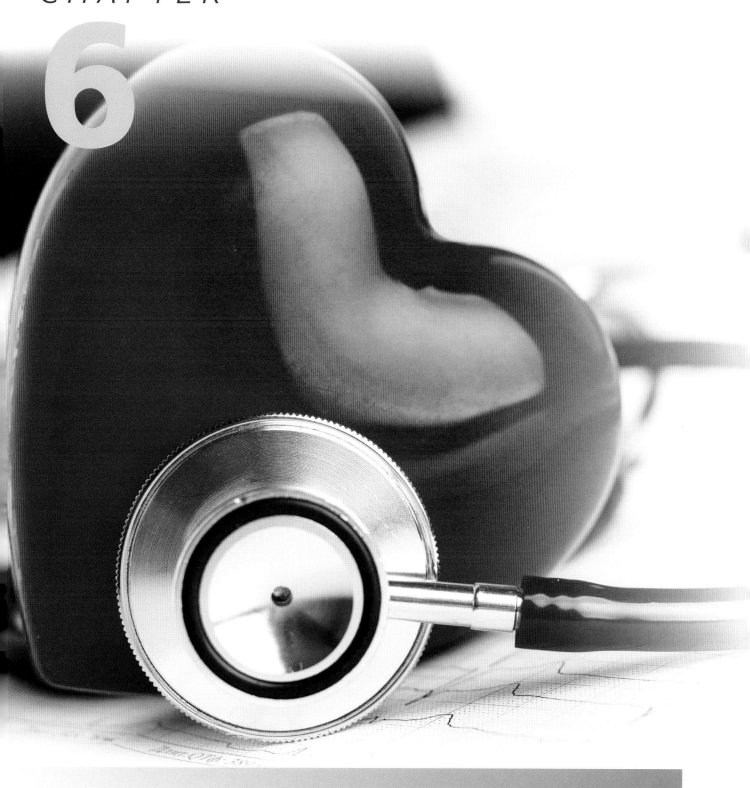

CHAPTER

6

HEALTH & DISEASE MANAGEMENT

Exercise and Diabetes

Kathy Faitel, RN
Susan Halley, RN

Medication, blood glucose management, and exercise are the cornerstones of diabetic management. Yet, only 39 percent of diabetic adults exercise regularly. The American Diabetic Association recommends 150 minutes per week of moderate intensity exercise (similar to a brisk walk, or an intensity corresponding to 50 to 70 percent of the maximum heart rate achieved during exercise stress testing). Aerobic activity five days per week complemented by resistance training is widely promoted for optimum blood glucose management.

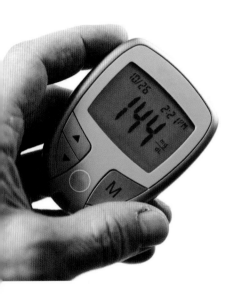

Before beginning a physical conditioning program, an initial evaluation is essential to ensure that there are no contraindications to exercise. Because exercise lowers blood glucose levels, it may be necessary to monitor your blood glucose more frequently and alter your meal times. The risk of hypoglycemia (low blood glucose) and hyperglycemia (elevated blood glucose) are significant among diabetics who exercise. Because exercise transiently reduces blood sugar, it is recommended that you do not exercise with a blood glucose below 100 mg/dl. In some diabetics, hormone shifts can transiently elevate blood glucose levels. This is why checking your blood glucose before you exercise and again after exercise is critical, especially when you start an exercise program. Following exercise your blood sugar can continue to drop for 24 hours. Accordingly, rechecking your blood glucose several hours after your exercise is strongly recommended.

Most diabetics know how they feel when their blood glucose level drops below 70 mg/dl: shaky, weak, tired, hungry, and irritable. Many patients complain of blurred vision. If you're a diabetic and you experience these symptoms, it's probably due to a transient drop in your blood glucose level and one of the following is recommended: three to four glucose tablets; 4 oz. of any fruit juice; 4 oz. of a regular soft drink; or, 8 oz. of milk. Recheck your blood glucose after 15 minutes. If it is still low or you do not feel any improvement, have another snack. Repeat these steps until your blood glucose is 90 mg/dl or higher and your symptoms are resolving. This is called the "Rule of 15." Each snack example above provides 15 grams of carbohydrate. After ingesting the snack wait 15 minutes and recheck your blood glucose level. These measures are expected to raise your blood glucose about 15 points.

After the first week of tracking your blood glucose levels, you should be able to anticipate any blood sugar modulations and adjust your diet/snacks accordingly. You should no longer require frequent blood glucose checks unless you substantially increase your exercise frequency, intensity, duration, or combinations thereof. For example, if you decide to progress from brisk walking to slow jogging, it is wise to go back to more frequent blood glucose monitoring until you know how your blood glucose will respond.

Home exercise guidelines include:

- Choose activities that you enjoy and that fit into your lifestyle.
- Invest in good exercise equipment, i.e., comfortable walking shoes.
- Start slowly and gradually increase frequency, duration, and intensity.
- Choose an exercise time of day to provide consistency.
- Exercise for longer duration and lower intensity to promote reductions in body weight and fat stores.
- Include a five to 10 minute warm-up and cool-down at the beginning and end of the exercise period.
  - ✓ Increase physical activity during lifestyle activities (park farther away from stores when shopping, use the stairs rather than taking the elevator, walk to co-worker's offices rather than e-mailing them).
  - ✓ If exercising alone, carry identification, a carbohydrate snack, and a cell phone.

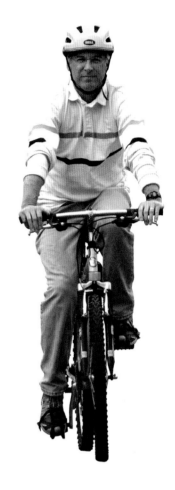

The number of diabetic patients in the U.S. is skyrocketing. Accordingly, the more fully patients understand the nature of the delicate balance that exercise has in treating diabetes, the greater the benefits they are likely to achieve. Without question, exercise is sound medicine. Consequently, regular exercise is widely considered an integral ingredient in a diabetic's recipe for a well-balanced, healthy life.

EVEN A LITTLE EXERCISE HELPS THE HEART

Even small amounts of physical activity each week will help reduce heart disease risk, and the benefit increases as the amount of activity increases, according to a widely-cited analysis. People who engaged in about 150 minutes or 2.5 hours of moderate-intensity activity a week, the minimum amount recommended in the U.S. Physical Activity Guidelines for Americans, had a 14 percent lower risk of heart disease compared to those who reported no exercise. Those who did more—about 300 minutes per week—had a 20 percent lower risk of heart disease. Interestingly, people who were physically active at levels lower than the minimum recommended amount also had significantly lower risk of heart disease. The 'take-home message' is:

If you are doing no exercise, do something. And, if you are doing some exercise, do more.

(*Circulation,* Aug. 2011)

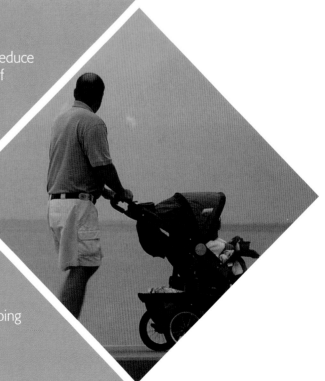

Get With the Program!
Cardiac Rehabilitation …
More Than Just Exercise!

Anne Davis, RN

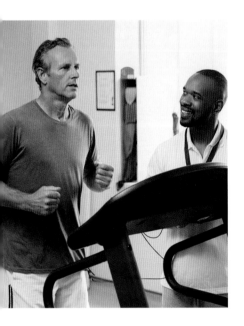

Cardiac rehabilitation is a multidimensional approach to maximizing physical fitness and reducing the risk of future cardiovascular events through exercise training, education, lifestyle modification, ongoing medical surveillance, and coaching. There are three phases to a contemporary cardiac rehabilitation program.

Phase I occurs in the hospital following a heart attack, coronary angioplasty, or heart surgery. It includes continuous monitoring of low level activities, such as grooming and bathing, range of motion exercises, and progressive walking. Prior to discharge, nurses and/or physicians may discuss a plan to identify and decrease or eliminate coronary risk factors, such as smoking, inactivity, high cholesterol, and hypertension. Patients should leave the hospital with a simple diet plan, prescribed cardioprotective medications and recommendations for progressive short walks and limited stair climbing, while maintaining a "fairly light" exertion level.

Following hospital discharge, Phase II is conducted at an outpatient rehabilitation center. It involves individually prescribed exercise at increased exertion levels, under close medical supervision. This surveillance allows for early detection and intervention in treating abnormal heart rhythms, dangerous blood pressure fluctuations, and other adverse signs or symptoms. There is opportunity for more in-depth education and counseling on topics such as cardiovascular disease, risk factors, diet, exercise and stress management.

Sometimes patients enter Phase II depressed and afraid to exercise, wondering if life as they knew it is over. As a clinician, it's exciting and rewarding to be a part of their growing confidence, as they make lifestyle changes and come to the realization that not only will they maintain their quality of life, they'll improve it! Currently, Medicare covers Phase II cardiac rehabilitation following a heart attack, cardiac bypass surgery, angioplasty, valvular heart surgery, and anginal chest pain. Patients graduate when they are stable (usually 18-24 visits) and have the option of continuing on their own or joining a Phase III program.

In Phase III, the patient learns to safely monitor his or her own prescribed heart rate and exertion level during exercise. Exercise physiologists and nurses are available for routine or emergent monitoring and continued education and counseling. Although the cost of Phase III is not generally covered by insurance, most patients find the benefits to be more than worth the investment. One dedicated Phase III patient writes: " … 18 years later, I am now in better shape than the day I started … I've been given more years to enjoy grandchildren, to make new friends, to travel all over the globe … in short, to enjoy life to its fullest!"

The benefits of cardiac rehabilitation include reductions in body weight and fat stores, systolic blood pressure, stress and cholesterol values as well as improved fitness levels. An organized program promotes a more active social life. The healing power of social support and friendships gained, among patients with common goals and interests, cannot be overestimated. Most important, participation is associated with a 20-25 percent decrease in one's risk for future cardiovascular events, and an increased longevity!

Ready to sign up? A physician referral is mandatory and a recent stress test may be required to begin an outpatient cardiac rehabilitation program. Should your physician prescribe cardiac rehabilitation, rest assured, you will gain an increased understanding of keeping your heart healthy, along with many useful tools to enhance the quality of your life.

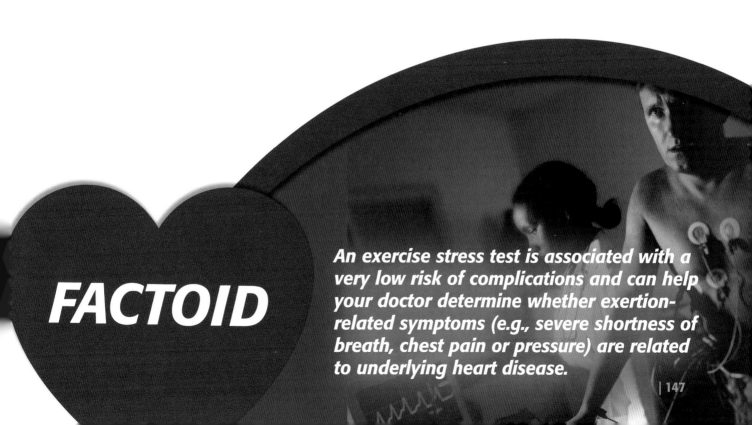

FACTOID

An exercise stress test is associated with a very low risk of complications and can help your doctor determine whether exertion-related symptoms (e.g., severe shortness of breath, chest pain or pressure) are related to underlying heart disease.

Treatment Options for Chronic Angina

Anne Davis, RN

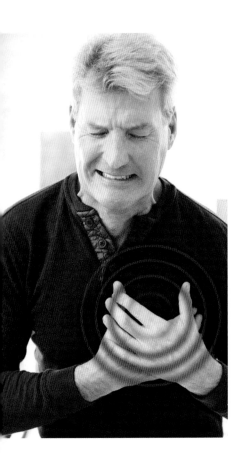

Angina is a symptom of heart disease, often presenting as chest pain, shortness of breath, or both. These symptoms result from inadequate blood flow or oxygenation to the heart, caused by partial obstruction or narrowing of the coronary arteries supplying the heart muscle. Treatment can be categorized into three options:

- Medical treatment includes lifestyle modification with appropriate cardiac medications to improve the blood supply/demand imbalance.
- Interventional treatment or revascularization techniques include coronary bypass grafting and coronary angioplasty, generally with stent placement.
- The third option, enhanced external counterpulsation therapy (known as EECP), is a non-invasive treatment series that transiently increases blood flow to the heart.

Risk factors, coronary anatomy, and the severity and acuity of symptoms, helps physicians determine the most appropriate course of action. In many cases, the above-referenced treatment options may be combined.

Medical therapy is generally considered the first-line treatment option. This includes aggressive lifestyle modification such as exercise or cardiac rehabilitation, a healthy diet, smoking cessation and cholesterol management. Standard cardiac medications are often prescribed to control angina, including nitrates, beta-blockers, calcium channel blockers and ranolazine or Ranexa. Nitrates such as nitroglycerin or isosorbide relax and dilate blood vessels, improving blood flow to the heart. Beta-blockers decrease the amount of oxygen needed by the heart muscle by reducing the heart rate, blood pressure and the force of the heart's contraction. Calcium channel blockers lower blood pressure and assist in reducing the heart's workload by dilating blood vessels. If a patient has been prescribed all these medications and continues to experience angina, ranolazine is another medication physicians are increasingly prescribing to relieve angina symptoms.

If anginal symptoms persist despite optimal medical treatment, your cardiologist may recommend an interventional or surgical treatment option. Cardiac catheterization or angiogram involves accessing the coronary arteries through a large artery in the groin or in the wrist. A catheter fed through the artery to the heart, followed by an injection of dye, enables your cardiologist to clearly visualize narrowed or blocked coronary arteries. In the case of a narrowed artery, he/she might insert the catheter and inflate a small balloon at the narrowing; pressure of the balloon, applied to the walls of the narrowed artery, helps to reopen it. This is known as angioplasty or percutaneous intervention. Usually angioplasty is followed by the insertion of a stent at the site to prevent it from re-occluding. In the case of angina, these interventions are used to reduce symptoms. Nevertheless, therapeutic angioplasty or coronary stents do not necessarily prolong life when done to relieve angina. Finally, coronary artery bypass grafting is the most invasive treatment option. A large incision of the chest cavity allows the cardiovascular surgeon to access the heart and a patient's own arteries or veins are used to bypass blockages or narrowed coronary arteries, thereby restoring blood flow to the area of the heart supplied by that particular artery. Despite a longer recovery period, up to 90 percent of patients remain angina free at one to three years after heart bypass surgery.

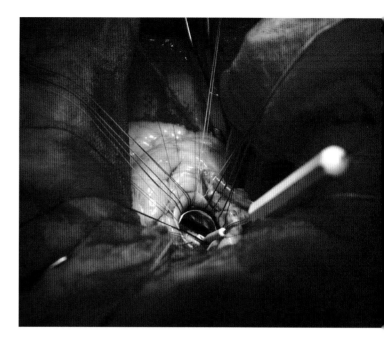

Unfortunately, up to 75,000 new cases of angina diagnosed each year do not respond to medical therapy or coronary revascularization techniques. In these cases, EECP may be prescribed. This non-invasive treatment consists of 35 one-hour sessions, where large blood pressure-like cuffs on the calves, thighs and hips inflate sequentially from the ankles up, between heartbeats, transiently increasing the pressure and flow of oxygen-rich blood to the heart.

EECP has minimal side effects and, in some cases, might even allow you to reduce or eliminate some of your antianginal medications. Unlike medication, EECP provides long-term symptom relief due to physiologic changes, similar to those of exercise. A large study done by the International EECP Registry reported that 70 to 80 percent of symptomatic patients noted a decrease in anginal symptoms, improved energy levels and activity tolerance with benefits lasting up to three or more years (*Clinical Cardiology,* April 2008).

If you are plagued by limiting angina symptoms despite optimal medical and interventional therapy, consider discussing EECP with your cardiologist. It may serve to increase your exercise capacity, reduce angina symptoms, and improve your quality of life.

EECP: A New Treatment Option for Disabling Heart Disease

Anne Davis, RN

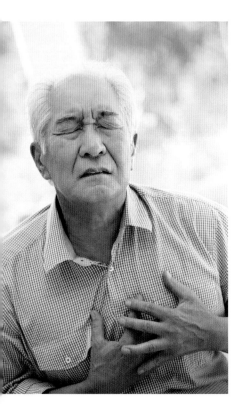

Each year, between 25,000 and 75,000 new cases of anginal chest pain, refractory to medical therapy (drugs) and standard coronary revascularization techniques, such as bypass surgery, angioplasty or stenting are reported. If you or someone you care about is one of these people, who has exhausted traditional treatment methods and still finds their life restricted with persistent chest pain and/or shortness of breath, there is hope.

Enhanced external counterpulsation (EECP) therapy has been studied for almost 50 years and is considered a safe, highly effective, non-invasive treatment, approved by the FDA to treat chronic stable angina, and congestive heart failure. The cost of treatment is covered by most health insurance companies. It is provided as an outpatient service and consists of 35 one hour sessions—usually 5 days a week for 7 weeks. Patients lie on a comfortable treatment table with large blood pressure-like cuffs on their calves, thighs and buttocks. Using a continuous electrocardiogram for timing, the cuffs inflate sequentially, from the ankles up, between heartbeats or while the heart is at rest. This is when the heart receives its major supply of blood and oxygen.

Symptoms of angina are caused by inadequate circulation to the heart muscle. EECP provides significant symptom relief to most patients (~70-80 percent) who complete their prescribed course of treatment. Most commonly, patients report a reduced frequency and intensity of chest pain, less shortness of breath, increased energy and improved exercise tolerance. Many patients are even able to decrease their cardiac medications. This therapy has improved the quality of life for many patients who had otherwise given up hope of an active life.

While it's evident the treatment works, it is still not totally clear why it works. Evidence strongly suggests, as EECP increases the coronary perfusion pressure, or the pressure of the circulation to the heart muscle, new tiny blood vessels called "collaterals" are formed around blockages, thus increasing blood flow to areas of the heart that were once deficient. Other studies suggest improved endothelial function, which is the tissue lining the inside of the blood vessel walls where atherosclerosis begins. This is similar to a benefit of exercise. Researchers have also noted an increase in plasma levels of nitric oxide after EECP. Nitric oxide is a natural potent vasodilator; therefore, increased levels may have a beneficial effect on the circulation to your entire body.

If you are plagued with persistent symptoms of angina and have tried conventional treatment modalities, including antianginal medications, coronary bypass surgery, or angioplasty without success, talk to your cardiologist about this treatment option. The risks are minimal and the results may be life changing!

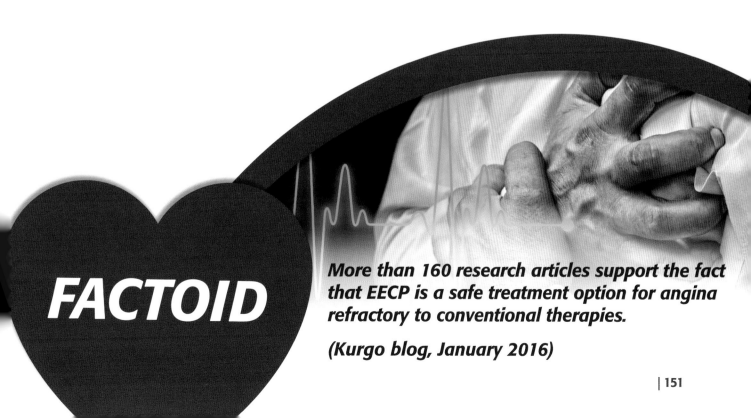

FACTOID

More than 160 research articles support the fact that EECP is a safe treatment option for angina refractory to conventional therapies.

(Kurgo blog, January 2016)

Rehabilitation Boosts Survival for Heart Patients

Barry A. Franklin, Ph.D.

An estimated 80 million Americans (nearly 1 in 3) have cardiovascular disease; in fact, coronary heart disease and stroke are currently the #1 and #4 causes of mortality, respectively. According to the American Heart Association (AHA), heart disease causes approximately 1 of every 4 deaths in the U.S. Moreover, 1.3 million coronary angioplasty procedures and 448,000 coronary artery bypass graft surgeries were performed in 2006, at a cost of over $100 billion.

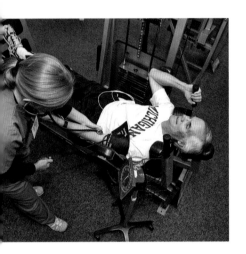

In 2010, an estimated 785,000 Americans experienced a new cardiac event, and approximately 470,000 had a repeat heart attack. Accordingly, for literally millions of previously affected adults in the U.S., interventions that have been shown to reduce the risk of recurrent cardiovascular events, collectively referred to as cardiac rehabilitation, are critically important. Core components include: patient evaluation; medical surveillance; psychosocial/vocational counseling; exercise training; lifestyle modification; and prescribed cardioprotective medications (e.g., aspirin, beta-blockers, statins), if appropriate.

Candidates for cardiac rehabilitation

Cardiac rehabilitation traditionally has been prescribed following a heart attack. Both the AHA and the American College of Cardiology clinical practice guidelines now recommend cardiac rehabilitation for heart attack survivors. However, many other patients may benefit from exercise-based cardiac rehabilitation programs. The Centers for Medicare and Medicaid Services also recognizes coronary artery bypass surgery, stable angina pectoris (chest pain/pressure), coronary angioplasty, heart valve repair or replacement, and heart transplantation as additional indications for cardiac rehabilitation. Evidence also supports cardiac rehabilitation for patients with heart failure. Currently, Medicare and most private insurers cover early outpatient cardiac rehabilitation programs; however, as with medications and other medical treatments, co-pays may be required.

Evidence for effectiveness

The most substantial benefits of exercise-based cardiac rehabilitation are summarized in the box. Added benefits include a reduction in anginal symptoms, decreases in exertion-induced signs or symptoms of coronary insufficiency, fewer recurrent cardiac events, a diminished need for subsequent coronary angioplasty or bypass surgery, and an increased exercise capacity. Such programs also provide referring physicians with valuable surveillance data to enhance the patient's medical management. Collectively, these benefits offer patients a distinct survival advantage.

A major systematic review of 48 well-designed trials of cardiac rehabilitation found that, compared with usual care, cardiac rehabilitation reduced all-cause and cardiac mortality by 20 percent and 26 percent, respectively (*American Journal of Medicine,* May 2004). Subsequently, researchers reported that among U.S. Medicare beneficiaries who were hospitalized for cardiac problems, coronary angioplasty or bypass procedures, mortality rates were 21 percent to 34 percent lower in cardiac rehabilitation users than nonusers (*Journal of the American College of Cardiology,* June 2009). Other investigators, using this patient subset (i.e., Medicare beneficiaries), reported that patients who attended the most rehab sessions demonstrated the greatest reductions in mortality and recurrent cardiac events (*Circulation,* Oct. 2010). Another analysis of outcomes from almost 2,400 patients who underwent coronary angioplasty procedures found that patients who participated in cardiac rehab programs reduced their risk of death by nearly 50 percent (*Circulation,* May 2011).

Referral and utilization of cardiac rehabilitation services

Despite it's proven benefits, less than one third of older coronary patients (i.e., Medicare beneficiaries) participate in outpatient cardiac rehabilitation programs, highlighting the vast underutilization of these services (*Circulation,* Oct. 2007).

Other groups who are underserved include poor/uneducated patients, women and minorities. The strength of the primary care physician or cardiologist's recommendation appears to be the single most powerful predictor of cardiac rehabilitation participation. Accordingly, physicians must take a more active role in promoting these programs. Nevertheless, many patients referred to cardiac rehabilitation do not enroll, suggesting that improving referral rates are only part of the solution. Other participation modulators include insurance coverage/co-pays, geographic accessibility, psychosocial variables, returning to work, spousal and family support, and patient motivation.

Conclusions

Physicians and their coronary patients must recognize that exercise-based cardiac rehabilitation is equally as beneficial and cost-effective as most contemporary technologies and drug therapies. This stance was underscored by an AHA policy paper addressing the cost-effectiveness of prevention (*Circulation,* July 2011). The message is a sobering one: BEAT STRONGER, LIVE LONGER.

Benefits of Exercise-Based Cardiac Rehabilitation

- increased exercise capacity/ fitness
- decreased anginal symptoms
- improvement in blood lipid/ lipoprotein levels
- reduction/elimination of cigarette smoking
- improvement in psychological status and functioning
- reduction in mortality

Cardiac Rehabilitation Extended to Congestive Heart Failure Patients

Amy Fowler, B.S.

There is excitement in the cardiology community regarding the Medicare extension of phase II cardiac rehabilitation coverage to include congestive heart failure (CHF) as a covered benefit for selected patients. Nearly 5 million Americans are living with diagnosed CHF. As the number one admission diagnosis in hospitalized patients older than 65 years, CHF is responsible for 11 million physician visits and more than 800,000 hospitalizations each year.

Congestive heart failure is a misnomer as it implies that the heart has "failed" and is no longer working or beating appropriately. In truth, CHF is a condition in which the heart is unable to pump as effectively as a healthy heart, which makes it difficult to supply adequate blood and oxygen to working muscles and organs throughout the body. Valvular disease, high blood pressure, coronary artery disease or previous heart attack(s) are common contributors to the development of CHF.

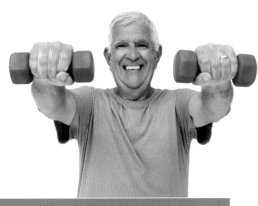

CHF is a condition in which the heart is unable to pump as effectively as a healthy heart, which makes it difficult to supply adequate blood and oxygen to working muscles and organs throughout the body.

Congestive heart failure is diagnosed following a physical examination (sometimes during a hospitalization), which may include a chest X-ray, echocardiogram (ultrasound of the heart), blood work and/or cardiac imaging studies. Common symptoms of CHF include weight gain, shortness of breath at rest or during low level activity, swelling of the lower extremities, unusual fatigue or combinations thereof. Treatment of CHF varies widely, depending on the severity of symptoms and extent of cardiac damage, but may include certain medications (e.g., diuretics, beta-blockers, angiotensin-converting enzyme inhibitors), lifestyle modification such as weight loss, salt restriction, and implantable devices such as a pacemaker or defibrillator.

Simultaneously, prescribed exercise in a supervised setting may prove beneficial in preventing rehospitalization, and help to improve functional capacity, symptoms and prognosis. In addition, comprehensive cardiac rehabilitation programs provide ongoing surveillance data which may help the referring physician to optimize their patients' medical care. For cardiac rehabilitation program participants, education specific to CHF is available that can help patients learn more about their heart disease, how to identify adverse signs or symptoms and potentially beneficial lifestyle changes.

With proper treatment and adherence to the prescribed medical regimen, many CHF patients can maintain and even enhance their quality of life. If you have received a recent diagnosis of CHF, talk with your primary care physician or cardiologist about whether participation in a structured exercise intervention program, is right for you.

Peripheral Arterial Disease: Walk the Talk and Talk the Walk

Amr Abbas, M.D.

More than 12 percent of patients greater than 70 years of age suffer from peripheral arterial disease (PAD), which involves a narrowing of the blood vessels that supply the lower extremities. Patients usually have occasional buttock, thigh or calf pain (claudication), occurring during walking, running and/or climbing. Complaints of discomfort, pain or fatigue in the legs generally improve by stopping the activity, referred to as intermittent claudication.

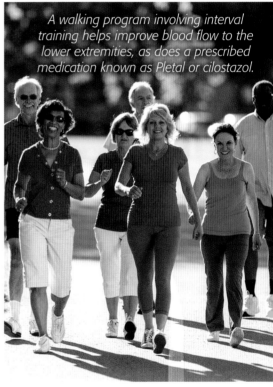

A walking program involving interval training helps improve blood flow to the lower extremities, as does a prescribed medication known as Pletal or cilostazol.

Since PAD is a form of atherosclerosis, it is not surprising that risk factors such as elevated blood cholesterol, cigarette smoking, hypertension, and diabetes, which are commonly associated with coronary atherosclerosis, are also associated with PAD.

Patients with PAD may subconsciously limit their activity level to avoid the pain; accordingly, they may skip their dance lesson, reduce the duration of their daily walk, and avoid taking their dog for long walks. Unfortunately, up to 50 percent of patients may not complain about their leg pain because "their doctor never asked about it."

Diagnosing PAD starts by obtaining a clinical history and conducting a physical exam. Telltale signs or symptoms of the condition may include less lower extremity hair growth, cooler feet and decreased pulses. A simple test known as the ankle-brachial index (ABI), which is the ratio between the ankle and arm blood pressure, is particularly helpful. PAD is considered to be present when the resting ABI is 0.90 or less (*New England Journal of Medicine,* March 2016). Other diagnostic tests may include ultrasound, a computed tomographic scan and/or magnetic resonance imaging.

Treatment includes a walking program involving interval training, where patients are counseled to walk to the point of significant leg pain or discomfort, rest until the pain subsides, and repeat this sequence several times each day. This helps improve blood flow to the lower extremities, as does a prescribed medication known as Pletal or cilostazol.

If symptoms continue to limit activity despite these interventions, an angiogram can be performed to determine the site of blockage, and a variety of treatments, including balloon angioplasty, stenting (both regular and drug-coated), laser, and blockage-shaving devices (atherectomy) may be effectively employed. Surgery is an option if the other treatments are not possible, or have failed.

Rarely, an acute vascular blockage of your lower extremities can occur causing leg pain, changes in your feet color, and absence of pulses in your feet. This is an urgent clinical condition that requires prompt medical attention and emergent angioplasty to open the blockage—in a manner similar to that of a heart attack.

If you think you have PAD, discuss your symptoms with your doctor. And remember, walking remains the initial exercise treatment of choice.

WALKING: MIRACULOUS BENEFITS?

Thomas Jefferson, the third U.S. president, who lived to be 83 years of age at a time when average life expectancy was about 40, walked four miles every day.

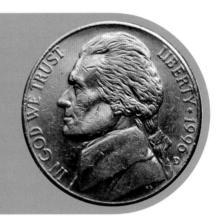

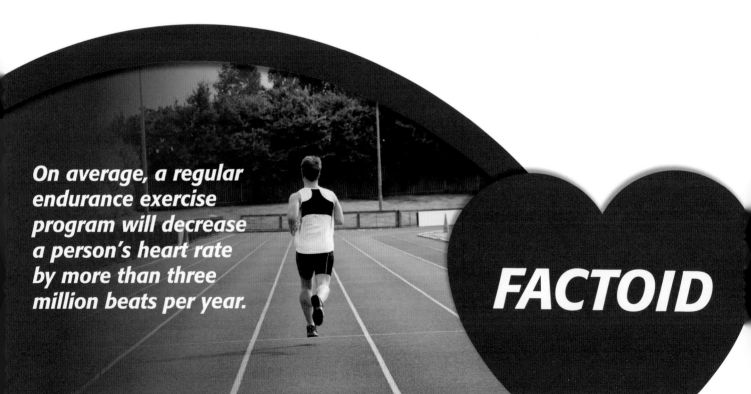

On average, a regular endurance exercise program will decrease a person's heart rate by more than three million beats per year.

FACTOID

Shifting From Disease Management to Health Promotion

Harold Friedman, M.D.

The costs of obesity and the medical conditions associated with excess body weight and fatness are on the rise worldwide, and especially in the United States. It also appears that the younger generation may be less healthy than their predecessors. As a result, health care organizations, government and employers are seeking to accelerate the accessibility and effectiveness of health and wellness programs. The basic goal of a wellness program is to create a "win-win" situation by keeping healthy people healthy.

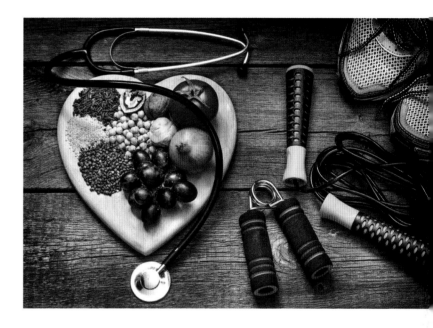

The benefits beside medical cost savings include an enhanced sense of well-being, increased productivity at home and work, and a reduction of skyrocketing health care service utilization, including prescribed medications.

In order to promote prevention in the current health care environment, worksite health promotion programs often begin by encouraging traditional screenings (breast cancer, colon cancer, prostate exam) and immunizations (flu, pneumonia). Typically, wellness programs may request the completion of a health risk assessment, often available online, creating a database of those risk factors and lifestyle behaviors closely associated with the development of chronic disease. Obesity, diabetes, hypertension, physical inactivity, high cholesterol and cigarette smoking are among the most predictive of future cardiovascular events. Filling out the assessment itself often initiates the process of self-awareness and the need for improvement. Importantly, many worksite wellness programs now include the spouse and dependent children.

Next, basic medical measurements, referred to as biometrics, including blood pressure, cholesterol, glucose, kidney function, height, weight and waist size are obtained. Based on these findings, individualized counseling for high risk conditions can offer a way to proactively engage people in comprehensive risk reduction interventions before they become ill, while simultaneously helping lower-risk individuals to maintain optimal health. The objectives are to break bad habits, address societal factors and reinforce healthier choices, both at home and/or at work. Health fairs that stimulate decision making, educational seminars that activate existing interests, professionally trained personal health coaches, and workplace group incentives that alter bad habits are among the most popular approaches.

Newer wellness programs designed to navigate the pathway to better health decisions range from optimal aging programs for seniors to group activities in grade schools, focusing on body weight, exercise, healthy food choices and smoking avoidance. Financial incentives and penalties in the new Affordable Health Care Act will further stimulate all of us to more closely examine our daily lifestyle choices. In addition, research studies from the University of Michigan have unequivocally shown that successful wellness programs can slow and, in some cases, completely halt the upward trend in annual employee health care expenditures.

As governmental health care policy reform shifts to reimbursement for healthy outcomes instead of medical procedures, and employers increasingly focus on employee wellness, there will be a shift toward a culture of health. Hopefully, we'll eventually see the old strategy of procrastination until sickness develops gradually fade into the past.

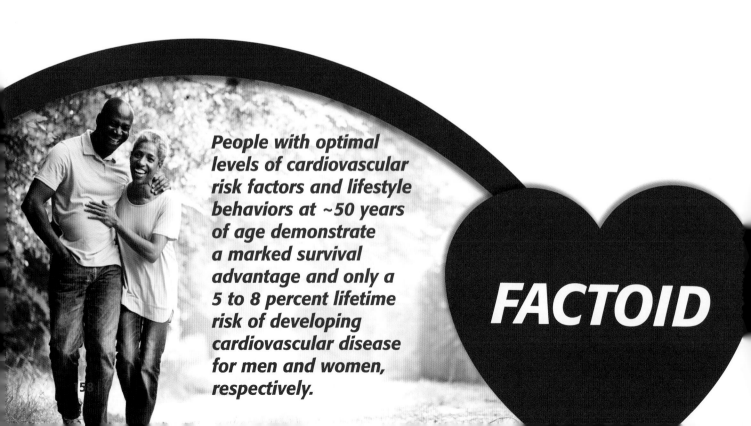

People with optimal levels of cardiovascular risk factors and lifestyle behaviors at ~50 years of age demonstrate a marked survival advantage and only a 5 to 8 percent lifetime risk of developing cardiovascular disease for men and women, respectively.

FACTOID

Taking Active "Steps" in Preventing and Managing Osteoporosis

Jenna Brinks, M.S.

Osteoporosis, a condition of diminished, porous bone structure, is an increasingly prevalent public health concern. An estimated 10 million Americans are afflicted with this "silent" disease, which often shows no outward symptoms until after an injury occurs. Osteoporosis most commonly affects the vertebrae (spine), hip and wrist bones, increasing their susceptibility to fracture. Unfortunately, recovery after fractures is often painful, long and expensive. Accordingly, efforts to halt and even reverse bone loss through proper nutrition, regular physical activity and pharmacotherapy, if appropriate, have become useful strategies for maintaining healthier, stronger bones.

Risk factors for osteoporosis

Although everyone should take an interest in maintaining bone health, some people are more vulnerable to bone loss than others. Female gender, Asian or Caucasian descent, post-menopausal status, smoking, poor nutrition, a sedentary lifestyle, small body frame, high caffeine consumption, and a positive family history for the disease represent common risk factors that may predispose an individual to osteoporosis. And, although you may not "fit the mold" for developing osteoporosis, you can still be at risk. According to the American College of Sports Medicine (ACSM), adults over 40 years of age lose 0.5 percent of their bone mass every year, regardless of risk factors, highlighting the need for everyone to take an active role in their bone health.

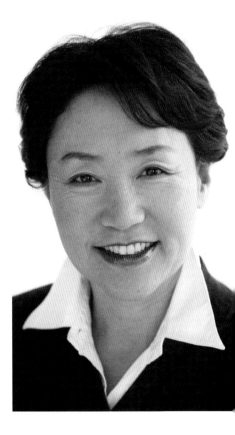

Understanding bone health

Bones are metabolically active, constantly remodeling structures that provide framework for our bodies. Two basic cell types determine bone density: osteoblasts, which build and replace bone, and osteoclasts, which dissolve bone. Osteoporosis occurs when an imbalance develops between the activity levels of these two cell types, with osteoclasts dissolving more bone than osteoblasts can build. The end result—a decreased bone density and increased susceptibility to fracture.

Prevention and management of osteoporosis

Fortunately, there are several research-based strategies for effectively maintaining bone health, including regular physical activity. A physical conditioning program with weight-bearing aerobic activity, resistance exercise and balance training is a simple (and literal) first "step" toward healthy bones. These interventions can effectively maintain bone density and/or decrease fracture risk for individuals with and without osteoporosis. Currently, ACSM recommends that adults perform weight-bearing aerobic exercise, such as walking, jogging and stairclimbing, three to five days per week for 30-60 minutes per session to preserve bone integrity. Additionally, a comprehensive program should also include strength training performed two to three times per week. These activities stimulate osteoblasts (bone builders) and provide the loading effect necessary for bone growth. Finally, balance training in the form of yoga, water aerobics and other balance-challenging activities, can reduce the risk of falling and minimize the likelihood of fractures. Always consult your physician before beginning an exercise program.

In addition to exercise, adequate dietary intake of calcium is another well established recommendation for maintaining and improving bone density. Calcium, a nutrient vital for several bodily functions (e.g., muscle contraction, bone growth), is the primary component of bone tissue. However, studies indicate that most middle-aged women consume less than 50 percent of the currently recommended 1,200 mg/day. To increase dietary intake of calcium, simply incorporate calcium-rich food choices, such as low-fat dairy products (e.g., yogurt, milk, and cheese), broccoli, and foods and drinks fortified with calcium. Calcium supplements are widely available and inexpensive, but should be approved by your physician before starting them.

Vitamin D is also a significant nutritional predictor of bone health. Without adequate vitamin D, calcium is poorly absorbed from our diet and is more easily excreted from the body. The current recommendation for vitamin D intake is 800-1,000 I.U. per day for middle-aged and older adults. Many foods are fortified with vitamin D; it is also found naturally in egg yolks and saltwater fish. Furthermore, our skin, when exposed to sunlight, makes vitamin D. However, because of the risk of skin cancer associated with excessive sun exposure, dietary intake and supplementation may be safer options for getting adequate vitamin D.

Knowledge and action are powerful tools for maintaining bone health. Through simple lifestyle choices, like beginning a weight-bearing exercise program and increasing dietary intake of important nutrients like calcium and vitamin D, we can take active steps toward preventing bone loss, decreasing fracture risk and increasing the quality of life as we age.

Pet Ownership: An Under-Recognized Strategy for Cardiovascular Risk Reduction?

Angela Fern, M.S.

According to the Humane Society of the United States web site, approximately 74.8 million dogs and 88.3 million cats are owned by Americans. For pet owners, coming home after a stressful day and seeing a furry, faithful companion waiting at the door can be a "heart warming" experience. Research has shown that humans respond positively when a "bond" has been formed with an animal. For example, blood pressure, heart rate and stress levels have been reported to decrease in pet owners (*Journal of Nursing Scholarship,* Sept. 1997).

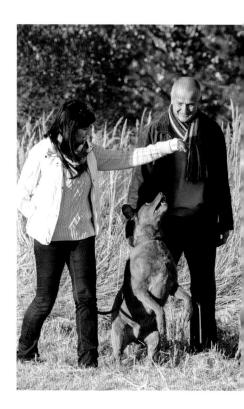

Several studies have investigated the relationship between animals and human health. Of particular interest, a study investigating social support and pet ownership revealed that following a heart attack, patients who owned dogs were significantly less likely to die within one year compared to those without pets (*American Journal of Cardiology,* Dec. 1995). The authors suggested that owning a dog may increase regular physical activity as well as the health status of the owner.

It appears that owning a pet can have a positive influence on decreasing some cardiovascular risk factors. It has been reported that systolic blood pressure and triglycerides are lower in pet owners aged 20-60 years and these individuals are more physically active than people who did not own pets (*Medical Journal of Australia,* Sept. 1992). The authors noted that owning a dog served to augment daily physical activity. A similar investigation found that adults over 65 years who owned a dog or cat demonstrated increased levels of daily physical activity as compared to those who did not own a pet (*Journal of the American Geriatric Society,* March 1999). It was suggested that caring for a pet created a sense of obligation and fostered physical activity. The study concluded that owning a cat or dog maintained or slightly improved the functional status of the owner.

Thirty-nine percent of American households have at least one dog and almost 34 percent have at least one cat. If you are part of this escalating cohort, you are likely reaping the benefits of pet ownership. If not, consider walking a neighbor's dog or volunteering at your local shelter for a "pawsitive" experience.

When to Consider Weight Loss Surgery

Kerstyn C. Zalesin, M.D.

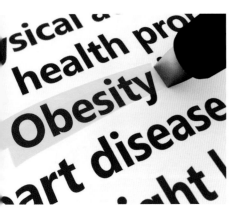

We are in the midst of an obesity pandemic. Although the burden of obesity is associated with huge economic costs, it can also adversely impact psychosocial well-being and heighten the risk of dying prematurely. Being overweight or obese increases the risks of chronic disease and associated complications such as: type 2 diabetes, high blood pressure, heart disease, obstructive sleep apnea, feeling breathless during mild-to-moderate activities, liver disease, arthritis, gallstones, and certain cancers.

Unfortunately, many individuals experience considerable weight gain throughout their lifespan, and effective treatment may be beyond conventional common sense advice like, "eat less" and "be more active." By the time an individual gains 80 to 100 additional pounds, it is rare to be able to lose this amount of weight without more drastic interventions. Accordingly, it may be reasonable to consider weight loss surgery to achieve your weight and health goals. Weight loss surgery, also known as bariatric surgery, is currently the best treatment alternative for producing lasting weight loss in selected obese patients for whom nonsurgical methods of weight loss, like calorie restriction and increasing physical activity, have been ineffective. Weight loss surgery may be an appropriate option when the following criteria are met:

- You have a body mass index (BMI) that is equal to or greater than 40 kg/m² (calculate your BMI online by searching a "BMI calculator," see explanation of BMI in the table).
- You have a BMI in the range of 35.0-39.9 kg/m² and are afflicted by other co-morbid conditions such as type 2 diabetes, hypertension, heart disease, fatty liver disease, sleep apnea or advanced arthritis at a weight bearing joint that impairs mobility.
- You have been either unable to lose or maintain weight loss through conventional methods (diet and exercise) in the past.

Classification of Disease Risk Based on BMI and Body Habitus

BMI (kg/m²)	Body Habitus	Disease Risk*
Under 18.5	Underweight	Increased
18.5 - 24.9	Normal	–
25 - 29.9	Overweight	Increased
30 - 34.9	Stage I obesity	High
35 - 39.9	Stage II obesity	Very high
Greater than 40	Stage III obesity or morbid obesity	Extremely high

*Relative to normal weight individuals

High remission rates of medical comorbidities (e.g., diabetes, hypertension, sleep apnea) are commonly reported in obese patients who undergo significant weight loss after surgical intervention. These individuals are often able to discontinue many of their prescribed medications, even insulin, and dramatically improve their health, longevity and quality of life (*Annals of Surgery,* Sept. 2004). Long-term success is of course dependent on the individual's ability to adopt the lifestyle changes that are required to keep the weight off.

Marathon Running And Immunity to Heart Disease

Justin Trivax, M.D.

Nearly four decades ago, Thomas Bassler, M.D., suggested marathon runners have immunity to coronary heart disease (*Physician and Sports Medicine,* April 1975). He emphasized that there had never been a documented case of a marathon finisher suffering from a heart attack and asserted that if you could finish a marathon, you wouldn't die from heart disease. This became known as Bassler's hypothesis.

Dr. Bassler compared athletes who participated in prolonged strenuous exercise to the heart disease-free Masai warriors and Tarahumara Indians. The Masai walk 10 or 15 miles per day while herding cattle and the Tarahumara take part in ceremonial distance running over courses of a hundred miles and longer. All are extremely active, eat healthy and, according to Dr. Bassler's theory, do not die of blockages obstructing the coronary arteries.

The 1970s contention that long-distance running could provide individuals with immunity from heart attacks may have contributed to a significant increase in marathon participation. For example, there were only 25,000 marathon runners in 1975. In 2010, more than 2 million participants completed a marathon.

But is the Bassler hypothesis valid? Jim Fixx was an avid runner who completed several marathons. He became an icon in the running world and was the author of the bestseller, "The Complete Book of Running." But Fixx was an ex-smoker with a strong family history for premature coronary artery disease. He would occasionally have angina (chest pain) while running, but believed in the Bassler hypothesis. In 1984, Fixx experienced a fatal heart attack during a long training run. An autopsy showed 100 percent blockage of one artery, which was likely the cause of his death, along with severe blockages in his other arteries. There was also evidence of prior heart damage or previous silent heart attacks.

Jim Fixx and many other runners who have died of coronary heart disease, including some while running long distances, have unequivocally proven that the Bassler hypothesis is incorrect. Some marathon runners have demonstrated more calcium build up around their coronary arteries than age- and gender-matched sedentary controls (*Missouri Medicine,* March/April 2014). And these runners, while participating in prolonged, strenuous exercise, are more likely to suffer from a coronary plaque rupture or heart attack, despite having an otherwise low-risk profile (low blood cholesterol, normal body mass index, non-smoker). Such endurance athletes can be symptom-free, whereas others, with high levels of fitness, may simply ignore the exercise-related chest pain or discomfort, rationalizing that because they are in such 'good shape,' it can't be heart disease.

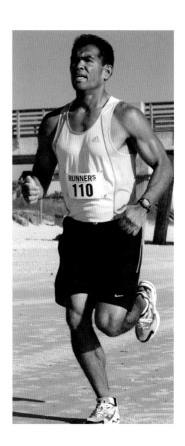

Flu Facts for the Cardiac Patient

Stephen Gunther, M.D.

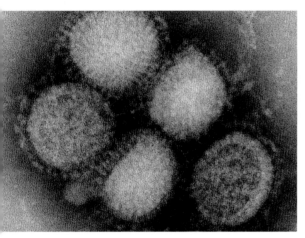

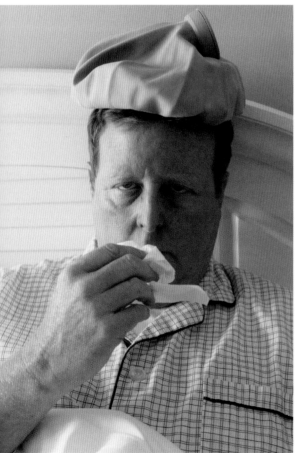

As we are out in the garden or on the golf course this summer, flu season is far from most of our minds. But it's not too early to prepare. Influenza is a major cause of death and hospitalization, and creates an enormous public health cost. Patients with cardiovascular disease are at especially high risk. The stresses of pulmonary infection, fever and dehydration are poorly tolerated by those with impaired cardiovascular function and can cause a much higher complication rate. In addition, the influenza virus directly destabilizes atherosclerotic plaque—increasing the risk of plaque rupture and blood vessel thrombosis. By triggering these causes of heart attack and stroke, influenza is potentially responsible for thousands of preventable deaths each year.

Cardiovascular events and mortality peak in the winter months, with the seasonal increase following one to two weeks after the spread of flu in the community. Early vaccination is critical and cardiac patients should know that the flu vaccine not only minimizes the inconvenience of flu symptoms and need for hospitalization, but saves lives. According to some reports, the rate of heart attack, stroke and out-of-hospital sudden cardiac death are markedly reduced in vaccinated individuals.

Despite its overwhelming benefit, less than 50 percent of persons at risk receive the flu vaccine every year. The Centers for Disease Control and Prevention recommends vaccination for everyone over the age of 50, and for anyone with cardiovascular disease, regardless of age. The current flu vaccines are safe and inexpensive and can help ensure you are able to enjoy next summer's pleasures.

The Flu Season: Reducing Risk in Older Adults

Jenna Brinks, M.S.

Influenza, more commonly referred to as "the flu," can occur at alarming rates in older adults during the late fall, winter and spring seasons. Onset of symptoms is typically sudden, and includes cough, fever, chills, body aches, sore throat, runny or stuffy nose, headache, fatigue, and less commonly, vomiting and diarrhea. Flu symptoms last anywhere from a few days to two weeks; however, complications such as pneumonia, bronchitis, and even death can occur. According to the Centers for Disease Control and Prevention (CDC), an estimated 80 to 90 percent of deaths related to the flu virus in recent years occur in adults 65 years and older. Because our immune systems weaken with age, older adults in particular are at an increased risk of severe illness if the flu is contracted.

The American Heart Association and the CDC recommend all older adults, including those with cardiovascular disease, receive the seasonal flu vaccine for protection against the flu virus (*Circulation,* Nov. 2011). Fortunately, there is no increase in cardiovascular event risk immediately after vaccination, whereas individuals who contract the flu are at increased risk for cardiac events (*New England Journal of Medicine,* Dec. 2004). Moreover, patients with established coronary artery disease who receive the flu shot demonstrate improved clinical courses and reduced frequencies of coronary ischemic events as compared with their non-vaccinated counterparts (*European Heart Journal,* June 2008).

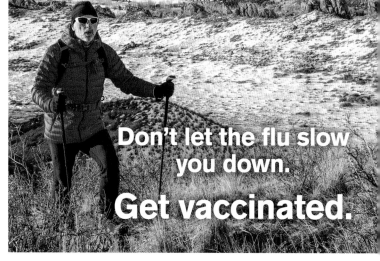

Don't let the flu slow you down.
Get vaccinated.

The efficacy of the flu vaccine fluctuates based on the prevalent flu strains circulating each season, and how well that season's vaccine 'matches' those strains. The flu vaccine is available as a shot, intradermal injection and nasal spray, and appropriately indicated delivery modalities are safe for most people over 6 months of age. For adults 65 years and older, a high-dose flu shot is recommended because it boosts immune reaction following vaccination, and is about 24 percent more effective at flu prevention than the standard vaccine (*New England Journal of Medicine,* Aug. 2014). The associated side effects are similar to those reported with the standard vaccine, although they may occur more often. Adverse responses in clinical trials were typically mild and temporary, and included redness at the injection site, pain, muscle aches, malaise and headache.

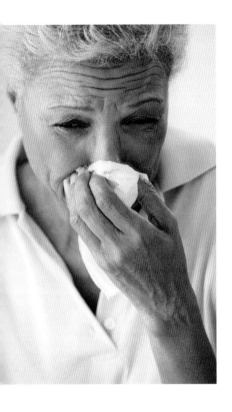

In addition to getting the flu vaccine, several other preventive actions can protect you from getting sick this flu season:

- Practice appropriate hand hygiene: Sanitizing your hands frequently reduces the transmission of germs, bacteria and viruses like the flu. Hands can be sanitized using alcohol-based sanitizers or the traditional "soap-and-water" method. Always choose soap-and-water over a hand sanitizer when your hands are visibly soiled. When washing your hands, lather soap vigorously for 20 seconds (try singing Happy Birthday twice through) before rinsing. And, encourage those around you to follow the same practice.

- Avoid others who have symptoms of the flu: If friends or family have symptoms of the flu or other viruses, stay away! Likewise, if you are sick, do your loved ones and coworkers a favor and stay home until your condition improves. Contact with others should be avoided (except when seeking medical care) until you are fever-free without the use of fever-reducing medications for at least 24 hours. If interaction with others can't be avoided, wear a protective mask to limit exposure.

- Cough into a tissue instead of your hands or the air: Viruses are often transmitted when infected individuals cough droplets into air that are subsequently inhaled by others, or through direct contact (i.e., shaking hands).

- Use the 'fist bump,' or simply omit any hand touching during greetings or introductions: The more we avoid hand shaking during the flu season, the less likely we are to transmit illness.

- Disinfect surfaces regularly: Regularly disinfecting commonly touched surfaces, such as door handles, tables, chairs and light switches, can reduce the spread of germs.

- Avoid touching your eyes, nose and mouth: The flu virus can enter your body via all of these access points if your hands are contaminated.

If you do get the flu, seek medical attention early. Anti-viral medications can be prescribed to reduce the duration and intensity of your illness. These medications work best when initiated within two days of getting sick, but may still be beneficial if started later (CDC).

The Bottom Line: *Get a seasonal flu vaccine, listen to your body, practice preventive measures, and take care of yourself and your family so we can all stay safe and healthy this flu season.*

Interested in learning more about influenza? Visit http://www.cdc.gov/flu/consumer/ for additional information.

The Future of Medicine

Steven Almany, M.D.

You may be surprised to know that the future of medicine may be as close as your pocket or your purse. Smartphones now are used on a daily basis in most civilized countries. These devices, whether they are Android or iPhone based, have more computing capability than the Apollo missions that landed the first man on the moon.

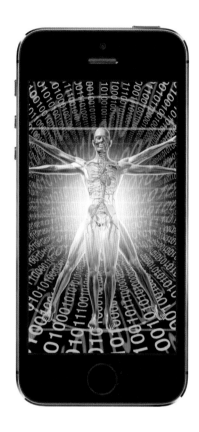

We live in an increasingly connected society. Over two billion people now use the internet on a daily basis. The average person with a smartphone checks their phone more than 150 times per day. Most U.S. physicians (86 percent) now use smartphones in practice every day and one in two clinicians use a tablet every day.

How will smartphones influence health care in the future? Health related applications are growing in an exponential manner for both iPhone and Android based phones. There are now nearly 100,000 health applications that are available. Most of these are in the fitness field, comprising about 31 percent of all applications. Others include: medical reference (17 percent); wellness (16 percent); nutrition (8 percent); medical condition management (7 percent); and, reminders and alerts (2 percent). At the current pace of smartphone adoption, 3.4 billion people worldwide will own a smartphone and one-half of them will be actively using health applications by 2017.

What does this mean for you? The future of medicine, particularly in regard to cardiovascular care, will increasingly rely on the use of biosensors. These sensors will either be external (and resemble a Band-Aid) or potentially even internal (as small as the tip of a pencil) and capable of relaying data back to your smartphone and then to a cloud application, respectively. Physicians will be able to immediately access these data and make appropriate changes in your medications, if necessary. A huge advantage of this technology will be the incredible amount of data (data mining) that we will be able to collect in regard to patients with chronic diseases. This should allow us to write standardized step-by-step procedures, depicted by algorithms, to immeasurably improve patient care.

Certain areas of cardiovascular care are particularly well-suited for this kind of innovation. Congestive heart failure, which is the number one cause for readmissions to hospitals, is sorely in need of new approaches to dramatically improve patient outcomes. Our ability to monitor a patient at home in regard to their blood volume, blood pressure, and heart rate and make real time changes in medical management should dramatically improve not only their well-being, but also limit rehospitalizations, markedly reducing health care costs and enhancing patient care.

Although the challenges of contemporary medicine are formidable, the opportunities are immense—particularly when one considers the potential impact of smartphones and related technologic advances.

CAUSES OF THE CURRENT OBESITY EPIDEMIC?

Although unhealthy eating habits are generally considered the primary factor underlying our national weight problem, a widely-cited report showed that over the last 50 years, work-related energy expenditure has decreased by more than 100 calories per day. The investigators concluded that this decrease alone largely accounts for the increased prevalence of obesity among men and women.

(*PLoS One*, May 2011)

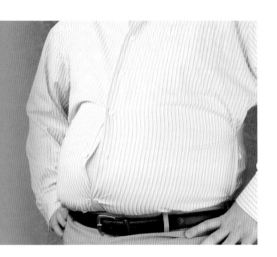

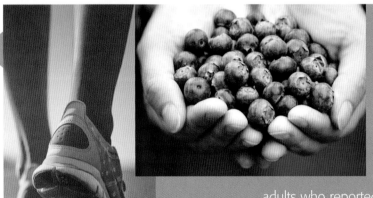

UNHEALTHY LIFESTYLES AMONG INDIVIDUALS WITH CARDIOVASCULAR DISEASE

In a survey of high-, middle- and low-income countries, the prevalence of three important healthy lifestyle behaviors (regular exercise, healthy eating practices, no smoking) was only 5 percent among adults who reported a history of cardiovascular disease.

(*Journal of the American Medical Association,* April 2013)

MEMORABLE HEART-HEALTHY QUOTE:

"If you stop exercising, start cigarette smoking, discontinue your prescribed cardiac medications, and increase your daily intake of high calorie and fatty foods, you'll definitely have enough retirement money to last you the rest of your life."

(An anonymous, 'health-conscious' financial planner)

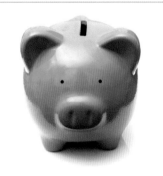

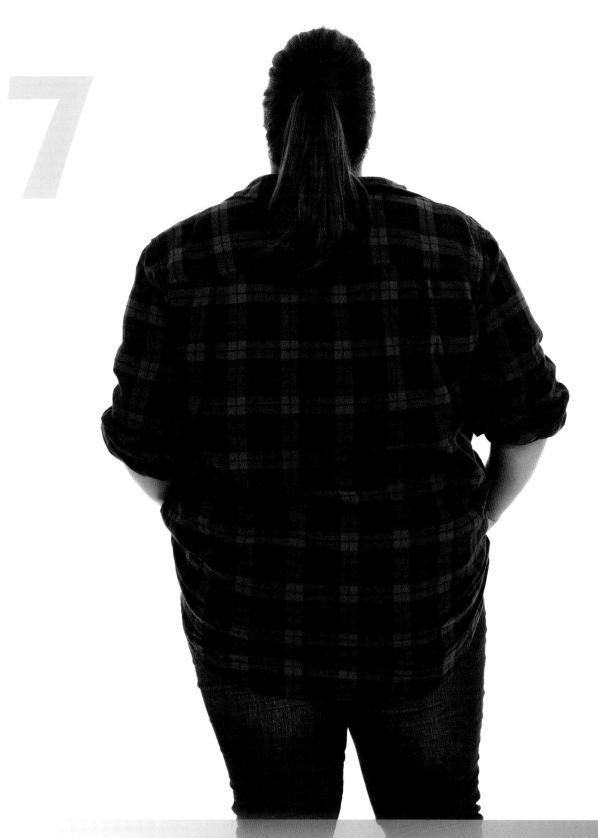

7

OBESITY AND LIFESTYLE MATTERS

Adverse Health Effects of Sleep Deprivation

Daniel Rothschild, M.D.

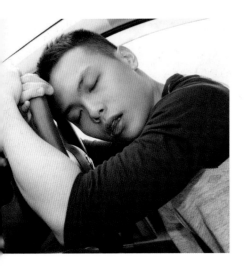

We spend more time doing it than perhaps any other activity—sleep! Up to a third of our lives are committed to getting our ZZZs, yet its purpose remains unclear. Some believe sleep was included in human evolution primarily for energy conservation, whereas others think it was to give our bodies a chance to restore and regenerate (http://healthysleep.med.harvard.edu/healthy/matters/benefits-of-sleep/why-do-we-sleep, Dec. 2007; *Nature,* Oct. 2005). What is clear, however, is that lack of sleep is harmful, both to cognition and overall health. Staying awake for 21 consecutive hours evokes a similar degradation of psychomotor performance as a blood alcohol level of 0.08, the legal driving limit in the United States (*Occupational and Environmental Medicine,* Oct. 2000). Prolonged sleep deprivation in animals leads to complete loss of immune function and death (http://healthysleep.med.harvard.edu/healthy/matters/benefits-of-sleep/why-do-we-sleep, Dec. 2007).

To clarify how much sleep the average American adult needs, a panel of 13 experts recently reviewed the relevant literature. They recommended seven to nine hours per night, but no fewer than six to be considered healthy (*Sleep Health,* Dec. 2015). A Gallup poll, however, noted that 40 percent of Americans get less than six hours of sleep per night (http://www.gallup.com/poll/166553/less-recommended-amount-sleep.aspx). What effects does sleep deprivation have on our health, and more specifically, on our cardiovascular health?

Many studies have reported that both short and long sleep durations (less than five or greater than 10 hours of sleep per night) are associated with a higher incidence of developing diabetes, hypertension and obesity. The risk of diabetes, for example, increases about 10 percent for each hour less than seven hours of sleep per night. Other studies have shown that, in addition to causing these cardiovascular risk factors, not getting enough sleep is also directly associated with cardiovascular disease. A study of over 30,000 survey participants showed that when compared to seven hours of sleep per night, those who get less than five hours have a 2.2 times higher risk of heart attack, stroke or angina (*Sleep,* Aug. 2010). This risk was independent of other factors associated with heart disease, including age, cigarette smoking or obesity. A larger analysis that combined data from 15 separate studies and included 474,000 subjects supported these results, finding about a 50 percent increase in the relative risk of death from cardiovascular disease (*European Heart Journal,* June 2011).

Even transient sleep disturbances such as daylight savings time and jet lag may have a significant impact on our hearts. One widely cited study found a 5 to 10 percent increased incidence of heart attacks the week after daylight savings time in the spring, and, in the autumn, a pronounced decrease in heart attacks on the Monday after the switch to standard time (*New England Journal of Medicine*, Oct. 2008). Another case report described a patient who developed a stress-induced syndrome mimicking a heart attack, called takotsubo cardiomyopathy, after severe jet lag and prolonged, disturbed sleep (*International Journal of Angiology*, Summer 2007).

How can sleep deprivation cause such profound effects? Acutely, it is thought that the release of stress hormones and pro-inflammatory compounds can serve as a trigger that destabilizes vulnerable coronary plaque, leading to a heart attack (*New England Journal of Medicine*, Oct. 2008). Long term, there are several possible mechanisms. It is postulated that hypertension caused by sleep deprivation accelerates atherosclerosis leading to cardiovascular disease (*Sleep*, Aug. 2010). Others suggest that lack of sleep alters circulating levels of the hormones leptin and ghrelin, responsible for regulating our appetite, adversely affecting our glycemic control and metabolism, leading to obesity and cardiovascular disease (*European Heart Journal*, June 2011).

Although diet, exercise, smoking abstinence and medication adherence are all critical to maintaining our cardiovascular health, adequate sleep is also important. The bottom line: *Don't get caught sleeping on getting a good night's ZZZs!*

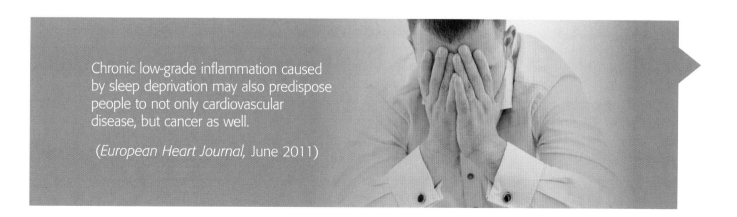

Chronic low-grade inflammation caused by sleep deprivation may also predispose people to not only cardiovascular disease, but cancer as well.

(*European Heart Journal*, June 2011)

Who Needs Sleep? Sobering Reasons to Get Your ZZZs

Monica Jiddou, M.D.

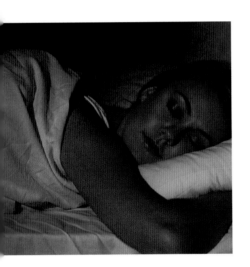

How often have you stayed up late to finish a project, woken up early to get a head start on the day or wished that there were more hours in a day? Likely, more times than you can count. Between work and play, there are too few hours to accomplish everything we would like in a single day. Because sleep is often considered a luxury, rather than a necessity, it is commonly sacrificed in order to accomplish more. Cutting back on hours spent sleeping or having disrupted sleep, however, can negatively affect overall health.

Sleep plays an important role in maintaining a positive mood, cognitive function and performance. On average, adults need seven to nine hours of sleep to function well. Over time, lack of sleep can lead to depression and anxiety, and a widely-cited survey revealed that patients diagnosed with depression or anxiety were more likely to sleep less than six hours a night.

Have you ever felt forgetful or absentminded after a night of poor sleep? If so, it's probably because the brain consolidates memories during sleep, allowing us to learn and think clearly. Sleep deprivation also can make you feel irritable and too tired to enjoy leisure-time activities that require sustained attention such as watching a movie or a child's softball game. With decreased sleep, concentration, reasoning, problem-solving skills and performance are impaired and can result in work-related injuries or automobile accidents. Drowsiness also negatively impacts reaction time, making driving in sleep-deprived individuals comparable to that of drunk drivers. According to the American Academy of Sleep Medicine, one in five auto accidents are due to driver fatigue, resulting in 100,000 to 250,000 accidents each year. Moreover, lack of sleep can decrease quality of life.

Sleep also provides the body time to recuperate after a long day. While we snooze, the body performs vital functions such as muscle repair, protein synthesis and tissue growth. Hormones that regulate our blood sugar and appetite are produced during sleep. With decreased hours of sleep, one's appetite is stimulated and cravings for high-fat, high-carbohydrate foods increase, potentially leading to obesity. People who sleep fewer than six hours a night are 30 percent more likely to be obese than their counterparts who routinely get seven to nine hours.

Chronic sleep deprivation also results in increased production of stress hormones and decreased insulin sensitivity. Consequently, sleep-deprived individuals may be more likely to develop diabetes, high blood pressure and cardiovascular disease. These medical conditions can then lead to other health issues such as kidney disease, heart failure and abnormal heart rhythms. Decreased sleep also affects our ability to fight infections. Interestingly, adults who sleep less than seven hours per night are about three times more likely to develop cold symptoms.

Difficulty sleeping can be related to unhealthy habits, such as eating before bedtime, or to an underlying health problem like obstructive sleep apnea. If you snore, wake up feeling fatigued, need frequent daily naps or have difficulty falling or staying asleep, see your physician.

Although general health is dependent upon many variables, sleep appears to be an important and often underappreciated requirement. It is important to develop good sleep habits to improve your overall health and well-being. So, if you ever ask "who needs sleep?" The fact of the matter is, you do!

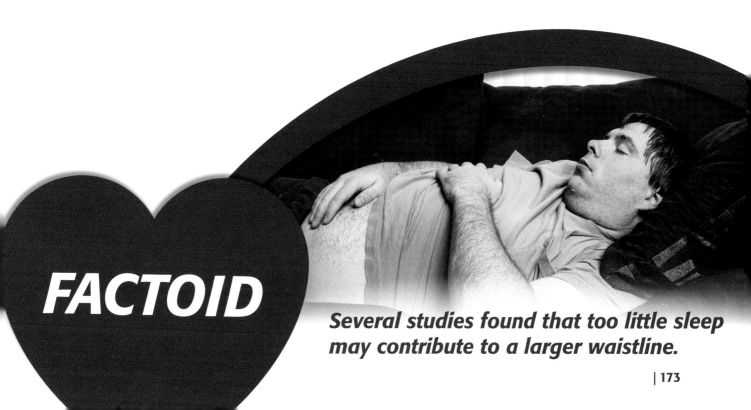

FACTOID

Several studies found that too little sleep may contribute to a larger waistline.

Please, Have a Seat … Maybe Not

Aaron Berman, M.D.

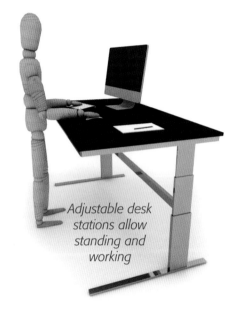

Adjustable desk stations allow standing and working

We all know that physical activity is good for us. Regular exercise helps us regulate our weight and avoid obesity, reduces our risk of cardiovascular disease, and increases our overall sense of well-being. Current recommendations indicate that at least 150 minutes of moderate intensity exercise a week can achieve these goals. But what about our behavior when we are not exercising?

Numerous observational and epidemiological studies from countries around the world have now linked prolonged sitting to adverse health outcomes. In a recent analysis of 47 separate studies (*Annals of Internal Medicine,* June 2015), investigators reported not only increased cardiovascular disease and death, but also higher rates of cancer and diabetes associated with prolonged sitting. The risk of developing type 2 or adult onset diabetes was almost twice as high in populations with the most sedentary (sitting) time per day. One provocative finding was that the risks of excessive sitting were noted even in people who engaged in structured exercise. This suggests that even if you exercise regularly, long hours at the desk without interruption are potentially harmful to your health.

The workplace is not the only place where sitting is harmful. The percentage of leisure time spent sitting (mainly at the computer or watching TV) has steadily increased. In a recent study, every hour of time spent sitting watching TV was associated with worsening quality of sleep, as well as an increased risk of developing sleep apnea. It also took longer for "TV sitters" to fall asleep at night (*Chest,* March 2015).

What can we do? The percentage of jobs involving prolonged sitting has exponentially increased in most industrialized nations. One group of scientists and clinicians in England has suggested that persons with sedentary jobs break up sitting with periods of standing and walking, and that efforts should be made to accumulate 2 to 4 hours of light activity (standing, walking) during the workday. Others advocate adjustable desk stations, which allow standing and working, or "treadmill-desks" which permit slow walking while you work. The health impact of these devices, however, has not been fully evaluated.

Other practical suggestions include (*Current Opinion in Cardiology,* Sept. 2011):

- stand and take short breaks from your computer every 30 minutes
- stand during phone calls
- drink lots of water during work; you'll end up taking more rest room breaks
- use the stairs, rather than elevators and escalators
- eat lunch away from your desk
- have conversations and meetings while standing

The take home message? Even if you consider yourself "physically active" by virtue of your thrice weekly gym visits, it's important to examine your daily physical activity habits and associated behaviors. Those hours in the gym may yield you less benefit if the rest of your time is spent sitting. Move more, sit less!

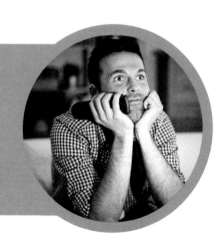

SITTING TIME AND MORTALITY FROM ALL CAUSES

A widely-cited study found that daily sitting time is associated with an increased death rate from all causes, independent of leisure time physical activity. The bottom line: move more, sit less.

(*Medicine and Science in Sports and Exercise,* May 2009)

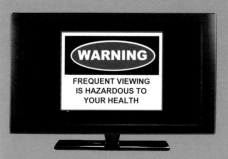

TELEVISION WATCHING INCREASES MORTALITY

A study of 8,800 adults showed that every hour per day spent watching television was associated with an increased risk of dying from heart disease, stroke or cancer. Reason: Researchers believe that the extended sitting time, often coupled with the consumption of high fat, high calorie snacks has a negative effect on blood sugar and cholesterol levels (*Circulation,* Jan. 2010).

Sitting Too Long, Too Often May Be Hazardous to Your Health

Amy Fowler, B.S.

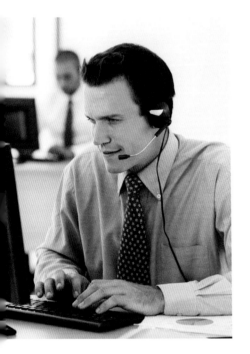

Those of us with sedentary jobs or hobbies have perhaps felt redeemed by our trips to the gym three to four times per week, our brisk evening walks with the family dog, and the fact that we usually take the stairs. Although the American public has known about the benefits of regular aerobic exercise for quite some time, we have been seemingly unaware of the harmful effects of prolonged sitting.

A few years ago, researchers reported on the leisure time and physical activity habits of ~100,000 U.S. adults over a 14 year period (*American Journal of Epidemiology,* July 2010). Time spent sitting was independently associated with total mortality, regardless of the amount of time individuals spent in recreational activity. In fact, those who spent greater than six hours per day seated (versus those who spent only three hours seated) had 20 and 40 percent higher all-cause mortality rates for men and women, respectively.

According to the *European Heart Journal* (Jan. 2011), data from the U.S. National Health and Nutrition Examination Survey demonstrated associations between prolonged sitting time and inflammatory biomarkers like C-reactive protein, which is associated with the development of coronary artery disease. Investigators also found that frequent breaks in sitting time were associated with a reduced waist circumference, a surrogate marker for abdominal obesity.

These studies highlight the need for Americans to take frequent breaks from the amount of time we spend sitting—to lessen the negative health impact of our increasingly hypokinetic lifestyle. This will be of critical importance as we navigate through the modern age of conference calls, webinars, texting, and instant messaging.

Tips to reduce time spent sitting:
- stand up frequently while talking on the phone
- walk to speak with colleagues rather than e-mailing them
- use the restroom or water fountains farthest away from your office
- take regular breaks from computer usage to stand, stretch, or walk a short distance

A Simple Way to Keep Ourselves and Our Kids Healthier? Just Stand Up!

Pam Marcovitz, M.D.

You may have heard that "prolonged sitting is the newest risk factor." The reason is that the more time we spend sitting, the greater the likelihood we will develop chronic disease. For the first time ever, the American Heart Association (AHA) has projected that the current generation of American children may not live as long as their parents. Because of the earlier development of heart disease, it is estimated that the average lifespan of children today may be five years less than their parents (*New England Journal of Medicine,* March 2005). This news seems paradoxical since we've heard that heart disease deaths are on the decline.

In fact, deaths due to heart disease have declined by about 13 percent in the U.S. population over the last decade. So, how do we explain the projection that younger people may be more likely to die prematurely of heart disease? Experts suggest that high blood pressure, cholesterol, diabetes, physical inactivity, and obesity, all of which lead to heart disease, are on the rise for kids as well as adults.

By the time children reach adulthood, subclinical heart disease may already be apparent. The reasons for this decline in our health and in the health of our children are likely multifactorial, beginning with the elimination of required physical education in schools and the lack of time families take to prepare and share regular meals. Lastly, but perhaps most important, is the estimated daily hours of "screen time," i.e., time spent sitting in front of a computer or TV. The AHA recommends engaging in at least 30 minutes of moderate-intensity exercise on most days of the week. For those who can't achieve this goal, sitting less may result in some surprising benefits. The renowned exercise physiologist, Dr. Steven Blair, has shown that very sedentary people are likely to die sooner from all causes. On the other hand, his studies have clearly demonstrated that habitually sedentary people have the most to gain by regularly performing even a little physical activity. Out of this list of unhealthy habits, time spent sitting may be among the easiest to change, and may have the greatest impact on our health.

The AHA recommends engaging in at least 30 minutes of moderate-intensity exercise on most days of the week.

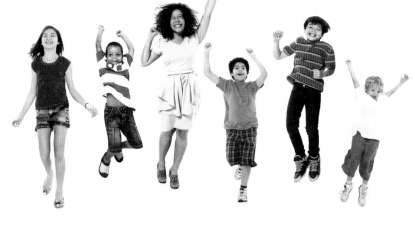

For adults and children, sitting has become our most common waking activity, averaging eight or more hours each day. Unfortunately, there seems to be something lethal about prolonged sitting. People whose jobs require them to stand upright—for example, workers who collect tickets on trains, or postal employees who walk to deliver the mail—generally live longer than their sedentary counterparts.

A classic study from Britain found that conductors on double-decker buses who stood to collect tickets all day lived longer than their co-workers who drove the buses (*Lancet,* Nov. 1953). Drivers were more likely to suffer heart attacks. Early on, it wasn't clear exactly why this was the case. However, recent studies may lend clues. For example, researchers in Sweden studied a group of sedentary, older adults, advising half of them to lose weight and become healthier in general terms. The other half was advised to sit less, and exercise more. (*British Journal of Sports Medicine,* Oct. 2014). Six months later, in those who reported less time sitting, blood cells appeared healthier, and actually resembled the cells of younger people. More youthful cells were generally seen in those who reported less sitting, regardless of how much structured exercise they performed.

Another study evaluated time spent standing versus sitting among Canadian adults (*Medicine & Science in Sports & Exercise,* May 2014). Those who reported engaging in activities that required more standing lived longer. Even more recently, a study among adolescent girls reported that prolonged sitting, even for a single session, led to detrimental decreases in leg blood flow (*Experimental Physiology,* Nov. 2015). These changes appeared similar to those in adults who ultimately develop high blood pressure. Fortunately, the harmful acute changes in vascular function demonstrated by these young girls was abolished by performing just 10 minutes of light activity each hour.

The take home message is: *Substantial health benefits may be gained simply by sitting less. In both children and adults, standing up or taking a brief stroll away from our desks and screens, may help reduce chronic disease and improve longevity. In other words, "if prolonged sitting is the newest risk factor," then standing may become the latest activity craze.*

CHRONIC DISEASE AND SITTING TIME

A sobering study of 63,048 men aged 45 to 64 years found that those who sat less than four hours per day were much less likely to report any chronic disease (cancer, diabetes, heart disease, high blood pressure) as compared with those who sat more. Men who sat at least six hours per day had a greater risk for diabetes. Take home message? If you have a desk job, make the effort to take frequent walk breaks—stand while you're on the phone, and wear a pedometer to motivate yourself to increase daily step totals.

(*International Journal of Behavioral Nutrition and Physical Activity,* Feb. 2013)

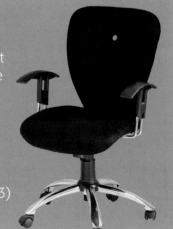

Healthy Hound or Fat Cat? Your Lifestyle Choices Affect Your Pet

Angela Fern, M.S.

Did you know that canines and felines share the human propensity to develop cancer, obesity, heart disease, diabetes, high blood pressure and high cholesterol? A 2014 USA Today article titled "Pet Health Crisis: Americans skimp on preventive care" highlighted the decreasing number of veterinary visits and increasing amount of obesity, diabetes and arthritis in dogs and cats (www. usatoday.com). Pet "parents" with poor personal exercise, eating or lifestyle habits may, unknowingly, be missing opportunities to provide their pets with proper health and medical care.

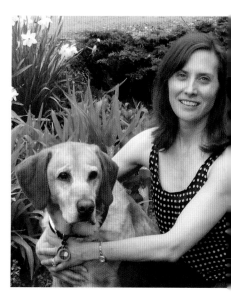

Consider that we have a modern day symbiotic relationship with our pets. Research has shown that during positive interactions between dogs and humans, blood pressure transiently decreases and neurochemicals (e.g., oxytocin) associated with bonding increase for both species (*The Veterinary Journal,* 2003). A study examining the health effects of pet ownership revealed that people with pets were happier, healthier and had greater personal well-being than those without pets, and that their pets provided social support and helped to reduce social isolation (*Journal of Personality and Social Psychology,* July 2011). Even the American Heart Association (AHA) recognizes the benefits of pet ownership (particularly dog ownership), including a decreased risk for cardiovascular disease (*Circulation,* June 2013). While not all conditions or diseases are preventable for both humans and animals alike, here are a few suggestions to lower the risk of disease for you and your pets.

❏ *Avoid cigarette (regular and electronic) and cigar smoking, and smokeless tobacco products.* Smoking is responsible for additional causes of death in smokers that were not previously realized, including renal failure, intestinal ischemia (lack of blood flow to the gut) and hypertensive heart disease among others (*New England Journal of Medicine,* Feb. 2015). The AHA's position on cigarette smoking is that it is the single most preventable cause of premature death in the United States. Additionally, the connection between secondhand smoke (smoke inhaled by people and pets that are in close proximity to smokers) and death and cardiovascular disability is strikingly clear (www.heart.org). A relatively new term, third-hand smoke, is "considered residual nicotine and other chemicals… that clings to hair, skin, clothes, furniture, drapes, walls, bedding, carpets, dust, vehicles and

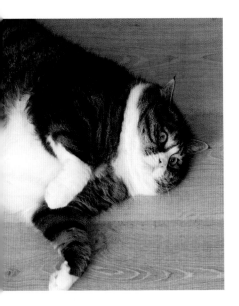

other surfaces, even long after smoking has stopped…and builds up on surfaces over time and resists normal cleaning" (www.mayoclinic.org). Consider the damaging effects that second and third-hand smoke have on your family and pets from exposure to toxins in the home, car or on clothing when breathing, sleeping, eating and playing. A Michigan-based study indicated that smokers who were made aware of secondhand smoke exposure risks for their pets were often motivated to quit smoking (*Tobacco Control,* Feb. 2009).

❏ *Avoid overfeeding yourself and your pet.* The current U.S. adult obesity rate is approximately 35 percent, affecting 78.6 million people (www.cdc. gov), whereas animal obesity rates are estimated at 57.9 percent and 52.7 percent for cats and dogs, respectively (www.petobesityprevention. org). Abdominal obesity in dogs has been linked to heart disease (*BMC Veterinary Research*, June 2014), as well as metabolic dysfunction (e.g., insulin resistance) (*BMC Veterinary Research,* 2012). Making conscious decisions about portion control for you and your pet can have livesaving implications. Banfield Pet Hospital has an overweight/obesity section on their interactive web site for portion sizes and visual examples of thin to overweight cats and dogs (www.stateofpethealth.com).

❏ *Exercise together.* Adults should aim for at least 20 minutes of daily aerobic exercise (150 minutes per week) (www.cdc.gov). Activity/exercise recommendations for dogs (breed dependent) include 30 to 120 minutes daily (www.petmd.com/dog). The People and Pets Exercising Together study resulted in weight loss for overweight people and their pets (*Obesity,* Oct. 2006). Furthermore, researchers reported that participants' dogs provided them social support, motivation and encouragement.

Only you can commit to the best lifestyle for yourself as well as for your pets. Make the years you have together the healthiest and happiest they can be!

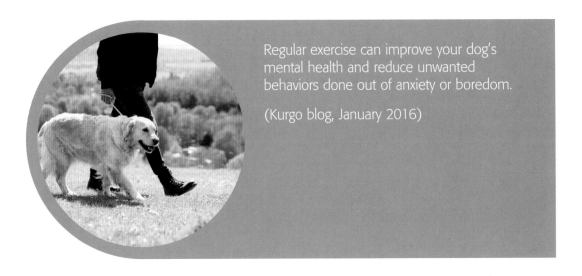

Regular exercise can improve your dog's mental health and reduce unwanted behaviors done out of anxiety or boredom.

(Kurgo blog, January 2016)

Treatment of Atrial Fibrillation: Fatness and Fitness Matter

Barry A. Franklin, Ph.D.

Atrial fibrillation, or AF, is a common disturbance of the heartbeat, during which the heart's two upper chambers, called the atria, may contract very fast (exceeding 300 beats per minute) and irregularly. This results in the loss of effective atrial contractions and typically a rapid ventricular response, usually in the range of 90 to 160 beats per minute. The incomplete contractions allow blood to pool and clots can form in an upper chamber of your heart. If a blood clot leaves your heart and enters the bloodstream, it can travel up to the brain and cause a stroke.

Today, AF is the most commonly treated cardiac rhythm irregularity in clinical practice, accounting for approximately one-third of U.S. hospital admissions for heart-related rhythm disturbances. Common risk factors for AF include increasing age, structural heart disease, high blood pressure, overweight/obesity, metabolic abnormalities (e.g., diabetes mellitus), excessive alcohol intake, and obstructive sleep apnea.

Today, AF is the most commonly treated cardiac rhythm irregularity in clinical practice, accounting for approximately one-third of U.S. hospital admissions for heart-related rhythm disturbances.

The good news is that a procedure called cardioversion (during which a synchronized direct current shocks the heart) can often normalize AF. Alternatively, a cardiologist with specialized training may perform an ablation procedure to abolish the AF using a special catheter. In addition, you may be prescribed an anticoagulant such as Coumadin to decrease the likelihood of blood clot formation. Other medications like beta blockers or calcium channel blockers are frequently used to control the associated fast heart rate. Over the last two years, however, three landmark studies have reported on the favorable impact of purposeful weight reduction, improved cardio-respiratory fitness, or both, in providing complementary interventions to prevent the development of AF and/or its recurrence.

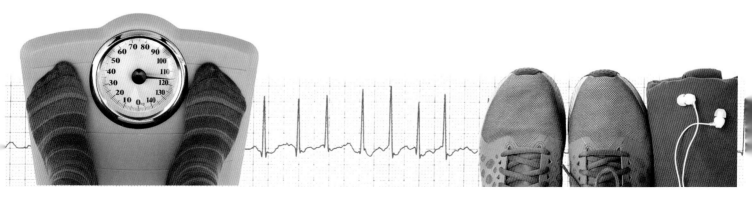

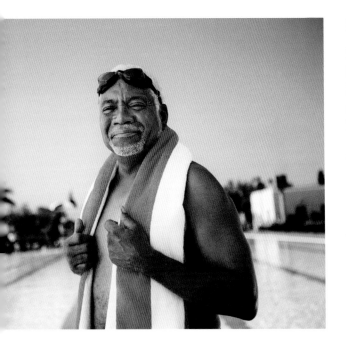

Nonpharmacologic or lifestyle interventions

In one report, after screening for exclusion criteria, investigators evaluated the long-term impact of weight loss in 355 overweight/obese patients with symptomatic AF (*Journal of the American College of Cardiology,* May 2015). Three groups were evaluated: group 1 (n = 135; 10 percent or greater weight loss); group 2 (n = 103; 3 to 9 percent weight loss); and, group 3 (n = 117; less than 3 percent weight loss or weight gain). Over a five-year follow-up period, those who lost greater than 10 percent of their body weight (group 1) had a six-fold greater freedom from AF. The researchers noted beneficial effects of weight loss on blood pressure, diabetic control, the cholesterol profile, and inflammation, all of which may have contributed to the reduction of the AF burden.

A second report, also by the above-referenced investigators, using essentially the same patient database, examined the role of baseline cardiorespiratory fitness, expressed as peak metabolic equivalents (METs) achieved during exercise testing, and the added benefit of fitness improvements in reducing the recurrence of AF (*Journal of the American College of Cardiology,* Sept. 2015). Over a four-year follow-up, those with the highest levels of baseline fitness were more likely to be free from AF without the need for medical or ablative therapy. Moreover, for every 1-MET increase in exercise capacity, there was a 9 percent decrease in AF recurrence. Collectively, these findings support the notion that improved cardiorespiratory fitness provided benefit beyond that provided by weight loss alone.

In a more recent study, researchers sought to determine the relation between baseline cardiorespiratory fitness and the risk of developing AF in 5,962 military veterans (mean age, 57 ± 11 years) over the next eight years (*Mayo Clinic Proceedings,* May 2016). Cardiorespiratory fitness, expressed as peak METs during exercise testing, was inversely related to the incidence of AF. For each 1-MET increase in exercise capacity, there was a 21 percent lower risk for developing AF. Moreover, the protective impact of fitness held, even after adjusting for concomitant beta-blocker and/or calcium channel blocker therapy. The investigators concluded that increased cardiorespiratory fitness independently lowers the risk of developing AF.

When interpreted in aggregate, these studies suggest that patients should be encouraged to lose weight and participate in moderate-to-vigorous exercise programs to achieve an improved fitness level when the goals are the prevention of AF and maintenance or enhancement of long-term cardiovascular health.

Can Obese People Be Healthy? New Insights

Wendy Miller, M.D.

The obesity epidemic persists, with more than one-third of adults and 17 percent of youth affected in the United States. It is estimated that 78 million adults and 12 million children are obese. Michigan generally ranks in the "top 10" most obese states, and approximately 32 percent of Michigan residents are currently classified as obese.

Obesity is often defined by body mass index (BMI), which is expressed as an individual's weight relative to their height [weight in kilograms (kg) divided by height in meters squared (m^2)]. In general, 35 pounds or more of excess weight typically places an individual in the obese category, which corresponds to a BMI at or above 30 kg/m^2. Although BMI is less accurate than measuring an individual's adiposity with an imaging scan, it has been shown to correlate quite well with body fat for most individuals. A physician or healthcare provider can determine your BMI, or there are several BMI calculators on the internet, such as the National Institutes of Health BMI calculator at http://www.nhlbi.nih.gov/health/educational/lose_wt/BMI/bmicalc.htm

It is well established that obesity increases the risk for heart disease, type 2 diabetes, high cholesterol, high blood pressure, stroke, obstructive sleep apnea, fatty liver and many other conditions. These diseases develop over time as an individual continues to carry excess weight. If a person became obese as a teen or young adult, these risk factors or chronic diseases often become evident when he/she reaches 30 to 50 years of age. However, for a small percentage of individuals, this is not the case. Such individuals may be obese for several years and yet they do not have type 2 diabetes, high blood pressure, high cholesterol or other medical conditions commonly associated with excess weight. The term "healthy obese" is often used to describe this population. What factors may help to temporarily prevent disease in the healthy obese group?

Will healthy obese persons continue to be healthy as the years go by?

Fat location plays a significant role in determining risk for chronic diseases, such as type 2 diabetes, high cholesterol and heart disease. Individuals with a substantial amount of abdominal fat will have a much higher risk for disease than those whose fat tissue is distributed more in the hips and thighs (*Journal of the American Medical Association,* Jan. 1993). Waist circumference measurement is the simplest way to assess abdominal fat content and

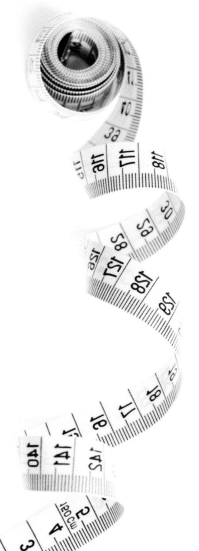

Reducing belly fat and health risk		
Waist measurement	Aim for a waist size of: • less than 40 inches for men • less than 35 inches for women	
Weight	If you are carrying excess weight: • weight loss is the most effective way to decrease belly fat • a 10 percent reduction in weight is often associated with health benefits If you are normal weight: • develop and maintain a healthy lifestyle to prevent weight gain	
Diet	Avoid or greatly limit: • refined grains (white bread, white flour, white pasta, white rice, baked goods) • fructose sweetened beverages (including high fructose corn syrup) • trans fats (partially hydrogenated oils)	Opt for this instead: • whole grains (whole-wheat bread and pasta, bulgur, oatmeal, whole cornmeal, and brown rice) • water, unsweetened tea/iced tea, coffee, infused water (add fruit, vegetable and/or herbs to water) • monounsaturated fat - found in olive, peanut and canola oils; Nuts, fish and seeds containing unsaturated omega-3 fatty acids
Exercise	Structured exercise, increased lifestyle physical activity, or both, particularly when combined with a reduction in calorie intake, can decrease belly fat. Consider wearing a quality pedometer to track daily step totals. It's also a great motivator!	

specified cut points are associated with a higher risk for disease. For men, a waist circumference of 40 inches or above, and for women, a waist measurement of 35 inches or above, increases risk. Obese individuals with a waist size below these cut points may be less likely to have the typical chronic illnesses associated with excess weight.

What determines the location we carry our fat? This is believed to be genetically determined, in part, which means that one or both of your parents may have experienced a similar fat distribution if they carried extra weight. However, there is also evidence that what we eat increases our belly fat. Specifically, fructose used as a sweetener in beverages, including high-fructose corn syrup, is associated with increasing belly fat (*Journal of Clinical Investigation,* May 2009).

High-fructose corn syrup is found in many sodas, energy drinks, sports drinks and juice blends, so check the list of ingredients on nutrition labels and avoid beverages with fructose or high-fructose corn syrup listed.

The type of grains you eat also can contribute to belly fat. Refined grains made from white flour or refined wheat flour may increase your waistline. A widely cited study found that those eating a higher amount of whole grains rather than refined grains had less abdominal fat (*American Journal of Clinical Nutrition,* Nov. 2010). Examples of refined grains include white bread, white pasta, white bagels, and white rice. Replacing refined grains in your diet with whole grains, such as whole-wheat bread and pasta, bulgur (cracked wheat), oatmeal, whole cornmeal and brown rice can help your waistline and your health. Look for the word "whole" listed on the food label, such as "whole wheat," or "whole grain oats," instead of just "wheat," "wheat flour" or "multigrain," which often are not whole grain foods.

Additionally, trans fats, which are found in some snack foods and fast foods, can cause your waistline to expand (*Obesity,* July 2007). The U.S. Food and Drug Administration has mandated that food manufacturers phase out trans fats in their product ingredients over time, which may take years. In the meantime, look for "partially hydrogenated oil" on the food label, which signifies trans fats, and avoid these foods.

A study of British government workers (*Journal of the American College of Cardiology,* Jan. 2015) sought to answer the question: Do obese individuals who are apparently healthy develop typical weight-related medical problems over time? Among approximately 2,500 participants in the study, 36 percent of them were healthy obese individuals at baseline. After following this group over time, approximately one-half of healthy obese adults became unhealthy obese, with the typical weight related medical issues. People who started out obese but healthy were eight times more likely than their healthy normal weight counterparts to develop medical problems over two decades. Thus, healthy obese individuals have a much higher risk of developing medical illness over time than their normal weight counterparts.

The bottom line? Obesity increases the risk for many chronic illnesses, including type 2 diabetes, high cholesterol, high blood pressure and heart disease. Even obese individuals who are apparently healthy are at significantly higher risk of developing risk factors and/or chronic diseases over time. Therefore, lifestyle changes that elicit gradual weight loss for all obese individuals are commonly recommended. Reaching an ideal weight is not necessary to achieve health benefits. A 10 percent weight reduction is often associated with improvement, resolution or prevention of weight-related medical problems. Recommended lifestyle changes include opting for a variety of vegetables, fruits, lean proteins, whole grains and water in your daily regimen rather than prepackaged foods, refined grains, sodas, sweets, baked goods, and high fat meat and dairy. Increasing daily physical activity level, when combined with calorie intake reduction, is also helpful for weight loss and particularly helps with maintaining lost weight. Other treatment modalities, in addition to lifestyle changes, may be necessary for long-term sustained weight loss, such as support groups, weight loss medications and/or weight loss surgery. Comprehensive medical weight management programs can empower individuals to achieve and maintain a healthier weight through a multidisciplinary team of professionals who provide education, support and a variety of treatment options.

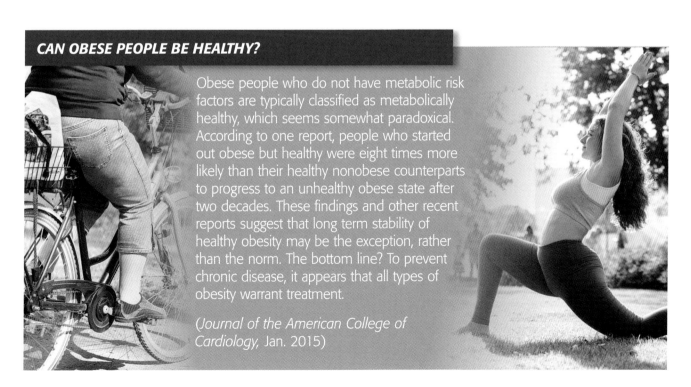

CAN OBESE PEOPLE BE HEALTHY?

Obese people who do not have metabolic risk factors are typically classified as metabolically healthy, which seems somewhat paradoxical. According to one report, people who started out obese but healthy were eight times more likely than their healthy nonobese counterparts to progress to an unhealthy obese state after two decades. These findings and other recent reports suggest that long term stability of healthy obesity may be the exception, rather than the norm. The bottom line? To prevent chronic disease, it appears that all types of obesity warrant treatment.

(*Journal of the American College of Cardiology*, Jan. 2015)

Being Heart Healthy and Overweight/Obese Are Incompatible

Barry A. Franklin, Ph.D.

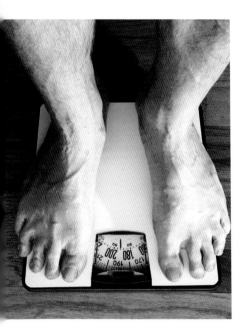

Overweight or obese middle-aged men are at a higher risk of experiencing a heart attack, stroke, heart failure or sudden cardiac death, even if they don't have other common risk factors for cardiovascular disease, according to one published report (*Circulation,* Dec. 2009).

Although modern-day advertisements and previous studies have promoted the existence of a "metabolically healthy" subgroup of obese individuals who are at no increased cardiovascular risk, these findings discount this notion. When previous studies have examined the occurrence of heart disease risk, obese people without the cluster of risk factors associated with the metabolic syndrome have not demonstrated an increased cardiovascular risk. These risk factors include: abdominal obesity, elevated blood pressure, low levels of "good" HDL cholesterol, increased fasting blood glucose and, high levels of blood fats called triglycerides. Persons with three or more of these risk factors are classified as having the metabolic syndrome. However, a recent study suggests that if you follow overweight and obese people long enough, there *is* an added risk of cardiovascular events.

The 30-year study involved 1,758 men born between 1920 and 1924 in Sweden, all of whom underwent a comprehensive health evaluation at age 50. All were classified as either normal weight, overweight or obese according to their body mass index. Those with known diabetes and heart disease were excluded. During the follow-up, 788 participants died and 681 suffered a cardiovascular event, including 386 fatalities. After adjusting for age, cigarette smoking and cholesterol levels, the researchers noted three major findings:

- overweight and obese men were at increased risk of having cardiovascular events, even if they didn't have the metabolic syndrome
- men with the metabolic syndrome were at greater risk of experiencing heart attacks and/or strokes, regardless of whether they were overweight or obese
- the highest risk cohort were obese men with the metabolic syndrome

Putting the findings in perspective

Although some researchers have suggested that heavy people without other risk factors don't need to lose weight, these data do not support this notion. Overweight and obese middle-aged men are at higher risk of having non-fatal or fatal cardiovascular events, even if they do not have metabolic syndrome.

Moreover, the investigators acknowledged that although their study was conducted in men, similar findings may apply to women. The bottom line? There appears to be no such thing as metabolically healthy obesity. Being heart healthy and weighing too much are incompatible.

Achieving a healthy weight

Numerous studies now suggest that a modest weight loss, even five to 10 pounds, can have significant health implications.

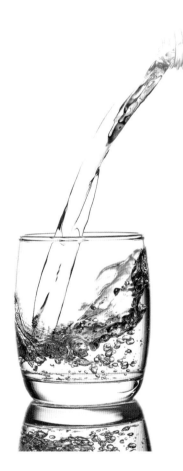

- *Set realistic goals and have them posted where you'll see them often* (i.e. computer screen, car visor or refrigerator). There is increasing evidence in the scientific literature that we become what we think about and we attract what we fear.
- *Move more throughout the day.* In addition to a structured exercise program, start tracking your daily steps with a quality pedometer. According to one review of numerous trials (*Journal of the American Medical Association,* Nov. 2007), pedometer users significantly increased their physical activity by nearly 2,500 steps per day as compared with their non-user counterparts.
- *Avoid the hidden calories in many drinks.* Alcoholic drinks, soda pop and even fruit juices can, over time, contribute to a "calorie imbalance" and weight gain. Even diet sodas with no calories have now been linked to a higher risk of developing obesity and other risk factors for heart disease (*Circulation,* July 2007). Why? Researchers now believe that diet sodas may promote a dietary preference for sweeter foods. Drink water instead.
- *Participate in group interventions.* Other studies (*Metabolic Syndrome and Related Disorders,* Oct. 2009) suggest that group obesity treatment is associated with greater weight loss and improvement in more cardiovascular risk factors than an individual intervention.
- *Visualize yourself at a lower weight.* Without question, visualization is one of the chief strategies in developing the subconscious mind's magnetic forces. You'll really start to lose weight when you give your subconscious mind a mental picture of a slimmer you.
- *Start exercising.* Exercise has been shown to be helpful in reducing body weight and fat stores and in preventing weight regain. Moreover, numerous studies have now shown that low fit individuals are approximately two to three times more likely to die during follow-up compared with their more fit counterparts, matched for age and body habitus (normal weight, overweight or obese). Thus, regardless of your weight, significant health benefits can be achieved by moving out of the least fit, least active subgroup.
- *Take action.* In many respects, humans obey the law of inertia: A body at rest tends to remain at rest, whereas a body in motion tends to remain in motion. The universe rewards action. By taking action, you overcome inertia and build momentum in achieving your goals.

The Obesity Paradox: Higher Weight = Lower Risk?

Barry A. Franklin, Ph.D.

In recent years, obesity has become much more prevalent—and highly demonized by society. We've been led to believe that excess body fat is bad, no matter what. Yet, using body mass index (BMI), calculated as weight in kilograms divided by height in meters squared, more than 70 percent of U.S. adults are now classified as overweight or obese. Consequently, the vast majority of Americans are preoccupied with losing weight to improve their health.

Causes of the obesity epidemic

Although unhealthy eating habits are often considered the primary factor underlying our national weight problem, research suggests that technologic advances and the associated reduction in physical activity is a major culprit. In fact, one sobering report showed that the dramatic drop in energy expenditure during work-related activities over the last 50 years largely explains the U.S. weight gain (PLoS ONE, May, 2011).

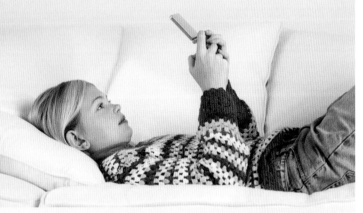

Research suggests that technologic advances and the associated reduction in physical activity is a major culprit in our national weight problem.

Let's face the facts. Increasingly we're paid to think, to provide specific sedentary skills, or to communicate or process information. Automobiles, elevators, escalators, moving walkways, remote controls and energy-saving devices such as washing machines, dishwashers, microwave ovens, self-propelled lawn mowers, automatic garage door openers, and on-line ordering/bill paying have engineered physical activity out of daily life. Smartphones and computers have become part of our vocational garb.

Impact of obesity on health

Admittedly, obesity is associated with a number of chronic diseases or medical conditions, including diabetes, insulin resistance, inflammation, high blood pressure and heart disease. Thus, purposeful weight reduction, especially in some people, is commonly recommended. Unfortunately, we've gotten so used to framing health issues in terms of obesity that we may be overlooking other potential causes of disease. Consider the following: you gain weight and, over time, develop heart disease. Your conclusion? Weight gain is the problem. However, correlations or statistical relationships between two variables do not necessarily imply causation. Other confounding variables (things that occurred simultaneously) may have also contributed to the development of disease. Perhaps during this timeframe you encountered escalating stress levels, increasingly relied on unhealthy fast food choices, started smoking again or became unfit due to technologies that made you more inactive throughout the day?

Being overweight or obese does not necessarily confer adverse health outcomes. Numerous studies have now shown that other variables can have a huge impact on the relationship between fatness and mortality. For example, consider the 'fat real estate' axiom: location matters. People with excess belly fat have the worst prognosis. Similarly, it's better to be fat and fit than thin and unfit. According to one report, fit obese men were half as likely to die over a 10-year follow-up as compared with their unfit, normal weight counterparts (*Journal of the American Medical Association,* Oct. 1999).

Extra pounds are OK?

Over the past decade, researchers have uncovered a startling and perplexing revelation: carrying a few extra pounds may not be as bad as once thought, and may actually be beneficial in some people. This finding is commonly referred to as the 'Obesity Paradox.'

In the early 1980s, the director of the National Institute of Aging, Reubin Andres, noted that older individuals were generally better off if they were overweight—a highly controversial statement at the time. In 2002, investigators reported that overweight or obese patients, as compared with their thinner counterparts, had roughly half the risk of dying within a year after undergoing an angioplasty procedure (*Journal of the American College of Cardiology,* Feb. 2002).

More recently, a blockbuster review of 97 different studies involving nearly 3 million people and more than 270,000 deaths, confirmed the obesity paradox (*Journal of the American Medical Association,* Jan. 2013). People who were overweight (BMI between 25 and 30) were at lower risk of dying than those in the moderately (BMI above 35) or morbidly obese (BMI over 40) or normal-weight (BMI, 18.5 to less than 25) categories. The mildly obese cohort (BMI between 30 and 35) had a slightly lower risk of dying. These findings persisted after adjusting for potential confounding variables.

Collectively, these studies, and other recent reports, indicate that being at the ends of the continuum, either morbidly obese or painfully thin (BMI less than 18.5) spells trouble. It's what clinicians refer to as a classic U-curve, and you don't want to be on either end of the spectrum.

Explaining the obesity paradox

Why is being overweight or mildly obese associated with a lower mortality risk? Some have suggested that such individuals may receive earlier and more aggressive medical treatment because of their 'unhealthy' weight. Others suggest that overweight persons may fare better than thinner ones because of superior genes, or because thinner persons may be more likely to be smokers or have underlying illness. Some studies suggest that modest amounts of body fat may actually be protective.

Take-home messages

Are the concerns about being overweight or mildly obese unwarranted? Clearly, obesity and its complications increase the risk for developing many diseases, including diabetes, heart disease and heart failure. However, in patients who already have these medical conditions, numerous studies have demonstrated an 'obesity paradox,' whereby overweight and mildly obese patients generally have better outcomes than leaner ones.

Perhaps Dr. Carl Lavie, a world-renown cardiologist, summed it up best when he stated that when it comes to BMI, 27 is the new 23. He suggests that it's not doomsday to have some extra fat on you, especially if you're reasonably fit. In fact, you don't have to fret about your inability to get your BMI below 25. With respect to long-term survival, you may actually be better off, he contends, maintaining a BMI of between 25 and 30, or even slightly higher.

THE OBESITY PARADOX AND HEART DISEASE: CAN HEAVIER REALLY BE HEALTHIER?

Overweight and mildly obese patients with heart disease appear to have a more favorable prognosis than their normal weight counterparts. In contrast, purposeful weight loss for long term health remains important, particularly for cardiac patients with more severe degrees of obesity (body mass index approaching or exceeding 35 kg/m²). Quite likely, their prognosis can be further enhanced if it is combined with increased lifestyle physical activity, structured exercise and improved cardiorespiratory fitness.

(*Heart*, June 2015)

Big Waist Doubles Risk of Premature Death

Barry A. Franklin, Ph.D.

Having a large waist is related to a host of potentially serious health issues, such as heart disease, elevated blood cholesterol, metabolic syndrome, type 2 diabetes and higher circulating levels of inflammatory markers (e.g., C-reactive protein). Belly bulge may be associated with these conditions because it suggests excessive fat stores in the cavities of the body. And, according to one study, it may also be linked to something else: early death.

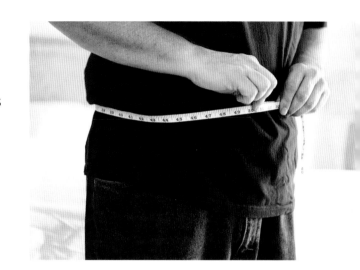

Researchers from the Epidemiology Research Program of the American Cancer Society used data from more than 104,000 men and women, 50 years or older, who were followed from 1997 to 2006. At baseline, all subjects were required to provide their height, weight and waist circumference. Nearly 15,000 people died during the nine-year follow-up.

After adjusting for body mass index and other risk factors, very large waists—47 inches or more in men and 42 inches or more in women—were associated with about a two-fold higher risk of early death in both sexes, as compared to those with the smallest waists. Four extra inches around the waist increased the risk of dying by approximately 15 to 25 percent. The three most common causes of death were lung diseases, such as chronic bronchitis and emphysema, cardiovascular disease and cancer, respectively.

Interestingly, the pattern of increasing risk with increasing waist size held true in every BMI category—including normal weight, overweight and obese. Indeed, among women, the association between waist size and mortality was strongest in those in the normal BMI category as compared with their counterparts who were overweight or obese.

"Even if your weight is considered normal for your height and you haven't noticed a big weight gain, if your waist size is starting to increase—if you're having to move into a bigger pant size—that's an important sign that it's time to start eating better and exercising more," said lead author Eric Jacobs, Ph.D.

Bariatric Surgery Reduces Cardiovascular Risk and Mortality

Wendy Miller, M.D.

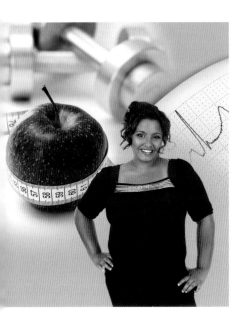

The prevalence of obesity in the United States has reached epidemic proportions. The majority of adults, 68 percent, are either overweight or obese, and one-third are obese (*Journal of the American Medical Association,* Jan. 2010). Along with escalating weight, there has been an unprecedented increase in obesity-related medical conditions, including type 2 diabetes, high blood pressure, elevated cholesterol, obstructive sleep apnea, stroke and heart disease. Unfortunately, most patients with severe obesity (body mass index greater than 40 kg/m^2 or approximately 100 lbs over ideal weight) are unable to achieve and maintain a healthy weight through non-surgical treatment (*Proceedings of the Nutrition Society,* Nov. 2010). Bariatric surgery, which includes gastric bypass, gastric banding, and gastric sleeve surgery, has been shown to be an effective tool for long-term weight reduction as well as resolution of obesity-related health problems (*British Medical Journal,* Aug. 2009).

Bariatric surgery is considered a relatively safe procedure, with less than 1 percent 30-day post-surgery mortality (*Journal of the American Medical Association,* Oct. 2005). Indeed, the procedure may soon exceed gallbladder surgery as the most common elective surgical treatment. Physicians within Beaumont's Division of Nutrition and Preventive Medicine were one of the first groups to quantify cardiovascular risk reduction after bariatric surgery (*American Journal of Cardiology,* Jan. 2007). We found a significant improvement in Framingham risk score, a tool that predicts cardiac risk, at 17-months post-bariatric surgery for both men and women. Meta-analyses summarizing data from numerous studies have shown resolution or improvement in cardiovascular risk factors following bariatric surgery, including resolution of type 2 diabetes in 77 percent of patients and resolution of hypertension in 62 percent (*Journal of the American Medical Association,* Oct. 2004; *Annals of Internal Medicine,* April 2005; *American Journal of Medicine,* March 2009). Subsequently, the American Heart Association published a scientific statement on bariatric surgery and cardiovascular risk factors (*Circulation,* Jan. 2011). The statement highlighted several studies that have reported increased survival in morbidly obese patients who have undergone bariatric surgery compared with those who have not. This was due specifically to mortality reductions related to heart disease, diabetes and cancer.

My Roller Coaster Ride With Obesity: Loving the Downhill Plunge

Kaylee Kaeding, B.S.

Over the years, my weight has been analogous to a roller coaster ride, with more uphill climbs than thrilling downhill plunges. Ultimately, after many years, I lost hope and felt I was past the point of no return. I've always been very private about my weight and tried to camouflage it with larger clothes, hoping people would not notice me. Ultimately, my motivation emanated from my intrinsic desire to take better care of myself and put my health first. Here's my story, and what worked for me.

As a young person, I stayed active on our farm and played sports. Over time, there was less opportunity for play and increasing demands to "grow up." I continued to gain weight, and began to feel hopeless. I struggled with what psychologists refer to as cognitive dissonance. My mental stress increased while my self-efficacy plummeted. Simultaneously, I was frustrated with conflicting beliefs, ideas and values (wanting to be a 'normal' weight).

Every day, every activity, every vacation revolved around my obesity. Unfortunately, on July 16, 2013 I was involved in a rollover car accident and suddenly life, love and family felt different. Later that year my husband, Trevor, received an alarming blood chemistry report. His hemoglobin A1C was markedly elevated and needed a drastic reduction. Collectively, these two events led us to change our attitudes toward better living and a healthier lifestyle.

In March 2014, my body mass index (BMI) was 47.6, which is considered "extreme obesity, class III." In just one year, I decreased my BMI by more than 13 points. How? I developed a plan that incorporated five simple steps, and took action.

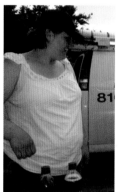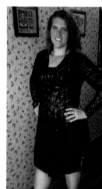

Before　　　　**After**

Step 1: Meal plan

The Daniel Plan: a healthy lifestyle program focused on the essentials: Faith, Food, Fitness, Focus and Friends (danielplan.com).

Our refrigerator went from unhealthy boxed food, jugs, meats and Styrofoam containers of left-overs from the previous night's carry out to looking like the produce section of a grocery store. It blossomed with greens, reds, oranges, yellows, and vibrant scents of vegetables and fruits. I then started packing all of my meals for work (breakfast, lunch and dinner). Now, I consume most of my calories by late afternoon—because I tend to be less active in the evening.

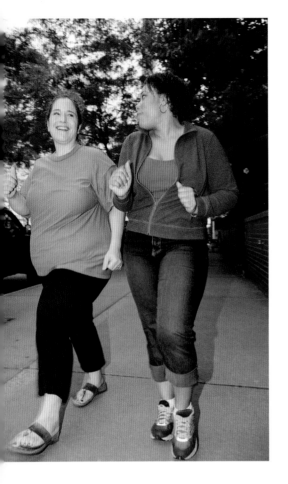

Step 2: Exercise

For successful weight loss, I needed more than just a healthier eating plan. Trevor and I also incorporated exercise/lifestyle activity to our daily routine. We invariably exercise at least four or five days a week for 30 to 60 minutes. Over time, we increased the exercise intensity to burn additional calories and improve fitness.

Step 3: Regularly monitor and measure

The hardest things about weight loss are not seeing the weight numbers you want to see, weight plateaus and setbacks. Your body doesn't always give you the "number" on the scale or the results you think you deserve. So, I did other things to track my progress and stay motivated. For example, a regular weigh-in with meticulous, standardized body measurements. I began to see the inches decrease, and clothes size reductions. In addition, I purchased a pedometer. This heightened my awareness of daily step totals and kept me honest. To help me track my weight, I downloaded an app on my phone to monitor my daily weight fluctuations, and now weigh-in regularly.

Step 4: Be smart and stay accountable

Holidays, birthdays and family gatherings, oh my! These are the biggest struggles that weight-conscious people deal with. It is simple math—calories in and calories out. Today, I am acutely aware of everything that I eat, which may be reflected by small fluctuations on the scale. For gatherings, I bring a large salad for the dish-to-pass so I know there will be at least one option I can rely on.

Step 5: Support

Trevor and I are now beyond the first year of our new lifestyle intervention. He has been with me all along the way as a supporter and experimental subject. His hemoglobin A1C decreased by more than half and is now in the healthy normal range. Both of us remain laser-focused on our goals. We struggled together and conquered together. It has allowed us to feel blessed, successful, and much more positive about a healthy lifestyle and all that it can offer. My uphill roller coaster climb has finally overcome inertia, and I'm now experiencing the exciting and accelerating downhill ride.

The most important message I have is make the choice! You cannot be successful without faith, will-power, support, love (for yourself and others), planning and motivation. I did it—and you can too.

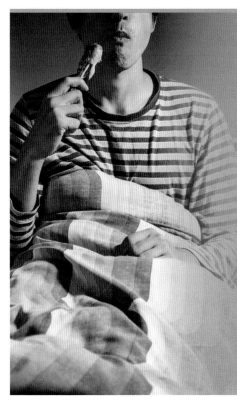

EATING TIMES AND ELEVATED CORONARY RISK

Eating habits, including skipping breakfast and late night eating, were assessed in 1992 in nearly 27,000 American men who had no history of cardiovascular disease and/or cancer. The men were all educated health professionals—like dentists, veterinarians, and podiatrists—and were at least 45 years of age. Over the next 16 years, 1,527 suffered fatal or nonfatal heart attacks. Men who skipped breakfast had a 27 percent higher risk of coronary events as compared with men who did not. Moreover, those who ate late at night had a 55 percent higher cardiac risk as compared with their counterparts who did not. These associations were related to differences in indices of overweight/obesity, high blood pressure, elevated blood cholesterol, and diabetes mellitus. The investigators suggested that if these findings can be replicated in women and other population subsets, the results support a recommendation of daily breakfast eating as well as the avoidance of late night snacking.

(*Circulation*, July 2013).

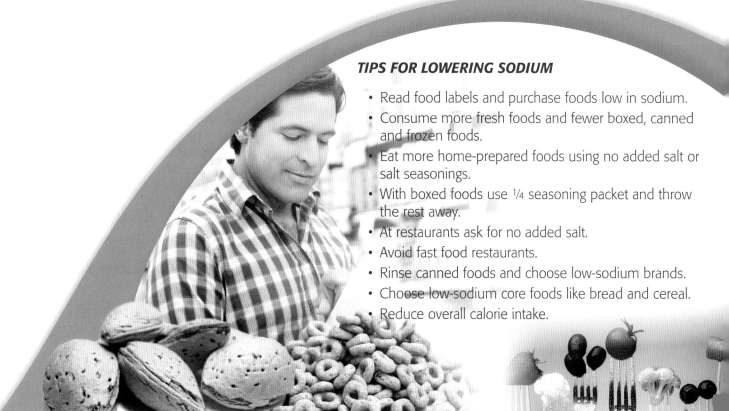

TIPS FOR LOWERING SODIUM

- Read food labels and purchase foods low in sodium.
- Consume more fresh foods and fewer boxed, canned and frozen foods.
- Eat more home-prepared foods using no added salt or salt seasonings.
- With boxed foods use ¼ seasoning packet and throw the rest away.
- At restaurants ask for no added salt.
- Avoid fast food restaurants.
- Rinse canned foods and choose low-sodium brands.
- Choose low-sodium core foods like bread and cereal.
- Reduce overall calorie intake.

8

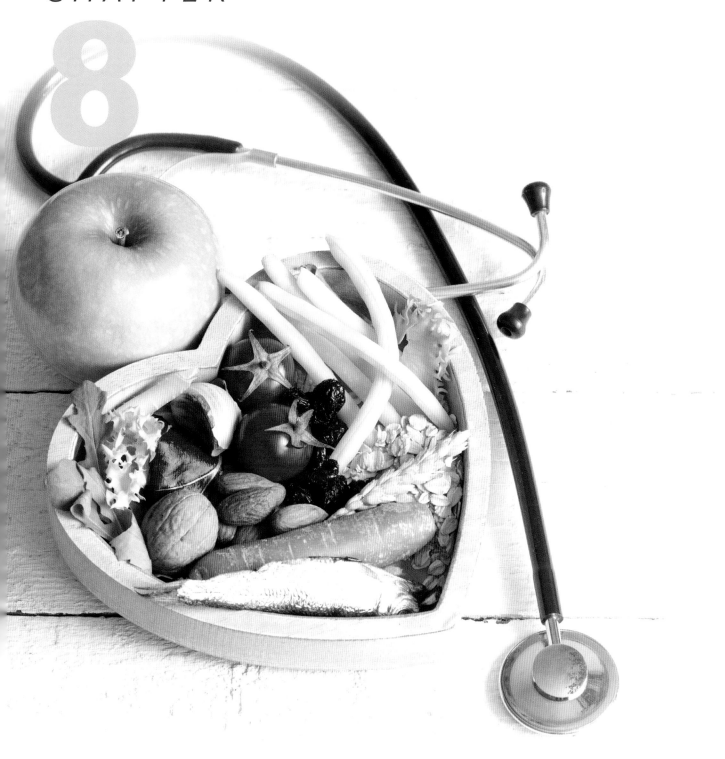

NUTRITIONAL CONCERNS

Unhealthy Eating: Cows, Pigs, and Chronic Disease

Barry A. Franklin, Ph.D.

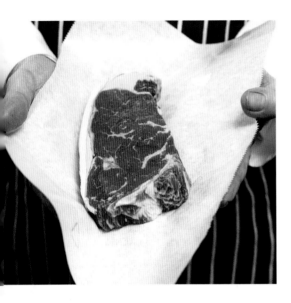

Also: Stop cigarette smoking and avoid secondhand smoke, reduce food portion sizes, limit prolonged sitting (i.e., extended TV watching or computer interactions), increase daily physical activity and get enough sleep.

A number of recent research studies show that certain dietary practices are associated with lower rates of chronic disease. In other words, what we include in our diet is as important as what we exclude. For example, "good" carbs (e.g., fruits, vegetables, whole grains) and fats (e.g., fatty acids found in fish oil, flaxseed oil) seem to be cardioprotective, whereas "bad" carbs (e.g., white bread) and fats (e.g., trans fats) are associated with a heightened risk of developing varied illnesses.

Why is this so important? Because more than 75 percent of the $2.6 trillion in annual health care costs are spent in treating chronic diseases such as coronary heart disease. Healthier dietary practices are likely to lessen the consequences of these unhealthy conditions, thereby reducing health care costs. This premise was substantiated by a widely cited European study (*Archives of Internal Medicine,* Aug. 2009), which showed that patients who adhered to healthy dietary practices had a 75 percent lower overall risk of developing a chronic disease.

Dietary and Lifestyle Priorities Associated with Cardioprotective Benefits	
Consume more:	**Consume less:**
• fish and shellfish • whole grains • fruits • vegetables • nuts • low-fat or non-fat dairy products • vegetable oils* • water	• potatoes, refined grains, sugars • processed meats • sweetened beverages, diet sodas • grain-based desserts and bakery foods • fats, oils or foods containing partially hydrogenated vegetable oils • salt • alcohol+
* Examples include flaxseed, canola, and soybean oil	+ For adults who drink alcohol, no more than moderate consumption (i.e., up to 2 drinks/day for men, 1 drink/day for women) should be encouraged, ideally with meals.

Is processed and unprocessed red meat bad for you? In a word, yes. Five years ago, the first large-scale prospective longitudinal study in men and women showed that regular consumption of red meat is associated with an increased risk of premature death from all causes including cardiovascular disease and cancer (*Archives of Internal Medicine,* April 2012). In a related study by the same investigators, red meat consumption was associated with an increased risk of developing type 2 diabetes (*American Journal of Clinical Nutrition,* Oct. 2011). Thus, substituting healthier foods for red meat provides a double benefit to our health.

A group of nutrition experts provided a series of recommendations for health practitioners, patients and policy makers to better understand contemporary issues related to the effects of diet on cardiovascular disease (*Circulation,* June 2011). Their dietary priorities for cardiovascular and metabolic health are summarized on the previous page.

In closing, I'd like to share a few relevant quotes that I've used in my teaching and presentations over the years with specific reference to healthy and unhealthy dietary choices. Enjoy!

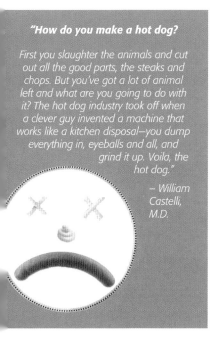

"How do you make a hot dog?

First you slaughter the animals and cut out all the good parts, the steaks and chops. But you've got a lot of animal left and what are you going to do with it? The hot dog industry took off when a clever guy invented a machine that works like a kitchen disposal—you dump everything in, eyeballs and all, and grind it up. Voila, the hot dog."

– William Castelli, M.D.

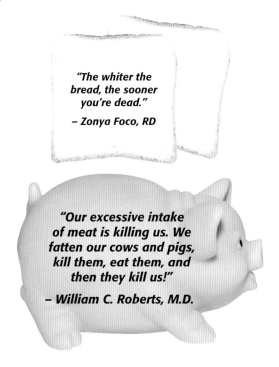

"The whiter the bread, the sooner you're dead."

– Zonya Foco, RD

"Our excessive intake of meat is killing us. We fatten our cows and pigs, kill them, eat them, and then they kill us!"

– William C. Roberts, M.D.

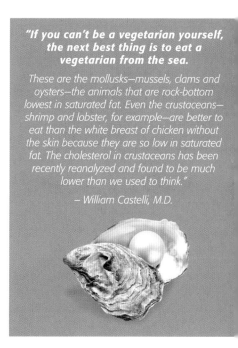

"If you can't be a vegetarian yourself, the next best thing is to eat a vegetarian from the sea.

These are the mollusks—mussels, clams and oysters—the animals that are rock-bottom lowest in saturated fat. Even the crustaceans—shrimp and lobster, for example—are better to eat than the white breast of chicken without the skin because they are so low in saturated fat. The cholesterol in crustaceans has been recently reanalyzed and found to be much lower than we used to think."

– William Castelli, M.D.

Americans Are Eating Too Much Salt—And It's Making Them Sick

Sue Haapaniemi, M.S.

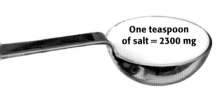

One teaspoon of salt = 2300 mg

High blood pressure is a real problem. It is the second leading modifiable cause of death and disability in the U.S., and globally, it contributes to half of all strokes and heart attacks.

The key word here is "modifiable"—which largely boils down to controlling our intake of salt. There is a clear connection between sodium intake and high blood pressure. What's more, even when blood pressure is in the normal range, excess sodium can, over time, harm the heart, kidneys and blood vessels in several ways. The American Heart Association (AHA) issued a call for Americans to reduce their intake of salt (*Circulation,* Jan. 2011).

Reducing one's sodium intake can lower blood pressure in adults, especially in those with elevated blood pressure, and has been shown to prevent hypertension in about one-fifth of the population. The "call to action" is part of the AHA's 2020 Strategic Plan to improve the cardiovascular health of all Americans by 20 percent while reducing deaths from cardiovascular diseases and stroke by 20 percent. The plan targets a reduction in sodium consumption to 1500 mg per day, which is enough to meet nutritional needs.

This is no small goal. Forty years of urging people to consume less sodium hasn't worked. The current U.S. dietary guidelines call for the consumption of less than 2300 mg of sodium per day. However, the average daily intake for Americans is 3400 mg, with studies reporting average intakes as high as 5000 mg per day or more in some population groups.

Part of the problem is the salting of our food. But the salt shaker is not the culprit that many people think. On average, it accounts for only 5 percent of total intake. The salt added in home cooking is just 6 percent of total intake. The real problem is with convenience foods (boxed, canned and frozen) and restaurant meals, which account for more than 75 percent of U.S. sodium intake. Until food manufacturers and restaurants take steps to lower the sodium content of their foods, individuals trying to cut back and stay within recommended guidelines will continue to face an uphill challenge. To a large extent, reduced sodium and salt-free foods are simply not available in the marketplace.

The AHA has set a goal of lowering the sodium content of prepared foods by 50 percent. Already, the city of New York is on board, having launched a nation-wide initiative for food manufacturers and restaurants to cut the amount of salt in their products. The city's goal is a gradual reduction of 25 percent, so that consumers can get accustomed to the flavor of foods with lower salt content. Currently, this program is voluntary, but many restaurants and manufacturers have joined in.

In the meantime, it's important for all of us to make the best choices possible to reduce our sodium intake. That means reading nutrition labels and avoiding high sodium content products. It also means preparing more meals at home, from scratch, so that you can have greater control over the amount of salt in your foods. By reducing the sodium content of your diet, you'll lower your blood pressure as well as the risk of heart disease and stroke. The potential health benefits are worth it!

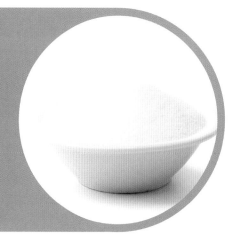

CARDIOVASCULAR DEATHS EACH YEAR LINKED TO HIGH SODIUM INTAKE

Approximately 1.65 million cardiovascular-related deaths per year can be attributed to sodium consumption above the World Health Organization's recommendation of 2,000 mg per day. These findings highlight the substantial global burden of high sodium intake and support population-based initiatives to reduce dietary sodium in our food products.

(*New England Journal of Medicine,* Aug. 2014)

Warning: Trans Fats Are Hazardous to Your Health

Barry A. Franklin, Ph.D.

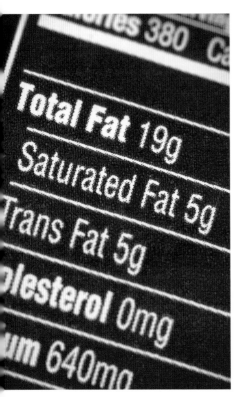

Trans fats (or trans fatty acids) are created in an industrial process that adds hydrogen to liquid vegetable oils to make them more solid for use in margarines, commercial cooking, and manufacturing processes. The average consumption of industrially produced trans fatty acids in the United States is 2 to 3 percent of total calories consumed. Major sources of trans fats include: fried foods; commercially baked goods; packaged snack foods; margarines; and crackers. Common questions include:

Why do some companies use trans fats?

Companies like using trans fats in their foods because they're inexpensive and easy to use, and may extend the 'shelf-life' of the product. Others emphasize that trans fats give foods a desirable taste and texture. Moreover, many restaurants and fast-food outlets use trans fats to repeatedly deep-fry foods throughout the day.

How do trans fats affect cardiovascular health?

Unfortunately, trans fats raise your "bad" low-density lipoprotein cholesterol (LDL) and a subcomponent of LDL cholesterol, lipoprotein (a), which has been identified as another cardiac risk factor. Trans fats also increase a number of inflammatory markers, including interleukin 6 and C-reactive protein. Moreover, these fats lower your "protective" high-density lipoprotein (HDL) cholesterol, and increase the risk of developing type 2 diabetes. The bottom line? People who eat foods rich in trans fat have a much higher risk of developing heart disease and stroke than those who don't (New England Journal of Medicine, April 2006).

How much trans fat can I eat each day?

In 2002, the Institute of Medicine stated that trans fat consumption should be as low as possible while consuming a nutritionally adequate diet. More recently, the American Heart Association recommended limiting the amount of trans fats you eat to less than 1 percent of your total daily calories. Accordingly, if you eat 2000 calories a day, no more than 20 of those calories should come from trans fats. That's less than 2 grams of trans fats a day.

A food labelling problem? Zero is not necessarily zero

The government (U.S. Food and Drug Administration) allows food manufacturers to say their product has no trans fats (0) if it has less than half a gram (0.5 g) per serving. A product that claims it has no trans fats can legitimately have up to 0.49 g of trans fats per serving. Thus, people who consume these foods may believe they are adding zero trans fats to their diet, when, in fact, there may be significant amounts of trans fats accumulated over the course of the day.

Avoiding trans fats—a simple rule of thumb?

To reduce trans fats in your diet, read food labels carefully before purchasing the item, including the ingredients. If the ingredients mention partially hydrogenated oil, hydrogenated oil, or shortening—the product is not trans fat free. Avoid these products!

Changing public policy: Trans fat ban in New York

New York was the nation's first city to ban artery-clogging trans fat at restaurants—from the corner pizzeria to high-end bakeries. A federal judge upheld a New York City regulation requiring calories to be posted on the menu boards of some chain restaurants. The Board of Health believes the regulation may help New Yorkers from becoming obese and developing diabetes. Hopefully, other major cities will follow their lead.

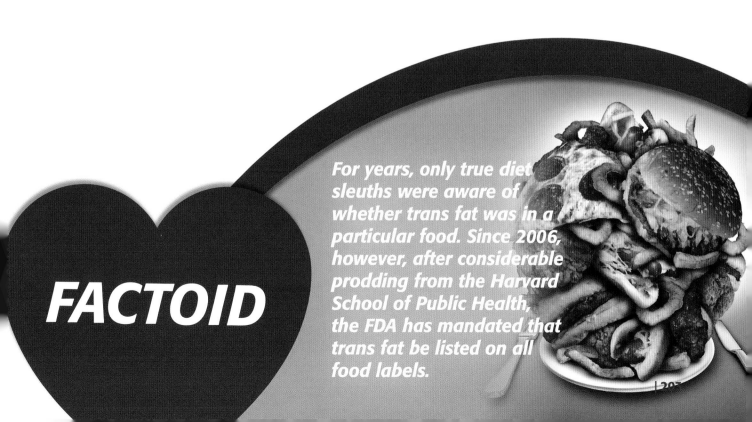

FACTOID

For years, only true diet sleuths were aware of whether trans fat was in a particular food. Since 2006, however, after considerable prodding from the Harvard School of Public Health, the FDA has mandated that trans fat be listed on all food labels.

Our Expanding Waistlines: A Soft Drink and Friends and Family Link?

Barry A. Franklin, Ph.D.

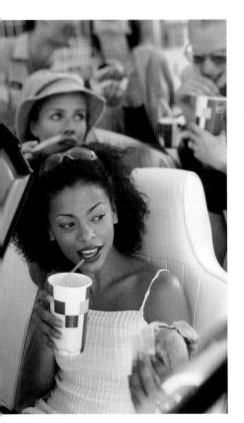

During a coast-to-coast flight to a scientific meeting, I was seated next to a pleasant 300+ pound passenger. I requested ice water, whereas he had a Diet Coke. Ironic, I thought. Consider the number of artificially sweetened beverages with "zero calories" that are now available—and yet, as a nation, we're getting fatter and fatter.

The latest figures show that approximately two thirds of all Americans are overweight or obese. This has created a major public health problem, because "excessive adiposity" is associated with several chronic diseases, including type 2 diabetes, heart disease, and metabolic syndrome.

What factors are responsible for the skyrocketing prevalence of obesity? According to one theory, our current high-tech milieu has increasingly emphasized comfort and convenience with the development of time-saving and labor-saving devices. In the current obesity-conducive environment, food has become readily accessible and, simultaneously, we have "engineered" physical activity out of our vocational and leisure-time pursuits. Interestingly, however, two widely publicized studies reported that other, seemingly innocuous factors, may be contributing to the spread of obesity.

Soft-drink consumption associated with chronic disease. Using the Framingham Heart Study database, researchers found that drinking more than one soft drink daily was associated with a higher risk of developing obesity and other risk factors for heart disease (*Circulation, July 2007*). Moreover, it didn't matter if the soda consumption was regular or diet!

The researchers speculated that middle-aged adults who regularly drink soda pop may tend to consume a greater number of calories as well as saturated and trans fat. They may also eat less fiber and have a more sedentary lifestyle. Previous studies also suggest that diet soda might induce a conditioning response in which the soft drink promotes a dietary preference for sweeter foods.

Spread of obesity in friends and family. Using the same Framingham Heart Study database, different researchers examined whether weight gain in one person was associated with weight gain in his or her friends, siblings, spouse, and neighbors. Interestingly, a person's chances of becoming obese increased markedly if he or she had a friend or family member who became obese in a given interval (*New England Journal of Medicine, July 2007*). Persons of the same sex had relatively greater influence on each other than those of the opposite sex. The investigators concluded that the spread of obesity in social networks appears to be a factor in the obesity epidemic.

Collectively, these reports suggest that consuming more than one soft drink daily, even sodas with "zero calories," is associated with increased health risks. Although obesity appears to spread through social ties, it may also be possible to harness the same forces to improve health outcomes. For example, health improvements in one person might spread to others. Thus, thin and/or physically fit friends and family, who refrain from regular soft-drink consumption, are "in."

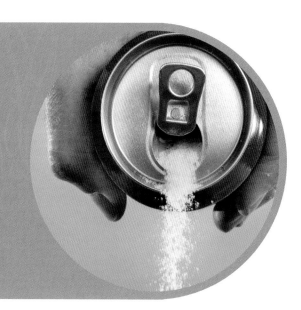

SUGAR-SWEETENED BEVERAGES AND RISK OF DEVELOPING TYPE 2 DIABETES

In an analysis of more than 25,000 residents without diabetes at baseline, regular consumption of sugar-sweetened beverages was associated with a higher risk of developing type 2 diabetes during an 11-year follow-up, even after adjusting for confounding variables, including body fatness. These findings suggest that reducing consumption of sugar-sweetened beverages, and promoting drinking water and unsweetened tea or coffee as alternatives may help curb the escalating diabetes epidemic.

(*Diabetologia,* July 2015)

DASH to a Healthier Heart and Weight

Silvia Veri, RD

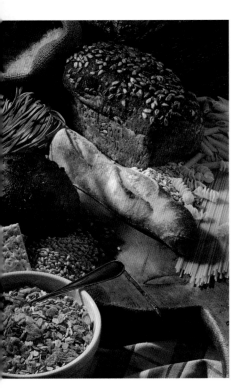

The million dollar question: Which diet is best for your heart, helps you to lose weight and maintain a healthy weight? Is it the low fat diet, low carb or one of the commercial diet plans? The role of a person's genetic makeup, the microbes in their gut, sleep patterns and more, may influence the answers to these questions. For right now, however, no one has found the magic bullet. Until we learn more, the DASH diet is heart protective and may promote weight loss.

DASH stands for *Dietary Approaches to Stop Hypertension*. It is a flexible and balanced eating plan that is based on research studies sponsored by the National Heart, Lung, and Blood Institute. These studies showed that DASH lowers high blood pressure and improves levels of blood lipids (fats in the bloodstream), which reduce the risk of developing cardiovascular disease. And, while the DASH diet is not a weight-loss program, you may indeed lose unwanted pounds, because it can help guide you toward healthier meals and snacks.

The DASH diet breakdown for a 2000 calorie diet is listed below. The number of servings can be adjusted to meet your calorie needs.

Food Group	Servings per Day	What a Serving Size Equals
Grains	6-8	1 slice whole-wheat bread, 1 ounce (oz.) dry cereal, or ½ cup cooked cereal, rice or pasta
Vegetables	4-5	1 cup raw leafy green vegetables or ½ cup cut-up raw or cooked vegetables
Fruit	4-5	1 medium fruit or ½ cup fresh, frozen or canned fruit or 4 ounces of juice
Low-fat or fat-free dairy	2-3	1 cup skim or 1 percent milk, 1 cup yogurt, or 1 ½ oz. cheese
Lean meat, poultry, & fish	6 or less	1 oz. cooked skinless poultry, seafood or lean meat or 1 egg
Nuts, seeds, or legumes	4-5 per week	⅓ cup (1 ½ oz.) nuts, 2 tablespoons seeds, or ½ cup cooked beans or peas
Fats and oils	2-3	1 teaspoon vegetable oil, 1 tablespoon mayonnaise or 2 tablespoons salad dressing
Sweets	Less than 5 servings per week	1 tablespoon sugar

DASH diet tips:

- Include at least three whole grain foods each day. Whole grains don't have fewer calories than refined grains, but they have more nutrients and fiber. The fiber makes the food more filling and satisfying. Although a serving of pasta is ½ cup, recognize that restaurants typically serve three to four cups of spaghetti.

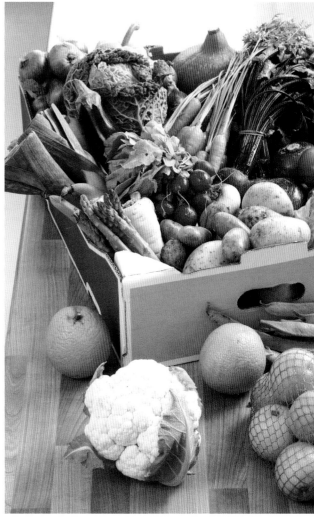

- With vegetables and fruit, variety is key. Different colors offer an assortment of vitamins, minerals, and phytochemicals including potassium. Potassium has been shown to lower blood pressure and reduce stroke by 30 percent. The National Academy of Medicine recommends 4700 mg potassium per day and a ½ cup of cooked spinach and one banana both have 420 mg of potassium. Keep your vegetables interesting by trying new raw veggies such as mini peppers, mini cucumbers, and sugar snap peas. Consider roasting broccoli, cauliflower, and Brussels sprouts. Add fruits and vegetables to your smoothies. And, eat fruit to curb your sweet cravings.

- Studies have shown that legumes, such as kidney and pinto beans, can lower LDL cholesterol. Consider having a vegetarian meal at least once per week. Add beans to a side dish, soup, salad or main dish. Make chili with lean meat and beans, bean burritos/tacos and bean dip. Go to www.meatlessmonday.com for additional recipe ideas.

- Nuts and seeds are a great source of magnesium. Higher magnesium intakes are associated with a lower incidence of type 2 diabetes and lower risk of stroke and heart disease. Women should aim for 320 mg of magnesium per day and men 420 mg. You can add nuts or seeds to your morning oatmeal, on a salad, or simply eat a serving for a snack. A ¼ cup of cashews and almonds have 90 to 95 mg of magnesium.

- Fruits, vegetables, whole grains and legumes all have FIBER in common. The American Heart Association recommends 25 to 35 grams of fiber per day. If we focus on this, we will naturally be eating healthier, and there won't be room for processed foods that are high in sugar, salt and fat.

We often hear what we need to cut out of our diet for a healthier heart and weight. It is encouraging to know that there are several foods and nutrients that we can add to our diet to help us reach our health goals.

Mediterranean Diet: An Easy and Flavorful Approach to Healthy Eating

Steven B.H. Timmis, M.D.

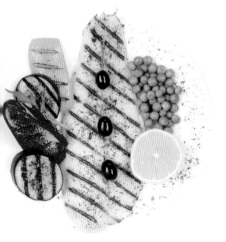

The word diet can make a person cringe. It harbors thoughts of measuring, counting, craving and sacrifice. Whether eating for better health or a thinner waist, diets are often faddish and unrealistic, with no real long-term hope for adherence or success. Imagine a diet that is easy to follow, flavorful and proven to improve health. Think of a diet that can be shared with a spouse, served to company and enjoyed by the whole family.

People along the coast of the Mediterranean Sea, from the shores of Spain to the seaboard of Greece, have enjoyed the benefits of healthy eating for centuries. Their Mediterranean diet has now garnered the intense interest of physicians and medical researchers, having shown in a number of well-conducted clinical studies to successfully reduce weight, cholesterol levels and cardiac risk. It has also been shown to lower the incidence of diabetes, cancer, Alzheimer's and Parkinson's disease.

The Mediterranean diet is not something you "go on" or "do." It is a long-term, preferably life-long, approach to eating. The Mediterranean diet is centered on eating foods that are fresh and unprocessed. It is rich in colored vegetables and fresh fruits. Nuts and legumes, such as beans and lentils, are prominently featured in this diet. Fish and lean meats replace steaks, burgers and fatty chicken. It includes whole grain breads and pastas. Extra-virgin olive oil richly enhances the many foods in this diet. A glass of red wine is another highlight. Absent from the Mediterranean diet are packaged and processed foods. Simple sugars, sweets and soda-pop are discouraged. Greasy and fatty foods are also avoided.

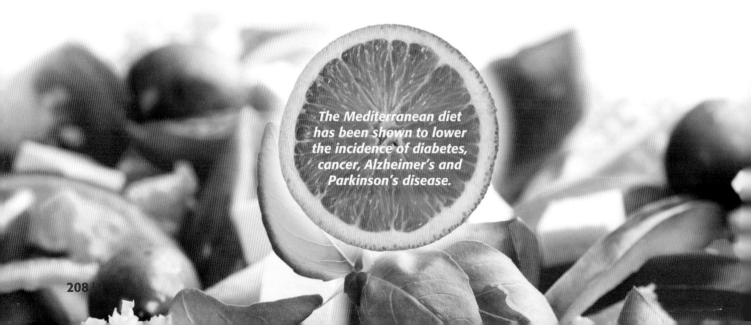

The Mediterranean diet has been shown to lower the incidence of diabetes, cancer, Alzheimer's and Parkinson's disease.

There are many reasons why the Mediterranean diet improves health and controls weight. The foods are rich in fiber, vitamins, minerals and essential nutrients. It is a practical diet, with foods that are available in any grocery store. The diet is not based on starvation and sacrifice. Rather, it focuses on smart and healthy food choices. Best of all, the Mediterranean diet is satisfying and tastes great. A diet works best when it is followed. The greatest advantage to the Mediterranean diet is not that it is easy to endure, but that it is craved and desired. It looks like you can have your baklava (but just a little) and eat it too!

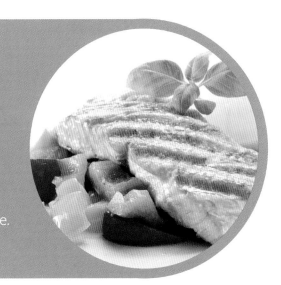

PREVENTION OF HEART DISEASE WITH A MEDITERRANEAN DIET

According to a widely-cited report, among persons at high cardiovascular risk, but with no cardiovascular disease at enrollment, a Mediterranean diet supplemented with extra-virgin olive oil or nuts reduced the incidence of major cardiovascular events by approximately 30 percent, as compared with a control group (advice to simply reduce dietary fat). These results support the benefits of the Mediterranean diet for the primary prevention of heart disease.

(*New England Journal of Medicine,* Feb. 2013)

How to Incorporate Plant-Based Nutrition Into Your Lifestyle

Megan Bowdon, B.S.

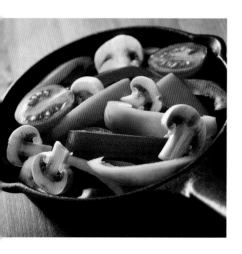

Heart disease is the number one killer of both American men and women. Although lifestyle clearly plays a role, unhealthy dietary habits in particular have been linked to the development of heart disease and the risk factors for it, including obesity, hypertension, hypercholesterolemia and diabetes (*The Permanente Journal,* Spring 2013). A diet loaded with excess calories, trans fats, saturated fats and processed foods is associated with an increased risk of developing these diseases. Remember the saying, "You are what you eat."

Moving towards a plant-based diet is a key intervention to prevent heart disease. According to the EPIC-Oxford cohort study (*American Journal of Clinical Nutrition,* March 2013), British vegetarians had a 32 percent lower risk of heart disease than did their non-vegetarian counterparts. Plant-based foods have been shown to decrease body mass index, waist circumference, blood pressure, total cholesterol and hemoglobin A1c (a key indicator of glucose metabolism and diabetes mellitus). Studies show plant-based nutrition leads to a longer lifespan, less chronic illness, a lower risk of cancer, decreased risk of cardiovascular disease and fewer bodily aches and pains (*Journal of the American Medical Association,* Dec. 1998).

Contemporary recommendations for lowering risk factors for heart disease invariably include increasing fruit and vegetable intake, while simultaneously decreasing processed and unprocessed meats and prepared foods.

Whether you're considering a pure plant-based diet or would simply like to add a few healthier meals per week, here are 10 tips to ease the transition:

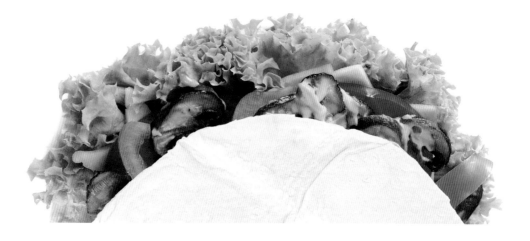

❏ State of mind

Before you can successfully adopt a lifestyle change, you must first be ready to make it. Start thinking about trying plant-based eating, and then begin your planning. Don't rush into major dietary changes. If you don't properly prepare yourself with the "principles and pluses" of plant-based eating, you'll likely fail. Prepare yourself with recipes and small changes in the kitchen. You can even order a complimentary vegetarian starter kit from www.pcrm.org before you start your journey.

❏ Clean out the pantry

If you have a kitchen full of unhealthy foods, you'll end up eating them. Get rid of the "garbage" foods in your pantry. If they're unopened, donate them to a local charity. Once you've done this, start buying healthier foods.

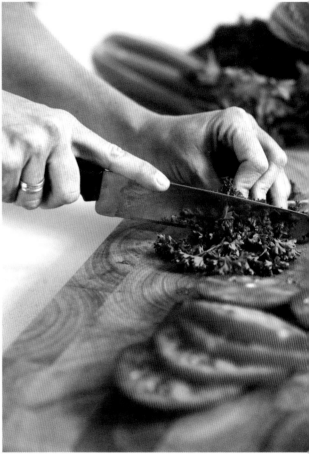

❏ Modify favorite recipes

This is an easy way to get started with plant-based eating. Love tacos? Next time, sauté onions, peppers and mushrooms, then add black beans and spices for your taco "meat." Love burgers? Marinate large Portobello mushrooms, grill and top with your favorite burger toppings. Chili? Load up on veggies, instead of meat. Veggies are equally delicious when done right and no one will miss the meat.

❏ Identify plant-based dishes you already enjoy

Regularly eat vegetarian meals you already enjoy, such as sushi, vegetable stir fry, minestrone soup, tomato soup, grilled cheese and pasta primavera.

❏ Meal plan

Plan your meals for the week—breakfast, lunch and dinner. Make a grocery list and stick to it. Using this approach, you'll have fewer excuses to deviate from your healthier, new meal plan.

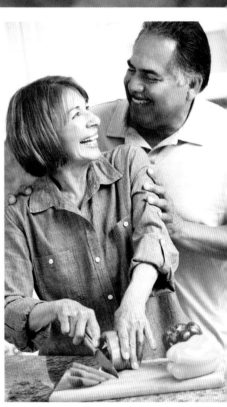

❏ Prep day

Set aside time, one day each week, to prepare your meals. Wash your fruits and vegetables. Cook rice or quinoa. Chop a large salad so it's ready when you are. Portion your snacks into snack bags. Preparing foods so they're ready to go will make you more likely to eat those foods.

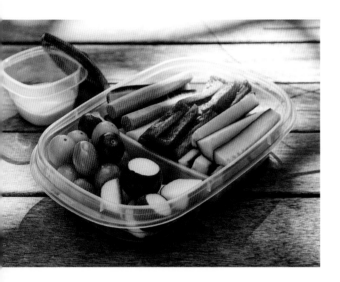

❑ Healthy 'last-minute' meals

With our busy schedules, have some immediately available meals planned for when you don't have time to cook. Here are some examples:

- Breakfast: Green smoothies, oatmeal topped with fresh fruit and nuts, whole wheat toast with peanut butter, egg sandwich.
- Lunch: Salad, left overs, Mediterranean pita, black bean wrap with veggies.
- Dinner: Vegetable stir fry, grilled veggie pasta, veggie fried rice, Portobello burgers, breakfast for dinner.
- Frozen meals are also available. However, look at the labels first. Choose the healthiest options (e.g., lowest sodium, non-genetically modified organisms, organic).

❑ Healthy snacks

Healthy snacks will keep you full throughout the day, helping reduce sugar crashes when you feel lethargic and tired. Ditch the chips, pop, ice cream and unhealthy crackers. Reach for vegetables and hummus, apple and peanut butter, a green smoothie, a handful of nuts, or fresh fruits.

❑ Try something new

When dining out, try a vegetarian meal or split two meals with a friend or spouse. Order stir fry without meat or add tofu (Don't be afraid of tofu, especially at a restaurant, because they've mastered it!). Start expanding your palate.

❑ Reach out for support

Communicate with your family and friends about your plan to eat healthier and explain the rationale behind your decision. If they're aware of your goal, they will likely be more supportive. Join an online plant-based community. You can sign up for newsletters with tips and recipes.

Whether you're looking to lose weight, reduce blood cholesterol or just add healthier foods into your lifestyle, these tips can help get you started. Take action. Start with one tip, master it, and then move to the next suggestion.

Coffee Consumption and Heart Disease: Ally or Adversary?

Barry A. Franklin, Ph.D.

Coffee is the most widely consumed beverage worldwide, second only to water. In fact, coffee is consumed by 83 percent of all U.S. adults. Despite its popularity, there has been a longstanding controversy regarding the association of coffee consumption with an increased incidence of cardiovascular disease, including the potential for triggering heart attacks.

More than a decade ago, researchers in Costa Rica examined the risk of experiencing a heart attack within one hour after drinking coffee (*Epidemiology,* Sept. 2006). The study population was relatively small, including approximately 500 incident cases. The relative risk of experiencing a heart attack soon after coffee ingestion increased slightly, as compared with other times throughout the day, especially among people with infrequent intakes of coffee (less than or equal to one cup per day), habitually sedentary individuals, or those with three or more risk factors for heart disease. The researchers concluded that in such individuals, coffee could transiently increase sympathetic nervous system activity, causing a heart attack.

Fortunately, the concerns raised by earlier studies like this one have been largely discounted by numerous major studies in recent years, unequivocally demonstrating that coffee consumption is not associated with an increased incidence of cardiovascular disease, and that it may actually have cardioprotective effects. A landmark study of more than 400,000 subjects showed a beneficial association of regular coffee consumption on all-cause and cardiovascular mortality after a 13 year follow-up (*New England Journal of Medicine,* May 2012). Another analysis of 36 different studies showed that moderate coffee consumption was associated with a decreased risk of cardiovascular disease, with the lowest risk among those consuming three to five cups per day (*Circulation,* Feb. 2014).

In a large sample of Korean men and women who were free of clinically evident cardiovascular disease, investigators reported that coffee consumption was associated with a lower prevalence of coronary artery calcium, a marker of early or subclinical coronary atherosclerosis (*Heart,* March 2015). Interestingly, participants drinking between three and five cups per day had the lowest coronary artery calcium scores.

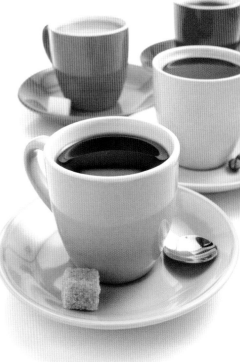

Collectively, these studies and other reports (*Circulation,* May 2006) indicate that drinking coffee in reasonable amounts is safe and does not increase blood pressure or the incidence of cardiovascular disease, stroke, and all-cause mortality. However, some studies have suggested that the potential cardiovascular dangers of coffee consumption, if any, were at the extremes, with the highest risk being in low coffee drinkers (zero to one cup per day) and high coffee drinkers (greater than or equal to 10 cups per day). It is what clinicians refer to as a U-shaped association, where it is preferable (and likely safer) to be in the middle of the distribution. In other words, it appears that the safest coffee consumption is in the three to five cups per day range, which probably represents the majority of coffee drinkers.

In summary, coffee consumption in reasonable amounts appears to be safe and is associated with more favorable health outcomes. Its apparent cardioprotective benefits may include antihypertensive effects, antioxidant actions, improved insulin sensitivity, reduced low density lipoprotein oxidation, and decreased risk of type 2 diabetes. Perhaps a recent analysis (*American Journal of Cardiology,* Sept. 2015) pertaining to coffee consumption and cardiovascular health summed it up best: "There is no reason for people to refrain from coffee drinking whether they are healthy or have preexisting high blood pressure or cardiovascular disease." When it comes to heart disease prevention, it appears that coffee is largely viewed as an ally, rather than an adversary.

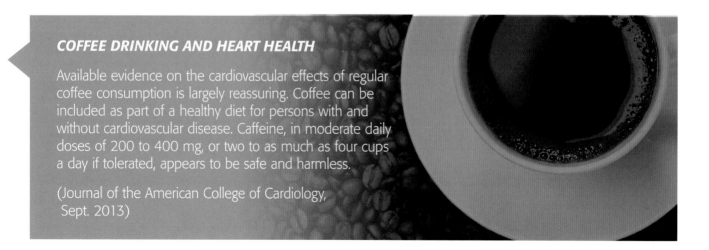

COFFEE DRINKING AND HEART HEALTH

Available evidence on the cardiovascular effects of regular coffee consumption is largely reassuring. Coffee can be included as part of a healthy diet for persons with and without cardiovascular disease. Caffeine, in moderate daily doses of 200 to 400 mg, or two to as much as four cups a day if tolerated, appears to be safe and harmless.

(Journal of the American College of Cardiology, Sept. 2013)

Alcohol and Heart Disease: To Drink or Not to Drink?

Rachel Sumner, MPH, RD

Many studies report a possible cardioprotective benefit of consuming alcohol regularly. However, one should consider the benefits and the risks of drinking alcohol. The American Heart Association recommends that if you drink alcohol, do so in moderation. Moderation is defined as up to two drinks per day for men and one drink a day for women; a drink is four ounces of wine, 1.5 ounces of 80-proof spirits, 12 ounces of beer or one ounce of 100-proof spirits.

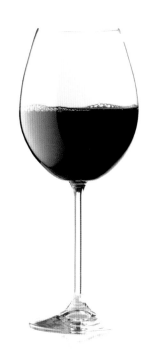

Several studies have investigated the potential cardiovascular benefits of alcohol consumption. One investigation reported that alcohol has a transient anti-clotting effect on the bloodstream (*American Journal of Cardiology,* June 2000). Another trial showed that alcohol consumption increased HDL ("good") cholesterol (*American Heart Journal*, March 2004). The beneficial effects of wine consumption in these studies was most likely due to resveratrol, an antioxidant that is found in red grapes. Nevertheless, the American Heart Association does not recommend that individuals begin drinking alcohol as a treatment strategy. A better option is to begin a regular exercise program under a doctor's supervision and to eat a diet rich in fruits, vegetables and low in saturated fats. Such lifestyle changes may serve to decrease the stickiness of the blood and increase HDL.

Alcohol consumption may also have a negative impact on one's health. In a study of 248 subjects who consumed alcohol, there was an associated increase in systolic blood pressure that was more pronounced in women (*American Journal of Hypertension,* Feb. 2006). Also, alcohol can add unwanted calories to your diet, making it difficult to achieve or maintain an ideal body weight. Eating or drinking too many calories can lead to a greater risk of obesity. For example, examine the calorie content of just one serving of these alcoholic beverages:

- 12 ounces beer = 153 calories
- 12 ounces lite beer = 103 calories
- five ounces wine (red) = 125 calories
- five ounces wine (white) = 121 calories
- 1.5 ounces liquor (80 proof or 40% alcohol) = 97 calories

Alcohol can also increase triglycerides as well as the likelihood of developing metabolic syndrome (*Tufts University Health & Nutrition Letter,* July 1997 and March 2005). When alcohol is consumed, the liver preferentially removes it from the bloodstream.

If alcohol is consumed frequently and in excess, insulin levels can be quickly depleted, resulting in an elevated blood sugar. Over time, the excessive and frequent use of alcohol may lead to an increased risk of liver disease as well as glucose intolerance.

To attain a healthier lifestyle, it is crucial to use the following guidelines. Never drink on an empty stomach. Moreover, never drink alcohol to satisfy your thirst and drink only in moderation. Finally, if you don't drink, don't start. Your doctor is the best resource on the benefits and risks of consuming alcohol and how it influences to your health.

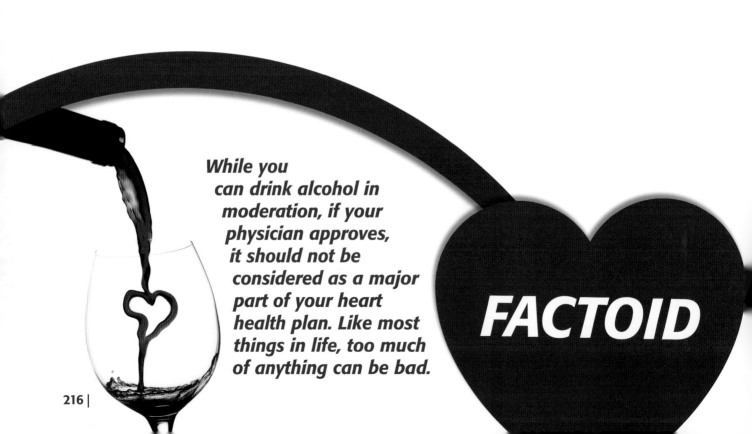

While you can drink alcohol in moderation, if your physician approves, it should not be considered as a major part of your heart health plan. Like most things in life, too much of anything can be bad.

FACTOID

Shedding Some Light on Vitamin D

Anne Davis, RN

Vitamin D has gained a lot of attention over the last few years. In 2010, the Food and Drug Administration, or FDA, increased the previous recommended daily allowances, known as RDA, of vitamin D. Recognize that the FDA does not make changes like this without considerable research and evidence. Is vitamin D the "wonder vitamin" of the decade? Let's look at some of the facts.

Vitamin D is a fat-soluble vitamin that can be stored in the body. It's most well known function is to support calcium absorption to aid in building strong bones. This was discovered in the early 1900s when rickets was a major epidemic in children. Why the recent hype? Adding vitamin D levels to routine blood chemistry studies has created a huge database of information, which scientists have now used to link low levels of this vitamin with many chronic diseases and medical conditions, including heart disease, asthma, depression and some cancers. The cardioprotective benefits of vitamin D may be related to reduced levels of inflammatory markers, like C-reactive protein (*American Journal of Cardiology,* Jan. 2012).

Natural sources of vitamin D are limited. The sun's ultraviolet or UVB rays enable our skin to make vitamin D. Moreover, fatty fish, such as salmon, tuna or mackerel are the best natural food sources. Orange juice, milk, some cereals and eggs are also fortified with vitamin D, but require four to six servings of each to meet minimal RDA requirements.

Several factors potentially increase our risk of vitamin D deficiency. Our geographical location is key. At least six months of the year, the sun's UVB rays, in latitudes north of Atlanta, Georgia, are not strong enough for vitamin D synthesis. As we age, our body is less able to convert the sun's UVB rays to vitamin D and while sunshine is truly our best option, most physicians prefer we limit our sun exposure, due to the increased risk of skin cancer. Adequate dietary intake of vitamin D is also challenging, due to the limited number of natural and fortified food options. Some people are more susceptible to vitamin D deficiency, including individuals with darker skin pigments, obesity, liver and kidney disease. Certain

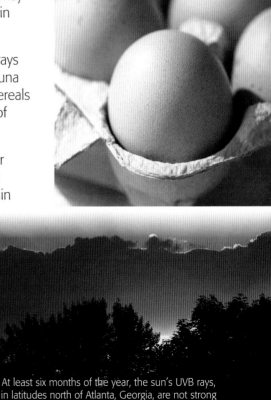

At least six months of the year, the sun's UVB rays, in latitudes north of Atlanta, Georgia, are not strong enough for vitamin D synthesis.

medications, such as steroids, dilantin, phenobarb and some cholesterol lowering drugs, also increase the risk of vitamin D deficiency.

Obviously, dietary and natural sources are preferred, but if the sun isn't a consistent or recommended source and our dietary options are limited, what is our next best option? For some people, a dietary supplement may be recommended. It is always best to check with your primary care physician, when considering any dietary supplement. A simple blood test can be done to determine your level of serum 25(OH)D or vitamin D. The following table lists the National Institute of Health's recommendations for vitamin D or 25(OH)D levels and provides a good starting point in gauging your need for supplementation.

nmol/L or ng/mL		Health Status
< 30	< 12	Associated with vitamin D deficiency, leading to rickets in infants and children and osteomalacia in adults
30 - 50	12 - 20	Generally considered inadequate for bone and overall health in healthy individuals
≥ 50	≥ 20	Generally considered adequate for bone and overall health in healthy individuals
> 125	> 50	Emerging evidence links potential adverse effects to such high levels, particularly > 150 nmol/L *or* > 60 ng/mL

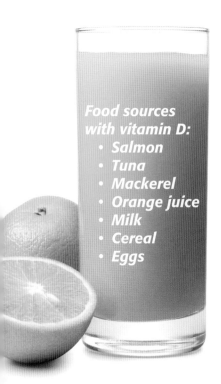

Food sources with vitamin D:
- **Salmon**
- **Tuna**
- **Mackerel**
- **Orange juice**
- **Milk**
- **Cereal**
- **Eggs**

If your levels are less than 50 nmol/L or 20 ng/mL, a supplement will probably be recommended. There are a few options. Cod liver oil provides 1360 international units (IU) per tablespoon and also comes in capsule form. This is the most natural supplement and also provides beneficial omega 3 fatty acids. Vitamin D3 (cholecalciferol) or vitamin D2 (ergocalciferol) come in tablet form and appear to be equally effective in raising serum vitamin D levels. Most multivitamins contain 400 IU of vitamin D. Because it is fat soluble, caution must be taken to avoid toxicity. Excessive sun exposure and food intake are highly unlikely to create toxic levels; however, inordinate amounts of vitamins D3 or D2 could be problematic. The threshold for vitamin D toxicity is high. The Institute of Medicine recommends a tolerable upper limit of 2500 IU per day for ages 1 to 3 years, 3000 IU per day for ages 4 to 8 years and 4000 IU per day for ages 9 to 71+ years.

Talk to your physician about assessing your serum vitamin D level, and then decide on a treatment plan together. By correcting vitamin D deficiency, improved cardiovascular health outcomes may occur. If you 'toast' to that objective, make it orange juice or vitamin D fortified skim milk.

Are My Calcium Supplements Putting Me at Risk for Heart Disease?

Dana Haddad, RN

Keeping bones strong throughout our lifespan is important to prevent osteoporosis, a condition in which bones become thin and are more prone to fracture as we age.

Research has shown that regular exercise, vitamin D and a diet rich in calcium are effective in preventing osteoporosis. However, many Americans find it difficult to get an adequate amount of calcium in their diet. Although doctors may recommend calcium supplements, the use of these supplements is now being questioned like others in the past. Why? Some studies have shown that calcium intake may increase the risks for heart disease and stroke in certain populations. These studies may leave you feeling unsure whether you should start or continue calcium supplementation.

Over the years, there has been confusion regarding the value of calcium supplements and their link to heart disease. One study (*British Medical Journal,* July 2012) reported that calcium supplements may increase the risk of heart disease, especially in women. The investigators suggested that the extra calcium may increase calcium levels in the bloodstream and, ultimately, in the arteries, increasing the likelihood of heart attack or stroke. However, this particular study tested calcium supplements alone, not with adjunctive vitamin D, which is normally recommended.

Another report involving the Women's Health Initiative (*American Journal of Clinical Nutrition,* Oct. 2011) noted that women taking 1,000 mg of supplemental calcium each day along with 400 IU of vitamin D showed no increased risk in cardiovascular events, including stroke and/or heart attack.

So now what? According to the American Heart Association, "calcium/ vitamin D supplementation neither increased nor decreased coronary or cerebrovascular risk in generally healthy postmenopausal women over a 7-year use period" (*Circulation,* Dec. 2007). The best way to get your intake of calcium is through foods; however, if you aren't able to do so, then

The best way to get your intake of calcium is through foods; however, if you aren't able to do so, then supplementation may be advised.

supplementation may be advised. Nevertheless, before throwing out all of your calcium supplements, talk with your cardiologist and/or primary care physician and follow their recommendations.

Always consult with your physician before starting and/or discontinuing any nutritional supplements pertaining to your daily health regimen. Following the guidelines for calcium supplementation (under the supervision of your doctor) coupled with regular exercise, heart healthy eating, and adherence to prescribed medications are especially important in preventing osteoporosis and cardiovascular disease.

THE NINE UNHEALTHIEST FOODS YOU CAN ORDER

When ordering a dinner entrée at a restaurant, few expect the waiter to return with a plate that exceeds their daily caloric requirement—or enough salt to meet their maximum daily intake for three days! Yet, according to a scathing report, "Xtreme Eating 2009," released by the nutrition and advocacy organization Center for Science in the Public Interest, there are an escalating number of choices right now that make it harder for Americans to eat well and watch their weight. Some of the unhealthiest foods you can order include: The Olive Garden: Tour of Italy; Chili's Big Mouth Bites; The Cheesecake Factory Fried Macaroni and Cheese; Red Lobster Ultimate Fondue; Chili's Half Rack of Baby Back Ribs; Uno Chicago Grill Mega-Sized Deep Dish Sundae; The Cheesecake Factory Chicken and Biscuits; Applebee's Quesadilla Burger; and, The Cheesecake Factory Philly Style Flat Iron Steak.

Daily Multivitamin Use May Not Reduce Cardiovascular Disease Risk in Men

Jenna M. Holzhausen, PharmD, BCPS

Multivitamins are currently the most common dietary supplement taken by U.S. adults, with 39 percent of Americans reporting multivitamin use between 2003 and 2006, an increase from 30 percent utilization between 1988 and 1994. The consumption of vitamins, minerals and/or herbs is commonly intended to promote adequate nutritional intake while preventing or correcting nutritional deficiencies. Several potential benefits to multivitamin use have been suggested, including reduction in cancer rates, infections, incidence of cataracts and risk of cardiovascular disease. Despite annual multivitamin sales in the billions, few data are available regarding the associated health benefits. A widely cited study (*Journal of the American Medical Association,* Nov. 2012), summarized below, suggested that there is no cardioprotective benefit from multivitamin use—at least, not in men.

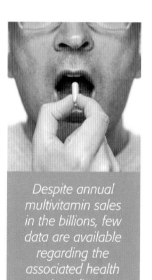

Despite annual multivitamin sales in the billions, few data are available regarding the associated health benefits.

The Physicians' Health Study II was conducted from 1997 to 2011 and enrolled almost 15,000 U.S. male physicians aged 50 years or older. Subjects were randomly assigned to receive a daily multivitamin or placebo and were followed for an average of 11.2 years, making it the first long-term study to examine the impact of multivitamin use on the incidence of chronic disease. The study demonstrated no significant cardiovascular benefit for men taking a daily multivitamin compared with those taking a placebo. There was no reduction in heart attack incidence, stroke, cardiovascular death or death from any cause with multivitamin use.

Additionally, no reductions in chest pain, heart failure or coronary revascularization rates were noted. Because only middle-aged and elderly (mostly Caucasian) men were included and only one multivitamin formulation was examined, it remains unclear whether these findings may be generalized to younger men, women and other ethnic groups. The investigators also suggested that physicians may lead healthier lifestyles than the average person, thereby decreasing the potential benefit of multivitamin supplementation.

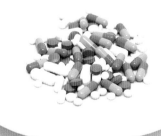

Despite the unremarkable results in preventing cardiovascular disease, there may be beneficial effects related to multivitamin use in specific patient populations. For example, the same study reported that daily multivitamin use was associated with an 8 percent reduced risk of cancer, although cancer-related deaths were not decreased. When asked about the differing results, Dr. Howard Sesso, the lead author and associate epidemiologist at Brigham and Women's Hospital, explained "The lack of effect for cardiovascular disease versus cancer benefit isn't necessarily inconsistent. There could be a difference in mechanism of effect."

Although multivitamins are associated with few adverse side effects (increased incidence of skin rashes and nose bleeds were reported in the trial), their use may discourage some people from engaging in other preventative health behaviors by providing a false sense of security. It is important to emphasize that the development of cardiovascular disease is known to be largely preventable through diet, exercise, smoking cessation and prescribed medications (if appropriate). Discuss with your doctor whether or not a multivitamin is right for you, but don't forget to also implement lifestyle modifications that have been proven to reduce the risk of cardiovascular disease.

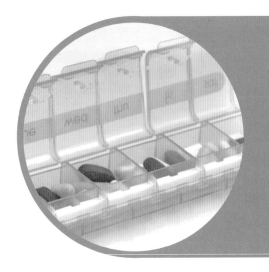

INEFFECTIVENESS OF MULTIVITAMIN SUPPLEMENTATION AFTER MYOCARDIAL INFARCTION

A widely-cited study examined the effectiveness of multivitamin supplementation in 1,708 heart attack survivors greater than 50 years of age. Patients were assigned to a high-dose multivitamin (six capsules daily) or to a look-alike placebo. Average follow-up was 55 months. The primary end point, death, was not significantly different in patients taking the multivitamin versus those in the placebo group.

(*Annals of Internal Medicine*, Dec. 2013)

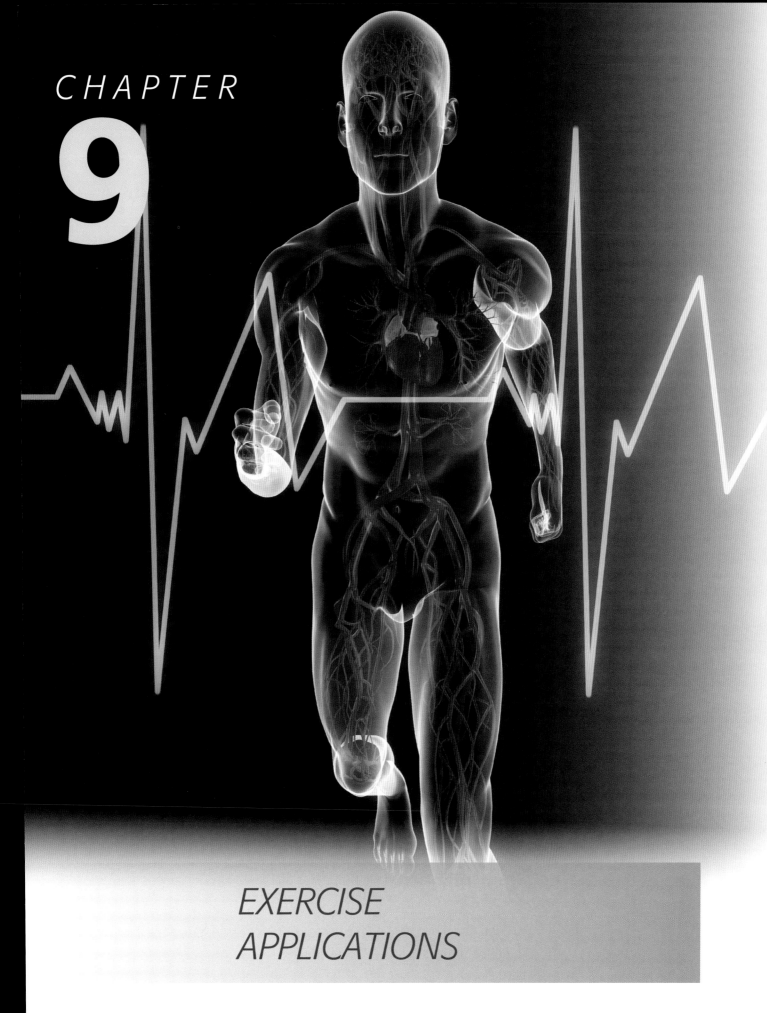

CHAPTER

9

EXERCISE
APPLICATIONS

Maintaining a Safe Distance From the Grim Reaper

Barry A. Franklin, Ph.D.

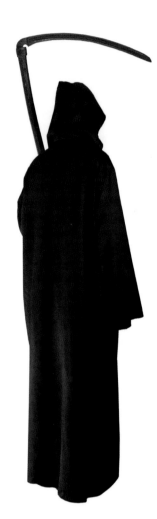

Walking speed is a commonly used objective measure of functional capacity or exercise tolerance in older adults, predicting survival in several studies (*Journal of the American Geriatric Society,* Oct. 2005; Sept. 2008; Feb. 2009). One widely-cited analysis found that being in the lowest quartile (bottom 25 percent) of walking speed compared with the highest quartile (top 25 percent) was associated with a three-fold increased risk of mortality (*Journal of the American Medical Association,* Jan. 2011). This finding was consistent across varied ethnic groups. Other reports, in persons with and without known heart disease, have also shown that walking speed and/or distance are powerful predictors of mortality (*American Journal of Cardiology,* May, 2008; *New England Journal of Medicine,* Jan. 1998; *Archives of Internal Medicine,* July 2012).

The Grim Reaper, the personification of death as a man or cloaked skeleton holding a scythe, is a well-known mythological and literary figure. Additional reported characteristics include a hooded black cloak and cachexia. Until recently, however, researchers had no idea of the ambulatory speed that may be synonymous with being 'caught' by the Grim Reaper, in other words, the walking pace that may be associated with a heightened mortality.

Data from the Concord Health and Ageing in Men Project, a cohort study of 1,705 men aged 70 and over living in several inner city suburbs in Sydney, Australia, were used to answer this question (*British Medical Journal,* Dec. 2011). At baseline, walking speed was carefully measured at the usual pace, documenting the fastest time from two trials. Follow-up averaged nearly six years. Using a sophisticated statistical model, the investigators determined the particular walking speeds that were most predictive of increased mortality and survival.

The findings were provocative– to say the least. A walking speed of 2 mph was most predictive of early mortality. Older men who walked at speeds greater than this were less likely to die during the follow-up. On the other hand, all men who initially walked at speeds of 3 mph or above were alive and well. These findings support the hypothesis that faster walking speeds appear to confer increased survival. The modest difference in walking speed associated with increased mortality (2 mph) and increased survival (3 mph) supports the notion that the primary beneficiaries of an exercise program are those at the bottom of the fitness/activity continuum.

Certainly, many variables beyond walking speed may be associated with early mortality and long-term survival. These include: age; severity of heart disease; coronary risk factors; the magnitude of heart damage after a cardiac event; associated co-morbid conditions (e.g., diabetes, hypertension); and adherence to prescribed cardiac medications. Although the mechanisms underlying the relationship between walking speed and mortality remain unclear, one explanation is that a slow walking speed may signify limited physical reserve and a decreased capacity to respond to stresses associated with aging and/or chronic disease. Another possible explanation is that a slow walking speed may serve as a surrogate marker for a high risk, inflammatory state, that may be less able to cope with major surgery or other potentially lifesaving medical interventions.

Over the years, exercise critics have rhetorically asked, "Fitness for what?!" Now, sobering new studies provide exercise enthusiasts with a compelling response: "Fit enough to stay at least a step ahead of the Grim Reaper."

FASTER WALK IN ELDERLY MAY PREDICT LONGER LIFESPAN

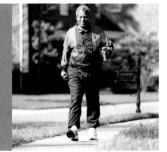

Older men who walk at a three-mile per hour or faster pace tend to outlive their counterparts who move along at slower speeds. The researchers suggest that older individuals who can pick up the walking pace are likely healthier and fitter than adults who move more slowly.

(*British Medical Journal,* Dec. 2011)

Survival of the Fittest

Barry A. Franklin, Ph.D.

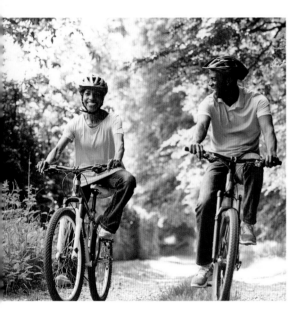

Doctors have known for a long time that regular physical activity plays an important role in promoting cardiovascular health. But new studies indicate that having a high aerobic fitness (or capacity) reduces one's risk of heart disease, and the reduction is greater than that obtained merely by being physically active.

New findings: Aerobic *fitness*, not merely *physical activity*, greatly reduces the risk of stroke and heart attack. A measure of aerobic fitness, called METs (metabolic equivalents), appears to be one of the most powerful predictors of cardiovascular health and longevity.

Understanding METs

One MET equals the amount of oxygen your body uses when resting. Walking at a leisurely pace uses about 2 to 3 METs. Singles tennis requires 6 to 7 METs. Jogging requires 8 to 10 or more METs, depending on the speed.

The average healthy young to middle-aged adult has an aerobic capacity of 8 to 12 METs. Heart failure patients and those who are elderly or morbidly obese could be as low as 3 to 4. On the other hand, elite endurance athletes such as Michael Phelps are usually in the range of 20 to 25 METs.

New studies indicate that for each MET increase in aerobic fitness, patients can reduce their chances of dying from a heart attack by approximately 15 percent. Thus, an inactive person who increases his/her MET capacity from 5 to 8 or 9 could reduce the risk of dying from heart disease by 45 percent to 60 percent.

High risk and cardioprotective fitness levels

Persons with high MET capacities generally live longer and have a lower risk of heart disease than those with lower levels. The Aerobics Center Longitudinal Study (ACLS), based in Dallas, Texas, represents the most comprehensive database to date regarding fitness and mortality. The tables for men and women illustrate low, moderate, and high fitness levels, expressed as METs, as a function of age.

The "low fitness" groups are at increased mortality risk (i.e., 2 to 3 fold), "moderate fit" groups are at average risk, and "high fit" groups are at lowest risk, regardless of existing medical conditions or underlying heart disease.

For example, a 55-year-old man with a 9.5 MET capacity would be considered in the moderate or average fitness category. A goal for him would be to achieve "high fitness" or greater than 10.9 METs. The 64-year-old woman with a 4.0 MET capacity would be classified in the "low fit category," which is associated with an increased mortality rate. An initial goal for her would be to increase her fitness to the moderate category (5.7-7.5), and higher (>7.5 METs), if possible, in the future.

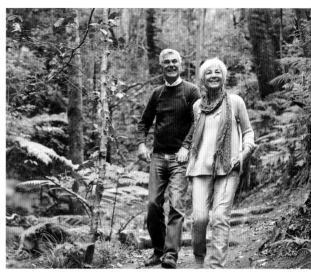

Determining your MET capacity

A treadmill test is the best way to accurately assess your MET capacity. Some patients with suspected or known heart disease get these tests routinely. Others may have a treadmill exercise test as part of their comprehensive annual physical examination.

If you undergo a treadmill stress test, ask your test supervisor (or your physician) to report on your MET capacity, along with such standard measures as heart rhythm and blood pressure responses.

Fitness and Mortality in Men, ACLS, Fitness Categories				
Fitness Group	Age Groups (years)			
	20-39	40-49	50-59	60+
LOW	≤ 10.5	≤ 9.9	≤ 8.8	≤ 7.5
MODERATE	10.6-12.7	10.0-12.1	8.9-10.9	7.6-9.7
HIGH	> 12.7	> 12.1	> 10.9	> 9.7
Table values are maximal METs attained during the exercise test				

Fitness and Mortality in Women, ACLS, Fitness Categories				
Fitness Group	Age Groups (years)			
	20-39	40-49	50-59	60+
LOW	≤ 8.1	≤ 7.5	≤ 6.5	≤ 5.7
MODERATE	8.2-10.5	7.6-9.5	6.6-8.3	5.7-7.5
HIGH	> 10.5	> 9.5	> 8.3	> 7.5
Table values are maximal METs attained during the exercise test				

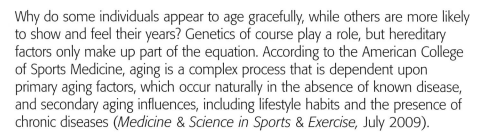

Exercise: The Antidote to Aging?

Cindy Haskin-Popp, M.S.

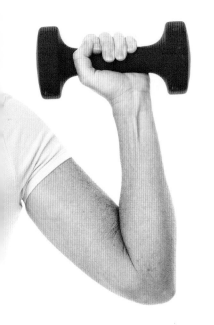

Why do some individuals appear to age gracefully, while others are more likely to show and feel their years? Genetics of course play a role, but hereditary factors only make up part of the equation. According to the American College of Sports Medicine, aging is a complex process that is dependent upon primary aging factors, which occur naturally in the absence of known disease, and secondary aging influences, including lifestyle habits and the presence of chronic diseases (*Medicine & Science in Sports & Exercise,* July 2009).

The body's physiological systems are inevitably affected by changes related to normal aging, but the extent to which deterioration occurs is, in part, related to the older adult's physical activity level. Common ailments that have been traditionally associated with aging, such as an increased prevalence of chronic diseases, decreased stamina, reduced muscular strength and endurance, loss of balance, increased risk for falls and bone fractures, cognitive dysfunction and loss of independent living are partially attributed to physical inactivity and disuse. Regular exercise can prevent, manage and largely reverse these effects, thereby improving the older adult's mental and physical function while maintaining his or her independence. According to the President's Council on Fitness, Sports & Nutrition, the most important components of fitness associated with healthy aging in older adults include muscular strength and endurance, aerobic endurance, flexibility and balance (*Research Digest,* June 2010).

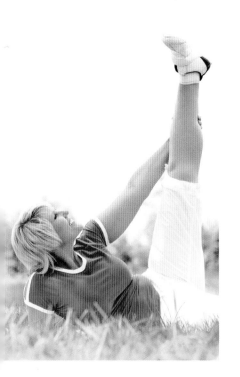

Strength training is particularly beneficial for older adults because of its role in increasing muscle mass, strengthening muscles and bones, improving balance, decreasing the risk for falls and bone fractures, mitigating the discomfort associated with arthritis and favorably modifying body weight and fat stores. Research has shown that resistance-based exercises can reverse the aging process by changing the gene expression of the mitochondria, the "powerhouses" of the muscle cells, to resemble the genetic profiles of younger people (*PLoS ONE,* May 2007). Fortunately, strength training benefits for the older adult can be achieved by a modest time commitment. Participating in resistance-based exercises that work the major muscle groups of the body (one set of 8 to 12 repetitions per exercise) on at least two days a week can enhance functional independence in older adults (*Physical Activity Guidelines for Americans,* 2008).

The incidence of chronic disease, such as cardiovascular disease, diabetes, arthritis and osteoporosis increases with age, with approximately 80 percent of older adults living with one or more of these conditions (*The State of Aging and Health in America,* 2007). Chronic illnesses can decrease quality of life by limiting the older adult's ability to carry out activities of daily living. Aerobic exercise, such as brisk walking or riding a bike, plays an instrumental role in preventing and controlling these conditions and their consequences (*Current Sports Medicine Reports,* June 2004). Older adults who participate in regular aerobic training can expect to reclaim and maintain some of their youth through positive effects on the cardiovascular, pulmonary and musculoskeletal systems. These include:

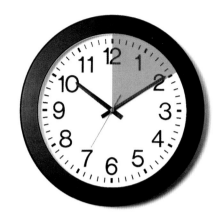

Older individuals who have not exercised in years or who are physically limited by chronic conditions can still get health benefits by exercising in 10-minute bouts accumulated throughout the day.

- *Increased stamina/endurance:* The oxygen requirement (amount of energy needed) for any given activity, such as vacuuming, is comparable among individuals, regardless of fitness level. Regular aerobic exercise increases the body's ability to transport and utilize oxygen per heartbeat. Therefore, fit older adults have a greater energy reserve, which allows them to perform more work with less fatigue.

- *Improved blood sugar control:* Cardiovascular training increases the body's sensitivity to insulin. Consequently, the older adult's muscles and body tissues are better able to extract and use sugar in the bloodstream, leading to normal circulating levels. Regular aerobic exercise also improves insulin's response to blood sugar.

- *Weight management/improved body composition:* The average inactive American adult will gain approximately 18 to 20 pounds between the ages of 18 to 55 years, with additional increases averaging 2 pounds per year over the next 10 years. This weight gain is primarily fat. Routine aerobic exercise helps to reduce body fat stores, particularly from the intra-abdominal area (*Medicine & Science in Sports & Exercise,* July 2009).

- *Blood pressure control:* The Centers for Disease Control and Prevention report that approximately 64 percent of men and 70 percent of women ages 65 to 74 years have high blood pressure. Hypertension is a risk factor for stroke, kidney disease and heart disease. Participation in regular aerobic exercise decreases the risk of developing hypertension and modestly reduces blood pressure values in individuals with hypertension.

- *Improved cholesterol profile:* The risk of developing elevated blood cholesterol levels increases with age. Routine aerobic training reduces this likelihood. Other studies have also shown (*Preventive Cardiology,* Fall 2005) that aerobic exercise can increase HDL cholesterol (the "good" cholesterol) by six percent. The results also indicated that cardiovascular training lowers the total cholesterol to HDL cholesterol ratio. Some exercise studies have reported that modest decreases in total cholesterol and LDL cholesterol (the "bad" cholesterol) can occur, especially with concomitant weight loss.

It is recommended that the older adult engage in moderate-intensity aerobic exercise (e.g., walking at a 2.5 to 4 mile per hour pace) for at least 150 minutes per week (*Physical Activity Guidelines for Americans,* 2008). This would equate to exercising approximately 30 minutes per day on at least 5 days of the week.

In addition to aerobic and resistance exercise, flexibility and balance exercises help to minimize the effects of aging and increase the likelihood that older adults can extend their years of independent living. Poor flexibility can impair mobility and negatively affect the older adult's ability to perform day-today tasks. Some studies suggest that range of motion exercises and stretching can increase the flexibility of the major joints (*Medicine & Science in Sports & Exercise,* July 2009). Flexibility exercises should be performed for varied muscle groups and each stretch should be held for 10 to 30 seconds and repeated four times (*Current Sports Medicine Reports,* June 2004).

Balance training and fall-prevention activities, such as tai chi, should also be included in the older individual's exercise regimen. Falls are the leading cause of death from injury in older adults (*The State of Aging and Health in America,* 2007). These accidents often lead to bone fracture, with a hip fracture being the most debilitating and life-threatening complication. Approximately 20 percent of hip fracture sufferers die within the year as a result of their injury. Thus, older adults should perform balance training exercises three to four days per week.

Older adults are highly encouraged to engage in structured aerobic exercise and increased lifestyle physical activity. Habitual physical activity can offset the negative impact of sedentary living on the aging process. Benefits can be obtained even if you haven't exercised in years. The bottom line? Regular physical activity is a 'time machine'—an antidote to the aging process. Use it, or lose it.

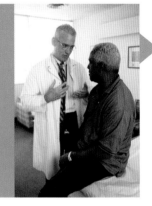

Perhaps Dr. Joseph Alpert, editor of *The American Journal of Medicine*, summed it up best. When asked by patients, friends, or family, "How often should I exercise?" he replied, "Only on the days you eat."

(*American Journal of Medicine,* Jan. 2011)

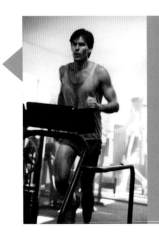

ANTI-AGING EFFECTS OF REGULAR EXERCISE

Several years ago, researchers in Germany compared the characteristics of circulating blood cells in young and middle-aged endurance athletes with age- and gender-matched inactive controls. The results were startling, showing that the athletes exhibited younger-looking cells with far less evidence of structural erosion. It was concluded that physical activity represents an anti-aging intervention and may be helpful in reducing the impact of age-related diseases.

(*Circulation,* Dec. 2009).

Fit for Surgery? Another Reason to Exercise

Barry A. Franklin, Ph.D.

More than 27 million non-cardiac surgical procedures are performed in the United States each year (*International Journal of Surgery,* Oct. 2011). Cardiac and non-cardiac complications can be a major source of morbidity and mortality in the postoperative period. Although age, body habitus and co-morbid conditions, including coronary artery disease, are likely modulators of these complications, several studies now suggest that preoperative levels of physical activity and/or cardiorespiratory fitness (CRF) are predictors of short-term surgical outcomes.

In addition to being a prognostic indicator of cardiovascular and all-cause mortality in both apparently healthy and clinically-referred populations, CRF may be especially helpful in the preoperative risk assessment of patients undergoing varied surgical procedures (*Anaesthesia,* Aug. 2009). These operations include abdominal aortic aneurysm repair, liver transplantation, lung cancer resection, upper gastrointestinal, intra-abdominal, bariatric (*Chest,* Aug. 2006), and coronary artery bypass surgery (*American Journal of Cardiology,* Oct. 2013).

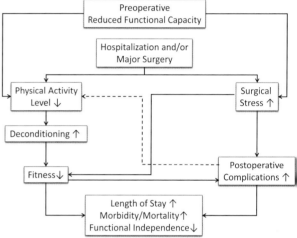

Although there is no firmly identified causal mechanism which directly links a higher CRF or physical activity level with reduced post-operative complications, one possible explanation is that physically active or fitter patients are simply better able to cope with the physical and cardiac demands created by the trauma of major surgery. A reduced level of CRF may also be associated with greater numbers and greater severity of unhealthy co-morbid conditions that, individually or collectively, may increase mortality.

Another reasonable explanation is that a low level of CRF identifies a patient subset that is more difficult to operate on, requiring longer operative and intubation times, or those characterized by a high-risk, proinflammatory state that may be related to the development of heightened post-operative complications. Interestingly, regular physical activity prior to hospitalization for heart-related symptoms appears to confer protection during the ensuing month relative to mortality and rehospitalization for recurrent cardiac events (*Journal of the American College of Cardiology,* May 2008). The potential impact of low preoperative physical activity and CRF on hospitalization and/or surgical outcomes is shown in the accompanying figure (*Current Opinion in Anaesthesiology,* April 2014).

Collectively, these data suggest that physical activity or fitness assessments may be helpful as part of the medical evaluation prior to major surgery.

Although it remains unclear whether increases in CRF will translate into lower surgical complication rates, regular exercise and a physically active lifestyle may represent a viable method of improving short-term outcomes associated with elective or emergent surgical procedures.

Over the years exercise critics have rhetorically asked, "Fitness for what?" Now, exercise enthusiasts can provide them with a sobering response: "Fitness for planned (or unplanned) surgery."

EXERCISE TRAINING IN PATIENTS WITH HEART FAILURE

A multicenter trial randomized 2331 clinically stable patients with heart failure (impaired heart pumping capacity) to exercise training or usual care. All were considered to be on optimal drug treatment regimens. The follow-up averaged three years. After adjusting for numerous baseline characteristics that could have affected outcomes, the exercisers demonstrated an 11 percent reduction in all-cause mortality or all-cause hospitalization. (*Journal of the American Medical Association,* April 2009).

Your Most Important Exercise Accessory? Athletic Shoes

Angela Fern, M.S.

Question: What do the following brands have in common? New Balance. Nike. Reebok. Asics. Brooks. Adidas. Puma. Mizuno. Saucony.

Answer: All are part of a billion dollar shoe industry. Men and women, teens and kids all wear athletic shoes, and not just because of their functionality. Fashion, popularity and value all play a role in the sale of athletic shoes, which include running, walking and cross trainers.

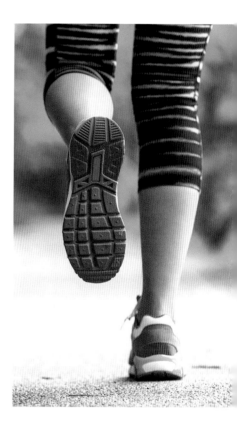

Exercise plays a significant role in many individuals' lives. In fact, considerable money is spent on home equipment and gym memberships, as well as exercise attire. Unfortunately, however, athletic shoes are sometimes at the bottom of the list. It is not uncommon for some people to wear their street shoes while exercising, or to wear the same pair of exercise shoes for several years. Shoes that are wearing at the heel or sole, and those that lack support or shock absorption, should be replaced.

Proper exercise footwear characteristics include foot and ankle support, a roomy toe box, and cushioned and non-skid soles. Ideal athletic socks are made of acrylic. Avoid flip-flops, sandals, high heels, slippers, moccasins or old sneakers when exercising.

The "anatomy" of an athletic shoe is critical when purchasing a new pair. The toe box is the front of the shoe, and there should be enough room to wiggle your toes. The vamp is the laced area of the shoe, and should not be too tight. The insole is the removable cushion inside the shoe, which should mold to your foot. The outsole is the hard area on the outside (bottom) of your shoe. It should be specific to your exercise activity. The midsole is the foam layer between the insole and outsole, which provides cushioned support. This is where the technical "bells and whistles" of the shoe are located. The heel counter wraps around the heel and acts as a stabilizer for your foot. Finally, the upper part of the shoe generally displays the company logo.

Your foot type and arch play a key role in your shoe purchase. An experienced salesperson at a shoe store can determine if you pronate (low arch, so foot rolls in), supinate (high arch, so foot rolls out) or have flat feet (very low or no arch). Bringing your old shoes with you can provide this information. A simple test to determine your foot type at home is to do a "wet test" by dampening your feet and stepping on a paper bag. If you can see most or some of your footprint, you likely have a low to average arch. If only the outside of your footprint is apparent, you likely have a high arch.

Tips to keep in mind when looking for athletic shoes: try on shoes with exercise socks in the late afternoon or evening when your feet are slightly swollen; get both feet measured while standing; choose shoes that feel snug but do not cause pain; and, shop a shoe specialty store for the best quality and properly fitted athletic shoes. Recognize that the "first step" in starting an exercise program is buying the right pair of shoes.

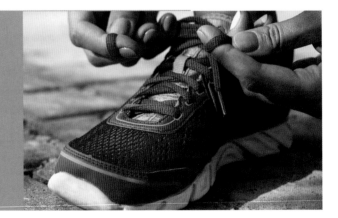

Medical professionals recommend that while every individual is different, changing the shoes you wear while running every 350-to-500 miles can help reduce your risk of injury.

(*Journal of the American Medical Association*, July 2014)

Pedometers: A Small Device With Big Benefits

Kristen Kubert, B.S.

Originally used almost exclusively by sports and physical fitness enthusiasts, pedometers have now become popular as an everyday exercise monitor and motivator. A pedometer is a portable battery-operated device that contains a mechanical sensor and software to record the number of walking steps you take on a flat surface. The 'counts' are triggered by the body's movement. Pedometers record step totals and distance covered when appropriately worn on your hip, at the belt line.

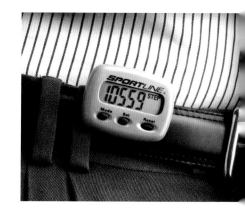

A total of 10,000 steps per day, which is equivalent to approximately five miles (distance = number of steps x average step length), is recommended as the benchmark for an active lifestyle according to the U.S. Surgeon General. One criticism of the 10,000 steps per day goal is that it may be too low for children and is not achievable for most older persons with mobility problems or people with chronic diseases. Although the pedometer doesn't track exercise intensity, you can make your step goals time oriented (e.g., 1,000 steps in 10 minutes would qualify as moderate intensity).

The cost of a pedometer generally ranges from $5 to $60; however, the most valid and reliable models average around $25. Many modern devices have built in step counters, including the Apple iPod Nano, iPod touch and a variety of cellular phones. Various websites now allow people to track their daily step totals, which can help you reach your fitness goals.

A pedometer is a great motivational tool for people who want to increase their daily physical activity. There are also cardiovascular benefits gained from the extra steps you take each day. According to one systematic review, pedometers are associated with significant decreases in body mass index and blood pressure (*Journal of the American Medical Association,* Nov. 2007). Moreover, pedometer users markedly increased their physical activity by an average of nearly 2500 steps per day more than their control counterparts.

Many people attribute the popularity of pedometers to the fact that this inexpensive device records the amount of exercise you do, without the use of expensive equipment and/or gym memberships. The good news is that, like deposits in a piggy bank, the steps accumulate throughout the day. And, the numbers can be motivating. You may just find yourself progressively increasing your daily step totals. Health-fitness goals begin with 'the first step'...

Do You Need a Fitness Tracker?

David R. Cragg, M.D.

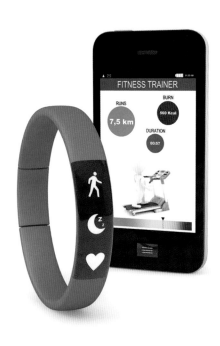

We all know that regular exercise is a vitally important part of staying healthy. Fitness trackers are one modern-day way to help you find the motivation to exercise and improve your lifestyle. Wearable fitness trackers are becoming more popular and there are numerous different products now available. In addition, many smartphones have free apps that have some of the same features as a wearable device. Smartphone apps today can monitor heart rate as well as measure ambulatory speed, distance and elevation by employing GPS. They can also keep track of progress, send encouraging comments and reminders, and estimate how many calories are burned.

Wearable fitness trackers are a combination of a sophisticated pedometer that counts the number of steps you take along with a mini computer that can tell you what time it is as well as your heart rate. In addition, you can get motivational updates from the device that makes it like having your own personal trainer urging you on. Each device on the market has its own unique capabilities. The most common features are:

Pedometer. These devices show how many steps you take each day. One widely cited study reported that pedometer users took, on average, an additional 2,500 steps each day, as compared with their counterparts who didn't use these tracking devices (*Journal of the American Medical Association,* Nov. 2007). Many products also track active minutes and stairs climbed. Setting a daily goal can be a great way to stay motivated to exercise. Comparing steps with co-workers can create a competition to be more active at work. Other research indicates that the exercise advice a doctor gives to his or her patients might be more effective if a pedometer were part of the prescription (*Sports Medicine,* Dec. 2009).

Sleep tracker. Adequate sleep is critical to staying healthy and monitoring it in the past has been nearly impossible. Moreover, several studies have now shown that sleep deprivation is associated with the development of high blood pressure, obesity and type 2 diabetes (see article by Dr. Rothschild in this book). With today's wearable technology you can keep track of the hours you sleep as well as the amount of time you are restless. This feedback can help you make better decisions about how to improve the quality and quantity of your sleep.

Calories burned. Using your weight and gender, it is possible to get a reasonably accurate estimation of the number of calories you burn each day. Combining this with a diet that has an approximate calorie number that doesn't exceed this daily amount is an excellent way to maintain or even lose weight.

Heart rate monitor. Using your heart rate to gauge how hard you are exerting yourself is a smart way to exercise. Having a heart rate goal, along with perceived exertion, can also keep you from under-or-overdosing your exercise. Most devices on the market provide accurate assessments of your resting and exercise heart rate, unless you are predisposed to significant heart rhythm irregularities (e.g., atrial fibrillation).

GPS monitors. For runners, a GPS tracker may be of interest since it can provide you with accurate feedback about distance covered, elevation, routes you ran as well as a summary of your workouts that include pace and splits.

Wearable fitness trackers are a new exciting way to help anyone improve their health. The technology is evolving and someday these devices will also likely tell us much more about ourselves. If you are not sure that you want to delve into a wearable device, simply try the apps already on your smartphone. Many of these are free and provide you with feedback on your heart rate, stairs climbed, as well as the number calories you have burned.

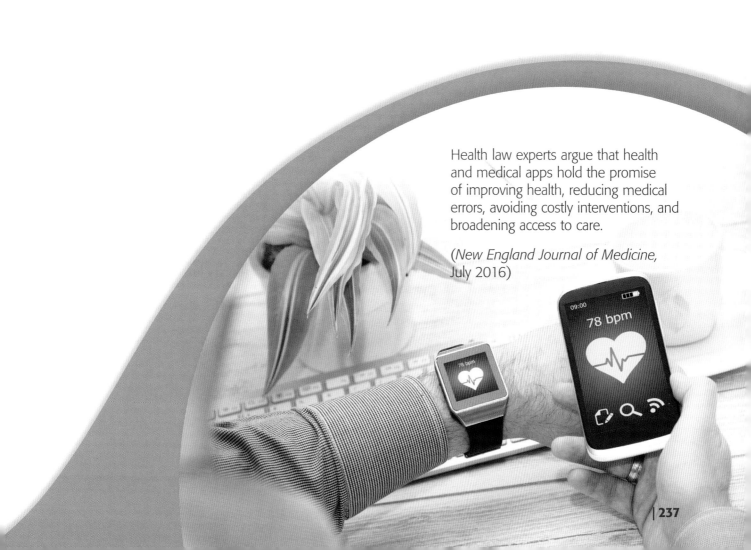

Health law experts argue that health and medical apps hold the promise of improving health, reducing medical errors, avoiding costly interventions, and broadening access to care.

(*New England Journal of Medicine,* July 2016)

Exercise Right With Proper Warm-up and Cool-Down

Roger Sacks, B.S.

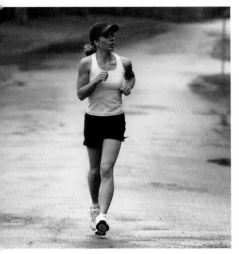

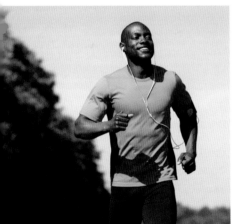

Exercise promotes good health and disease prevention. Regular physical activity also makes activities of daily living seem easier. Leisure activities that many of us take for granted, such as walking up stairs or doing yard work, can become challenging if we become increasingly sedentary. Exercise has been shown to increase bone density and/or decrease the rate of bone loss, especially by performing weight bearing activities such as walking and resistance training. Accordingly, many people don't do as much exercise as they should, and, even worse, do the exercise improperly.

Proper exercise includes three important components: warm-up, endurance activity and cool-down. The warm-up consists of a gradual increase in workload (speed, incline, resistance) for about 10 minutes to achieve a moderate exercise intensity. Why is a warm-up so important? The bottom line: it increases blood flow. The arterioles throughout your body that supply blood to your muscles and tissues are inherently small. When your body senses increasing levels of physical exertion, blood vessels dilate or "open up" which allows more oxygen-rich blood to flow to muscles. The result? Energy (called adenosine triphosphate, or ATP) is produced. Now, you may wonder, "Is a ten minute warm-up really necessary?" The answer is, "yes." Blood vessels don't dilate instantaneously. Knowing this one simple fact is especially important for people with heart disease.

Several years ago, researchers discovered that a preliminary warm-up serves to decrease the occurrence of electrocardiographic abnormalities that are suggestive of heart strain and irritability—abnormalities that may be provoked by sudden strenuous exertion. Warm-up also has the added benefit of reducing the potential for muscle injury. Why? After a preliminary warm-up, muscles become more elastic and stretch easier. Thus, warm-up has preventive value and enhances performance capacity.

Following the warm-up, exercising in a prescribed intensity level for at least 30 minutes is commonly recommended to achieve cardiovascular benefits. The exercise intensity is generally regulated by monitoring heart rate, perceived exertion, or both. Normally, the perceived exertion during exercise should be between fairly light and somewhat hard.

The third and final component to exercise is the cool-down. This phase of exercise allows you to gradually lower your heart rate and blood pressure and return to a resting state. Your heart rate and blood pressure will gradually return to normal after stopping exercise, but you are more likely to experience dizziness or lightheadedness if you don't cool down. If you've ever walked on a treadmill really fast, stopped abruptly, and experienced a momentary dizziness, this is the sensation you want to avoid. What happens is that blood tends to pool in the lower extremities—dramatically decreasing blood flow to the head and heart. Abnormal heart rhythms can also occur by abruptly stopping exercise.

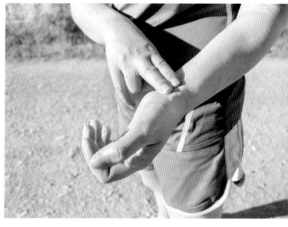

Exercise has been called the "elixir of life." It can prevent, treat, and cure many diseases and illnesses. However, there is a safe and proven method to gain the most benefit, and this includes performing a warm-up and cool-down. These two components (bookends to the endurance phase) are vital, but many people ignore them. If you can find time to be physically active, you can certainly find 10 to 15 minutes to do a proper warm-up and cool-down to achieve the benefits that a safe and effective exercise program can provide.

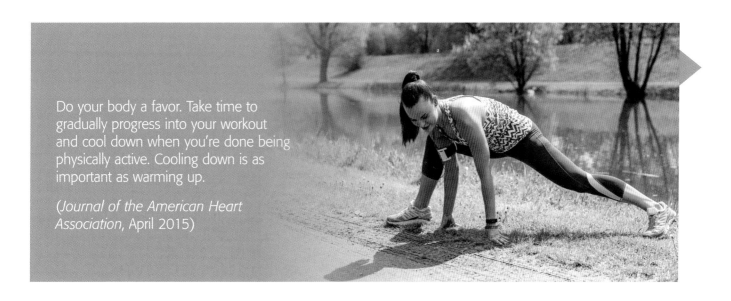

Do your body a favor. Take time to gradually progress into your workout and cool down when you're done being physically active. Cooling down is as important as warming up.

(*Journal of the American Heart Association*, April 2015)

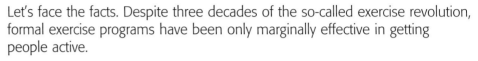

Disguise Your Exercise

Barry A. Franklin, Ph.D.

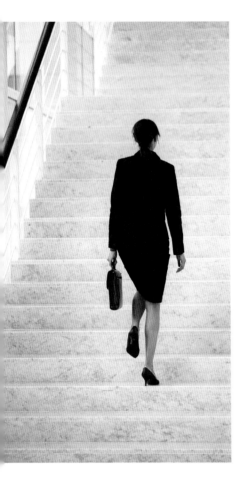

Let's face the facts. Despite three decades of the so-called exercise revolution, formal exercise programs have been only marginally effective in getting people active.

Why? Perhaps it's because planned exercise may extend the day or compete with other valued interests and responsibilities of daily life. According to one report, new members of health/fitness clubs typically use these facilities less than twice per month! In another study, heart patients undergoing exercise therapy spent more time in their cars going to and from the rehabilitation facility than they did on the equipment.

In the past decade, researchers have reevaluated the scientific evidence linking physical inactivity with chronic diseases. These analyses suggest that frequent bouts of moderate-intensity activity—like brisk walking, stair climbing, household chores, gardening, and recreational sports—can be as effective as vigorous exercise if the daily energy expenditure is comparable.

In other words, the desk-bound executive who jogs at the lunch hour may not be any better off than the person who does less-intense, periodic activity throughout the day.

Health professionals now encourage people to integrate multiple short bouts of physical activity into their daily lives. Here are some simple ways to fit exercise into your daily life, without signing up for an expensive health club membership.

Stop circling! Forget about driving laps around parking lots looking for the "closest" possible spot when you head out to the shopping mall, local pharmacy, grocery store or doctor's office. Park the car in the spot farthest from the door and use this opportunity to get your legs moving and your arms pumping.

Find the stairs! Forget about the elevator or escalator and move from floor to floor the old-fashioned way—climb the stairs. Using the flights of stairs in office buildings and shopping malls is a great calorie burner and helps build strong leg muscles.

Leave your desk/computer! Occasionally replace e-mails or phone calls to colleagues down the hall with person visits. Avoid sitting for prolonged periods and break up your workday with short walk-breaks, deliveries, and other errands.

Wear a pedometer! They're easy to use and can be worn on the belt, at the midline of the thigh, to track your daily step count. Inactive people take 2,000 to 4,000 steps per day, moderately active people take 5,000 to 7,000 steps per day, and active people take at least 10,000 steps per day. Glancing down at the pedometer and checking progress can provide the motivation needed to go for an extra walk when you're short of your goal.

Although lifestyle exercise is not being suggested to replace more traditional workouts, it's a wonderful complement to any health and fitness program. Try working calorie-burning and muscle-building activities into your everyday living.

LIFESTYLE INTERVENTIONS IN PATIENTS WITH HEART DISEASE

An interesting analysis of previously published randomized controlled trials showed a significant risk reduction of 18 percent in fatal cardiovascular events in patients undergoing multifactorial lifestyle interventions (e.g., diet, exercise, smoking cessation) aimed at improving modifiable risk factors.

(*American Journal of Preventive Medicine,* Aug. 2013)

Work Out With Your Canine Companion!

Angela Fern, M.S.

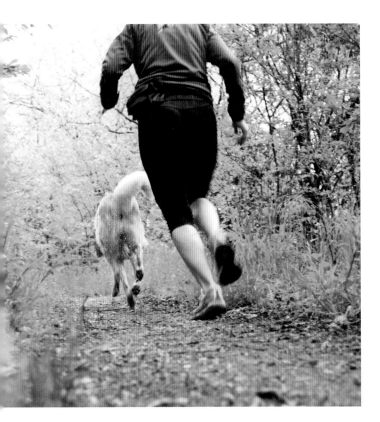

Looking for ways to spruce up your activities? Consider including your dog in your exercise plan, and you will both reap the benefits of cardiovascular conditioning and calorie burning. According to the Centers for Disease Control, 35.7 percent of adults are obese in the United States. Additionally, one fifth of dogs (and cats) are obese per the Association for Pet Obesity Prevention. So, if you and/or your pooch haven't been very active, check with your physician and your dog's veterinarian first. Then, start with walking short bouts (e.g., 10-15 minutes) and gradually building up to longer durations. One Michigan based study found that "dog walking was associated with more walking and leisure time physical activity" in adult dog owners (*Journal of Physical Activity & Health,* March, 2011).

While exercising outdoors in warm weather, keep in mind these tips from the Humane Society of the United States and the Michigan Humane Society: exercise in the early morning or late evening, bring water for both of you to be well hydrated, and avoid pavement or asphalt that is too hot for your dog's pads. If you are looking for more variety or a challenge activity with your four legged friend, ponder the following suggestions from the web site Petside.com: hill walking, trail running (ideally on dirt or grass), stair climbing, swimming, disc/Frisbee, rollerblading, cycling, Doga (yoga inspired), and agility/obstacle training. Always keep safety a priority in choosing the right exercise for you and your dog. Enjoy the weather and have fun with your canine companion!

Exercising Outdoors: Tips to Beat the Heat

Jenna Brinks, M.S.

During the summer months, many regular exercisers gravitate to the great outdoors. In 2013, almost 143 million Americans reported participating in outdoor activities, with nearly 25 percent exercising two or more days per week (*Outdoors Participation Report,* 2014). Walking, jogging, biking, hiking, swimming, tennis and golf are appealing activity options that are associated with an improved sense of well-being (*Environmental Science and Technology,* March 2011). Interestingly, when researchers equipped older exercisers with accelerometers to track their activities, those exercising outdoors accumulated more physical activity than their indoor counterparts (*International Journal of Behavioral Nutrition and Physical Activity,* July 2012).

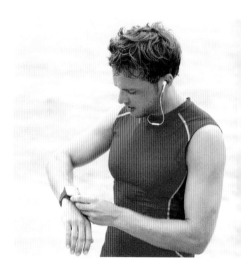

If you participate in outdoor activities this summer, mind the heat! Under hot/humid conditions, the body cools itself by increasing blood flow to the skin. This redistribution may disproportionately increase heart rate to maintain oxygen delivery to working muscles. Evaporation of sweat on the skin also serves as a powerful mechanism to cool the body. However, with high humidity, very little sweat is actually absorbed by the moisture-laden air, and the sweat merely rolls off the body. The heat stress can increase body temperature to dangerous levels, causing heat syncope (fainting), muscle cramps, heat exhaustion, and even heat stroke.

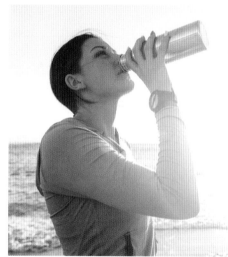

The good news? There are several ways to stay safe and reduce the likelihood of heat stress when exercising outdoors this summer:

- *Moderate your activity according to environmental conditions.* To decrease the likelihood of heat stress, consider modifying your exercise routine. For example, when exercising in extreme temperature and/or high humidity, you may need to slow your pace, shorten your distance, re-route to more shaded paths, or take frequent breaks. Avoiding exercise during peak heat hours (late morning through early evening) can reduce the potential for heat stroke and related complications.
- *Hydrate, hydrate, hydrate!* An average person sweats 27 to 47 ounces per hour while exercising. Without adequate fluid intake, one cannot effectively dissipate heat or maintain blood pressures necessary to oxygenate body tissues. If you are planning to exercise outdoors in the heat, drink plenty of cold fluids (preferably water) not only during exercise, but before and after as well. On the other hand, if you will be exercising at a vigorous intensity for more than 60 minutes, consider a sports drink to replace critical electrolytes like sodium, potassium and chloride lost in sweat.

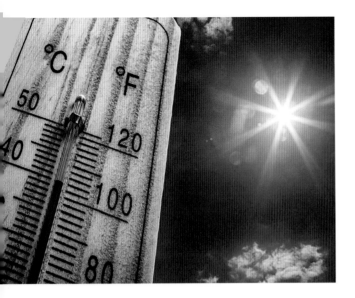

- *Dress appropriately.* Wear minimal amounts of clothing to facilitate cooling by evaporation. Porous, light-colored, lightweight clothing that wicks moisture from the skin helps to facilitate heat dissipation and your body's natural cooling mechanisms.

- *Gradually adjust to exercising in the heat.* For safety reasons, the first activity session should be limited to 10 to 15 minutes and gradually increased to 20 to 60 minutes as the body's heat dissipation mechanisms become more efficient over time. It takes most healthy people 10 to 14 days to fully acclimate to hot environments.

- *Don't forget ultraviolet (UV) protection!* Many water-resistant sunscreens are now available, offering UV skin protection. You still need to re-apply regularly, as sunscreen is not water-proof and eventually wears off. A hat or cap made from moisture-wicking fabric keeps your scalp protected, and UV-rated sunglasses prevent harmful rays from damaging your eyes.

- *Plan ahead.* Many weather 'apps' are now available for download directly to smartphones, and allow for quick and convenient heat advisory checks. Pack thoughtfully, based on your planned activity, location and duration. For example, if you are planning a two-mile hike in the woods, pack a small backpack with water bottles, protein- and complex carbohydrate-packed snacks, insect repellent and extra sunscreen. Keep extra clothes and supplies in your car.

- *Carry identification and your phone, and notify others of your 'solo' plans.* While no one expects to fall, break an ankle, or experience exertion-related chest pain, unfortunate events can occur. By informing others where you plan to be and when you expect to be home, your support network can activate the appropriate emergency response if you do not reconnect as scheduled.

Although exercising outdoors this summer can enhance physical and mental well-being, the likelihood of heat illness or injury may be especially high in some persons, including older adults, those who are hypertensive, diabetic, or obese, and patients taking prescribed medications such as diuretics, beta-blockers and vasodilators. Alcohol use, which enhances dehydration, can also be problematic. By planning ahead, making subtle changes in your routine, and listening to your body, you can increase the likelihood of safe exercise this summer. See you out there!

Making a Splash for Better Heart Health

Jenna Brinks, M.S.

If you are looking to supplement or adjust your current exercise program with effective and enjoyable alternatives, you are not alone. Adhering to a regular exercise program can easily be sidetracked by busy schedules and boredom with the "same old routine." Accordingly, it is important to vary exercise modalities and programming to remain committed to and excited about exercising regularly for cardiovascular health and fitness. To enhance compliance and satisfaction with cardiovascular conditioning regimens, athletic clubs and cardiac rehabilitation programs increasingly offer varied activities, including water-based exercise. When performed with appropriate instruction and monitoring, activities like shallow or deep water aerobics, stretching, walking/jogging, strength and balance training, and swimming can be safely added to most exercise regimens—even yours!

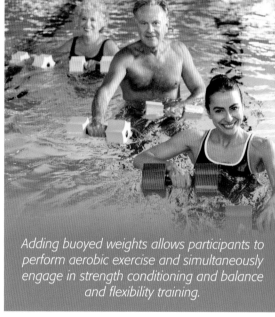

Adding buoyed weights allows participants to perform aerobic exercise and simultaneously engage in strength conditioning and balance and flexibility training.

Similar to land-based exercise, aquatic exercise can enhance multiple measures of cardiovascular health. Participants who engage in varied forms of water exercise, including shallow and deep water aerobics, can achieve appropriate intensity levels for improving health and fitness (*Journal of Strength and Conditioning Research,* Feb. 2001; *Medicine and Science in Sports and Exercise,* April 2003). Furthermore, longitudinal studies have now shown that regular participation in water-based exercise can improve cardiorespiratory fitness, muscular strength, body composition and agility (*Medicine and Science in Sports and Exercise,* March 2002; *European Journal of Applied Physiology,* Sept. 2006; *American Heart Journal,* Sept. 2007).

Participants with certain health conditions may find water exercise more appropriate than land-based exercise because it eliminates many common barriers to physical conditioning.

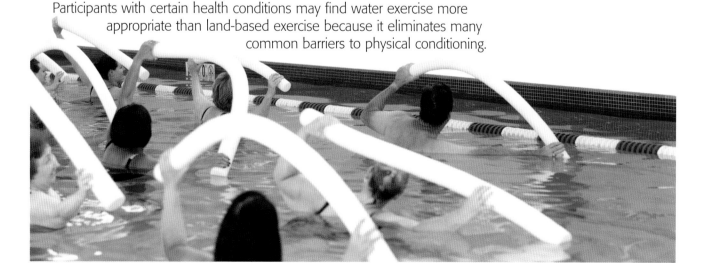

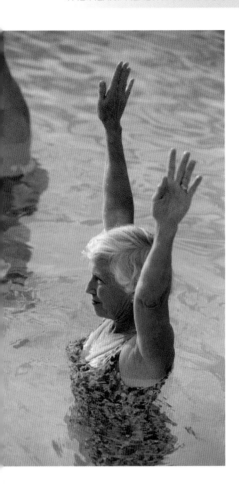

Aquatic exercise provides an environment that reduces impact forces, allows for easier control of positioning and intensity and aids in balance. Those with chronic conditions such as fibromyalgia, obesity, osteoarthritis, rheumatoid arthritis, selected musculoskeletal injuries, orthopedic limitations and post-stroke status may experience improved exercise tolerance in water.

Although aquatic exercise can be safe, beneficial and enjoyable, people with medical issues should consult a physician. For example, if you have congestive heart failure and have decreased cardiac function, water submersion exercise may be too taxing. In addition, exercising in cold water can mask anginal symptoms indicating inadequate blood flow to the heart muscle. Because of these potential issues, patients considering water-based exercise should consult with their physician for guidelines before starting.

If you are considering a water-based exercise regimen, all of the basic recommendations for exercise still apply. Each session should include a warm-up to increase blood flow and stretch muscles, an aerobic phase to achieve the health and fitness benefits of exercise, and a cool-down period. Water exercise can be easily modified to accommodate individual limitations and goals (e.g., using buoyed handweights for strength conditioning, adding wrist or ankle weights to increase resistance and intensity during aerobics and jogging, or using fins and kickboards to vary swimming drills). This allows participants to perform aerobic exercise and simultaneously engage in strength conditioning and balance and flexibility training. Another consideration when participating in a water-based program is how exercise intensity is regulated. Most heart rate monitors are now water-resistant, and can be worn during water-based activity. However, due to differing physiological responses to submersion in water, the heart rate response is often lower as compared with performing similar activities on land. Therefore, using target heart rate ranges developed from land-based treadmill testing as the sole indicator of pace or work rates may result in excessive exercise intensities. Accordingly, perceived exertion is a valuable adjunctive intensity modulator during aquatic exercise. In general, if you rate your effort level as "fairly light" to "somewhat hard," you are likely achieving a safe and effective exercise intensity.

In summary, aquatic exercise can provide an enjoyable alternative for most participants, and may be particularly useful for patients with neurologic and musculoskeletal disorders. Special aquatic exercises may include torso and extremity movements in shallow water, thus taking advantage of the water to minimize orthopedic trauma and the resistance of the water to augment the work load. Moreover, if performed at an appropriate level of perceived exertion, it can provide health and fitness benefits comparable to land-based activity. Whether you prefer group-based exercise classes or exercising alone, water-based exercise offers something for everyone. So get started—go "make a splash" for better heart health!

Walking the Dog for Better Health

Angela Fern, M.S.

According to the American Heart Association (AHA), most Americans do not engage in enough structured exercise and regular physical activity to achieve health and fitness benefits. The Centers for Disease Control and Prevention (CDC) suggest that adults need at least 150 minutes a week of moderate-intensity aerobic activity like brisk walking to improve health. For those who are able to engage in vigorous-intensity aerobic activity like jogging or running, the recommendation is *at least* 75 minutes a week. Despite these modest health-based recommendations, challenges to meet this exercise dosage remain.

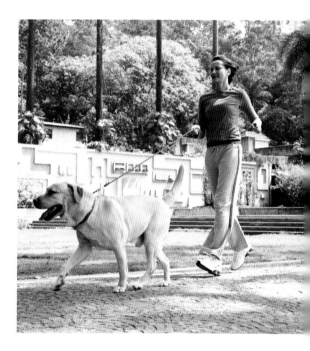

Perceived barriers to exercise often include lack of time, motivation, enjoyment, encouragement and social support. The CDC suggestions for overcoming common physical activity barriers include identifying daily times for brief exercise bouts, exercising with family or friends and walking the dog. In fact, one study suggested that "dog walking can contribute to a physically active lifestyle and may address several important barriers to physical activity in humans" (*Preventing Chronic Disease,* April 2006).

An estimated 107.4 million Americans walked three days per week in 2005, according to a survey conducted by the Federal Highway Administration. Another survey, administered by the National Highway Traffic Safety Administration, reported that exercise and health were the top reasons that people walked, at 27 percent. To achieve this goal, dog walking was commonly reported, and the average walking distance was approximately 1.2 miles.

Several studies support the positive influence of dog walking on exercise behavior. One report revealed that dog walkers were more likely to achieve 150 minutes of walking per week and were twice as likely to achieve recommended exercise levels as compared with people who didn't own dogs (*Journal of American Geriatrics Society,* September 2006). Americans are not the only ones to benefit from dog walking. Canadian dog owners participate in more moderate physical activity, walking an average of 300 minutes per week, than their counterparts without dogs (*American Journal of Preventive Medicine,* February 2006). In another study, Australians who became dog owners within the previous 12 months increased the amount of time they spent walking, averaging 130 minutes per week. The authors suggested that "dogs may have a significant role in the maintenance of owner walking behavior" (*The International Journal of Behavioral Nutrition and Physical Activity,* March 2008).

The AHA supports walking "as the single most effective form of exercise to achieve heart health" and encourages activities such as a short walk before breakfast or dinner, walking the dog and parking further away in the mall parking lot and walking the extra distance.

If you are inspired to walk a dog, whether it is your own, a neighbors' or one at a local animal shelter, consider these recommendations from the Michigan Humane Society to start off on the right "paw:"

- The dog should be leashed and wearing a collar with a current ID tag and license.
- Take short walks and gradually build up to longer durations.
- Limit or forego walking time during hot or cold weather or choose indoor play.
- In the summer, choose dirt or grass pathways instead of hot pavement.
- In the winter, wipe the dog's paws after walking to remove salt.
- Watch the dog for signs of limping or labored breathing.
- Always have water available for the dog to keep hydrated any time of the year.

EVEN SHORT BOUTS OF EXERCISE IMPROVE FITNESS

A recent study found that even short bouts of physical activity—just 10 minutes a day—can improve cardiorespiratory fitness levels in previously sedentary, overweight women. The researchers also found that while short bouts of exercise were beneficial, more exercise boosted fitness levels even higher (*Journal of the American Medical Association, May 2007*).

Heart Rate Increases Improve Fitness: A Common Misconception?

Barry A. Franklin, Ph.D.

I vividly recall a participant in our cardiac rehabilitation program who approached me with an intriguing question: "If the object of the exercise program is to increase my heart rate to a certain level, and hold it there for 30 or 40 minutes, why can't I just sit in a steam room or sauna to raise my heart rate? Wouldn't I get the same benefits I get from exercise if my heart rate was similarly elevated for the same period of time?"

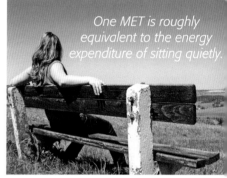

One MET is roughly equivalent to the energy expenditure of sitting quietly.

I realized that his logic probably reflects a common misconception; the increase in heart rate causes the body to become physically fit. Unfortunately, becoming physically fit is not that easy. If this was the case, high-strung, nervous individuals would be among the most physically fit people in the world!

Although a regular, sustained increase in heart rate is generally recognized as important to achieving improved cardiovascular fitness, the heart rate response merely serves as an indicator for the real training stimulus, which is increased body metabolism or oxygen consumption.

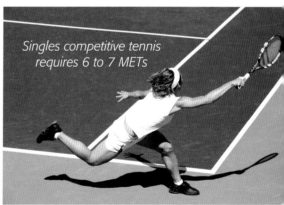

Singles competitive tennis requires 6 to 7 METs

Aerobic activities can be characterized in terms of a standardized energy unit known as "metabolic equivalents" or METs, which refers to the ratio of the exercise metabolic rate to the resting metabolic rate. It is a measure of how much incremental energy is expended during the activity as compared with rest. One MET is roughly equivalent to the energy expenditure of sitting quietly. Walking at a leisurely pace uses about 2 to 3 METs. Brisk walking approximates 4 to 5 METs, depending on the pace. Singles competitive tennis requires 6 to 7 METs, whereas jogging approximates 8 to 10 or more METs.

Exercisers should recognize that even though many real-life situations can evoke abrupt increases in heart rate, our breathing and energy expenditure (METs) remain essentially unchanged. The steam room and sauna are good examples. Giving a speech is another example. Several years ago, we monitored a lecturer during his presentation to a large audience. His heart rate ranged from 108 to 144 beats per minute. Was he getting the equivalent of a moderate intensity exercise session during the talk? Of course not. If we become extremely anxious or upset, or are subjected to certain environmental stressors (e.g., heat, humidity, altitude), our heart rate may remain elevated for some time, even though we are not getting the benefits of an exercise session.

Another way of disproving the notion that pronounced increases in heart rate are needed to enhance aerobic fitness is to study patients who are taking beta-blockers. These drugs can markedly decrease the heart rate at rest and during exercise. As a result, some patients have resting heart rates in the 40s or 50s and exercise heart rates in the 80s or 90s. Despite the fact that people who are taking beta-blockers achieve blunted exercise heart rates, they show normal improvements in cardiovascular fitness.

Hopefully it's obvious that an increase in heart rate alone does not cause the body to become physically fit. Instead, it is the rise in oxygen consumption and energy expenditure with exercise that results in the favorable adaptation and improvement. The increase in heart rate that occurs during exercise is simply a marker for the real training stimulus—a transient increase in metabolism or METs.

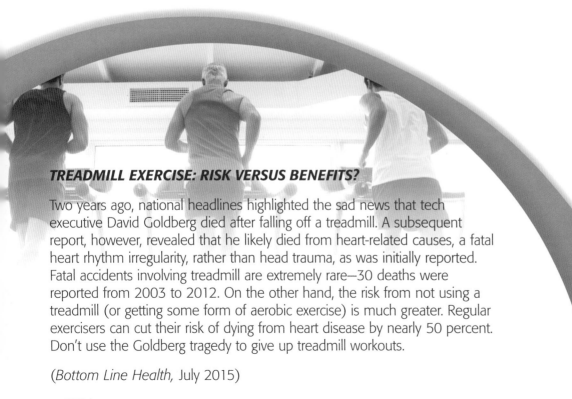

TREADMILL EXERCISE: RISK VERSUS BENEFITS?

Two years ago, national headlines highlighted the sad news that tech executive David Goldberg died after falling off a treadmill. A subsequent report, however, revealed that he likely died from heart-related causes, a fatal heart rhythm irregularity, rather than head trauma, as was initially reported. Fatal accidents involving treadmill are extremely rare—30 deaths were reported from 2003 to 2012. On the other hand, the risk from not using a treadmill (or getting some form of aerobic exercise) is much greater. Regular exercisers can cut their risk of dying from heart disease by nearly 50 percent. Don't use the Goldberg tragedy to give up treadmill workouts.

(*Bottom Line Health,* July 2015)

Hazards of Sudden Strenuous Exertion

Joyce Said Hansen, M.S.

Novice and experienced exercisers alike often shrug off the importance of a warm-up prior to aerobic exercise. Sudden strenuous exertion, however, is associated with potential cardiovascular and musculoskeletal complications. This article focuses on these risks and the rationale for a preliminary warm-up period.

By definition, a warm-up allows the body to transition from rest to exercise by promoting increases in the rate of nerve conduction and muscle elasticity, a rise in muscle and core temperatures, and gradual circulatory adjustments. Additionally, warm-ups reduce the likelihood of musculoskeletal injury by increasing blood flow to active muscles, improving connective tissue extensibility, and enhancing range of motion and muscular performance.

Research indicates that sudden strenuous exertion may place excessive demands on the heart that cannot be matched immediately by its circulation, leading to electrocardiographic (ECG) abnormalities, heart rhythm irregularities, or chest pain. The benefit of a warm-up was demonstrated in a classic study of healthy men with normal ECG responses to progressive, maximal exercise testing. Each subject was asked to run on a treadmill for 10 to 15 seconds at an intense workload without a prior warm-up. Nearly 70 percent of the men developed an abnormal ECG pattern, suggesting inadequate oxygen supply to the heart muscle. However, these abnormalities were generally abolished by a preliminary warm-up exercise (i.e., jogging in place).

Warm-up also allows internal body temperature to rise, and promotes arterial vasodilation. Blood flow is diverted from less vital organs (i.e., kidneys and digestive tract) to more active skeletal muscle to provide needed nutrients and oxygen, while reducing the formation of lactic acid, which is associated with muscle fatigue. Thus, the warm-up has preventive value and enhances performance.

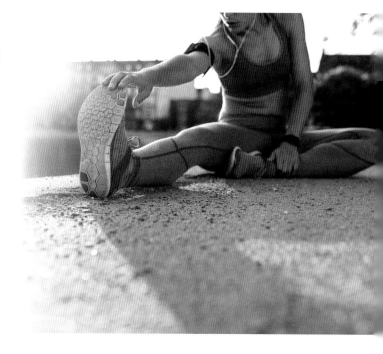

An effective warm-up should include 5 to 10 minutes of stretching and low intensity aerobic exercise sufficient to approach the lower end of the prescribed target heart rate range. Activities similar to the aerobic exercise, but done at a more moderate pace (i.e., brisk walking before jogging), are considered a good warm-up. Stretching activities can also be used as part of a warm-up and should focus on major muscle groups. The stretching exercises should utilize static movements to facilitate enhanced flexibility. This technique provides a lower risk of injury to tendons, ligaments, joints, and the muscles themselves.

Remember, sudden strenuous exertion may be hazardous to your health. To reduce the risk of cardiovascular and musculoskeletal complications, take time to warm-up.

HEALTHY LIFESTYLE AND RISK OF SUDDEN CARDIAC DEATH

A low-risk lifestyle (not smoking, exercising regularly, having a prudent diet, and maintaining a healthy weight) is inversely associated with the risk of sudden cardiac death in women. Women at low risk for all four lifestyle factors had a 92 percent lower risk of sudden cardiac death compared with women who had none of these healthy lifestyle characteristics. These findings suggest that widespread adoption of a healthy lifestyle in the population may make a substantial impact on reaching the American Heart Association's 2020 impact goal of further lowering cardiovascular disease mortality.

(*Journal of the American Medical Association,* July 2011)

Exertion-Related Acute Cardiac Events

Troy Silverthorn, B.S.

A Fennville, Michigan basketball player drives to the basket to make a game winning lay-up in overtime to cap off a perfect season. He makes the lay-up, his teammates hoist him in the air, fans rush the court and the celebration begins. It was a moment of pure happiness for the Fennville basketball team and its fans.

Yet, moments later, elation turned to tragedy as Wes Leonard, the 16-year-old Fennville player that made the game winning shot, collapsed on the court. An ambulance was called and paramedics started cardiopulmonary resuscitation. Two hours later, Leonard was pronounced dead at a local hospital. An autopsy revealed that he died of a previously undiagnosed heart condition called hypertrophic cardiomyopathy (HCM), also known as an enlarged heart.

Although exertion-related fatalities in athletes rarely occur, when they do, it sends shockwaves throughout the community.

What is sudden cardiac death (SCD)? Lethal cardiovascular events may result from intense physical training or competition in an athlete who has an underlying cardiovascular abnormality, triggering a potentially fatal heart rhythm irregularity. Although the number of athletes that experience exertion-related SCD each year is quite small, the exact number remains unclear due to the fact that a comprehensive athletic death registry does not exist.

In contrast, accurate data on the risk of marathon running are available. In reviewing marathon and half-marathon races in the U.S. from 2000 to 2010, researchers reported on the incidences and outcomes of cardiac events among 10.9 million registered marathon runners. Of 59 cases of cardiac arrest, 42 (71 percent) were fatal—indicating an average of 4 to 5 marathon running deaths each year (*New England Journal of Medicine,* Jan. 2012). Nevertheless, because distance runners are often viewed as invincible, that is, one of the healthiest population subsets, these deaths often generate sensationalized media headlines.

There are many different cardiac abnormalities that could potentially contribute to an athlete experiencing an exertion-related SCD, including congenital coronary artery anomalies, myocarditis and HCM. Nevertheless, the most common cardiac abnormality associated with SCD in young athletes is HCM, which is characterized by a larger than normal heart, primarily involving the left ventricle. Because of the left ventricle enlarging without compensatory dilation of the heart chamber, cardiac function during high-volume, high-intensity exercise may be compromised,

The deaths involved in athletes with HCM are most common in start-stop sports such as basketball and football, and less likely during endurance sports such as cycling and cross country running.

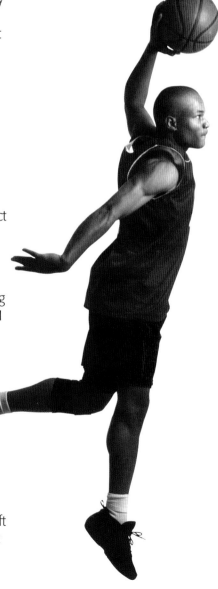

leading to threatening heart rhythm irregularities. Ventricular tachycardia and/or ventricular fibrillation are often the first symptomatic manifestation of HCM—arrhythmias that can trigger SCD.

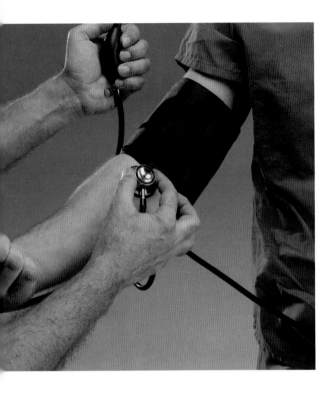

The deaths involved in athletes with HCM are most common in start-stop sports such as basketball and football, and less likely during endurance sports such as cycling and cross country running. HCM is typically diagnosed using an electrocardiogram (ECG) and echocardiogram, along with a comprehensive health history. About 90 percent of patients with HCM have an abnormal resting ECG. Echocardiographic findings that can help identify HCM include an asymmetric left ventricular wall thickening and a diminished left ventricle chamber size.

In the United States, if a middle school or high school student wants to compete in an athletic sport, they generally undergo a pre-participation screening (PPS) which may include a symptom assessment, family history and a physical examination. If, in younger athletes, HCM is most often associated with exertion-related SCD, why not make an ECG and echocardiogram mandatory for every athletic screening?

In Italy, there has been a protocol in place for the past 25 years that includes a resting ECG as part of the PPS. This methodology reduced the incidence of exertion-related SCD due to HCM by 90 percent! With such a profound impact, you would think that the United States would also adopt a PPS that routinely included an ECG. Although a more comprehensive cardiovascular screening may be a part of athletics in the future, as of now, the most appropriate screening tests remain controversial.

Despite the above-referenced evidence for including an ECG in a PPS, the American Heart Association does not support the routine use of ECG screening in athletic populations at this time. Some of the arguments against its use include concerns over false-positive readings, the cost-effectiveness of implementing the protocol, and related adverse psychological concerns for athletes and their families when abnormalities are detected. Some estimates suggest that up to 200,000 individual athletes would need to be screened in order to identify a single athlete at risk of dying suddenly during training or competition. However, since most SCDs occur without prior symptoms, a PPS protocol that includes a 12-lead resting ECG is certainly worth considering.

Exercise and Sudden Cardiac Death: Common Causes?

Justin Trivax, M.D.

We have all read the headlines: "Young Female Dies Running Marathon; Details Unclear," "60-Year-Old, Father of 4, Long-Time Runner, Collapses and Dies at Mile 5 During Marathon."

Or perhaps you recall the Detroit Free Press/Flagstar Marathon in 2009 where three runners died in a span of 16 minutes?

Marathon running has increased in popularity over the last three decades, with participation increasing from 25,000 runners in 1976 to approximately 2 million in 2010. With increased participation, there has been a rising occurrence of exercise-related fatalities. The risk of sudden cardiac death while participating in a marathon is one per 259,000 participants (*New England Journal of Medicine,* Jan. 2012).

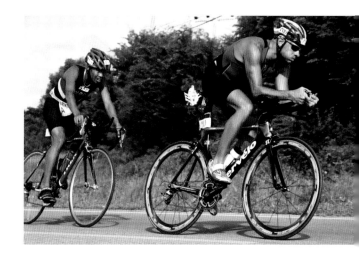

Sudden cardiac death in runners aged 40 years old or less is almost always due to a structural abnormality of the heart, most notably, hypertrophic cardiomyopathy. Because the heart muscle is abnormally thickened, it may have difficulty pumping blood, especially during vigorous physical activity. Abnormal heart rhythms may result, leading to cardiac arrest (sudden cessation of the heartbeat). Hypertrophic cardiomyopathy typically runs in families but may occur sporadically. Several high-profile athletes have suffered from this disorder including college-basketball star Hank Gathers (collapsed and died during a basketball game), Boston Celtics All-Star Reggie Lewis (collapsed and died during basketball practice), and Detroit Red Wings defenseman Jiri Fischer (resuscitated sudden cardiac death during National Hockey League game). Therefore, screening for this disorder is highly recommended prior to embarking on an intense exercise regimen or high-level athletic participation. This abnormality may be detected with a good history and physical exam, a 12-lead electrocardiogram, echocardiogram (cardiac ultrasound), and/or maximal exercise testing.

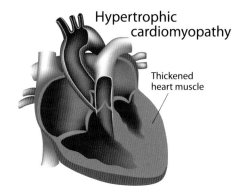

Hypertrophic cardiomyopathy

Thickened heart muscle

In athletes older than 40 years, the most common cause of exertion-related death is clogged coronary arteries or coronary artery disease. Vigorous exercise in persons with known or occult heart disease can trigger plaque rupture or threatening heart rhythms, leading to heart attack or cardiac arrest, respectively. Reduction in the most common risk factors for atherosclerosis is considered a first-line treatment strategy, including blood pressure control, lipid lowering, and smoking cessation. However, for reasons not clearly understood, endurance athletes often have an increased incidence of coronary artery calcification as compared with age-matched participants of similar atherosclerotic risk.

James Fixx, the author of "The Complete Book of Running," an avid runner who was one of the earliest advocates of long-distance running and its health benefits, died of a heart attack at the age of 52 during a training run. The cause of death was heart attack and autopsy findings revealed severe diffuse coronary artery disease. Presumably, he had been experiencing exertion-related symptoms in the weeks before his death. Did Fixx see a physician to clarify the cause of his symptoms; did he have blood work performed, an exercise stress test or an echocardiogram? Would he have benefited from a calcium score? Technologic advances now suggest that we may be able to prevent some of these occurrences with appropriate screening.

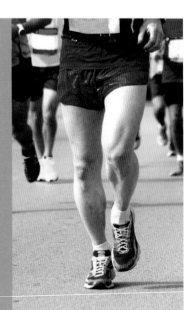

MARATHONS POSE MODEST RISK TO HEART

To clarify the cardiac risk associated with long-distance running races, researchers assessed the incidence and outcomes of cardiac arrest associated with marathon and half-marathon races in the U.S. from January 1, 2000 to May 31, 2010. Among nearly 11 million runners who participated, only 59 went into cardiac arrest during a race, for an incidence rate of just 0.54 per 100,000 participants. Forty-two of these were fatal. Men were more likely than women to have cardiac arrest and sudden death. Although the authors concluded that long distance running races are associated with a low overall risk of cardiovascular complications, they suggested that preparticipation exercise testing may be useful for identifying some persons at high risk.

(*New England Journal of Medicine,* Jan. 2012)

Exercise: Too Much of a Good Thing?

Justin Trivax, M.D.

There's always time during the year to revisit your New Year's resolution, especially if it involves exercising. In fact, the most common New Year's resolution is to start an exercise routine (www. associatedcontent.com). In 2009, my New Year's resolution was to complete a marathon, and I am happy to report that I completed the 2009 Chicago Marathon on a frigid October day. As a cardiology fellow, many patients, co-workers, family and friends have asked about my experience running the marathon. In particular, after 3 deaths in the 2009 *Detroit Free Press* marathon, many people have asked if marathon running or prolonged strenuous exercise is dangerous.

Participation in endurance sports has increased significantly in the United States over the past 30 years. In 1975, only 25,000 runners completed a marathon. By 2009, more than 400,000 runners completed at least one marathon, and many of those runners participated in multiple events in a year. With a 1 in 50,000 chance of dying from a heart attack during a marathon, this increased participation has accordingly led to an increased number of reported deaths in connection with marathon running. In 1975, there were no reported deaths associated with marathon running; but in the past year alone, there were nine deaths, with five of those occurring during a half-marathon. Despite this increased number of deaths, the risk of dying while participating in marathons remains unchanged. But the question remains: why are one out of 50,000 apparently healthy marathon runners dying while participating in these events?

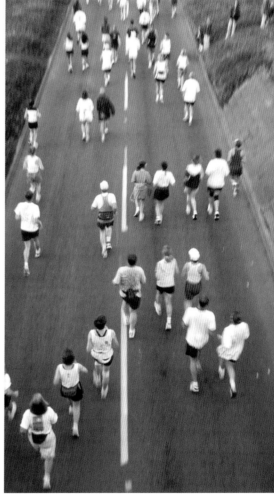

During the past 30 years, researchers have been studying the effects of prolonged strenuous exercise on the heart. We have learned that prolonged strenuous exercise results in elevation of blood enzymes known as cardiac biomarkers—the same enzymes that are released during heart attacks and heart failure. Immediately after running marathons or participating in triathlons, athletes develop dilation of the chambers and weakened pumping function on the right side of the heart, lasting up to three weeks. In addition, using cardiac magnetic resonance imaging, we have found that otherwise healthy marathon runners have an unexpectedly high rate of scar tissue in places where we would expect normal-appearing heart muscle.

Several minutes prior to lining up at the starting line, a cascade of events is triggered, setting the perfect environment for heart damage. Natural hormones—often referred to as adrenaline—are released, causing the heart to speed up, potentially causing spasms in the heart's arteries. During the race,

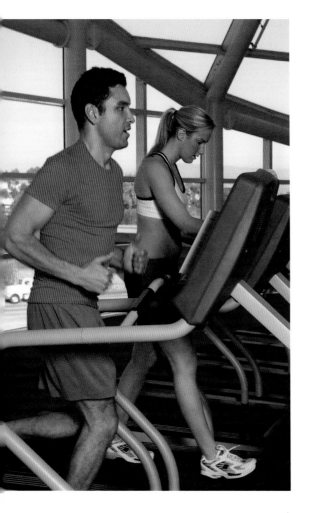

changes in metabolism occur, electrolyte imbalances ensue, and acid builds up in the muscles and in the blood. Blood returning to the heart increases markedly and pressures in the lungs are at least doubled, causing the heart to become stretched and overloaded. Some runners adapt to these changes without any problems, but for others, this strain on the heart may result in abnormal heart rhythms, causing collapse and, in extreme cases, sudden death. Invariably, those who die during or immediately after vigorous exercise have some form of underlying heart disease.

Reading these facts, one might wonder why anyone would engage in an activity that potentially increases one's risk of dying. Is it time to choose a different New Year's resolution? Not necessarily. Although the risk of a heart attack or sudden cardiac death increases transiently during periods of strenuous exercise—some studies have reported a two- to six-fold increase—such statistics should not be misinterpreted. For individuals who do not regularly engage in physical activity, the risk of having a heart attack increases more than 100 times during vigorous exercise. In contrast, there are significant benefits to regular physical exercise. The overall risk of a heart attack for individuals who are physically fit is half of that for individuals who are unfit and habitually sedentary. The bottom line is that the benefits of moderate aerobic exercise clearly outweigh the risks. As for the risk-reward balance for marathon running, the jury is still out.

EXERCISE IS 'GOOD' MEDICINE

A progressive treadmill exercise test is the best way to determine your exercise capacity or heart-lung fitness, expressed in units called metabolic equivalents or METs. Each 1-MET increase in exercise capacity is associated with an 8 to 35 percent (average, 16 percent) reduction in mortality, which compares favorably with the survival benefit conferred by low-dose aspirin, cholesterol-lowering statins, beta-blockers, and angiotensin-converting enzyme inhibitors after a heart attack.

(*Journal of the American Medical Association*, Jan. 2013)

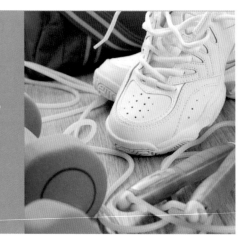

Exercising for Health and Longevity or Peak Performance?

Barry A. Franklin, Ph.D.

Endurance athletes are generally lean, have very favorable risk factor profiles, and superb cardiac performance (or fitness levels). These characteristics, coupled with other investigations suggesting that regular exercise has anti-aging effects (*Circulation,* Dec. 2009), have probably contributed to the skyrocketing increase in vigorous exercise participation, and the notion that "more exercise is better." Although this may be true when it comes to peak physical performance, with respect to health and longevity, new research suggests that it's not necessarily so.

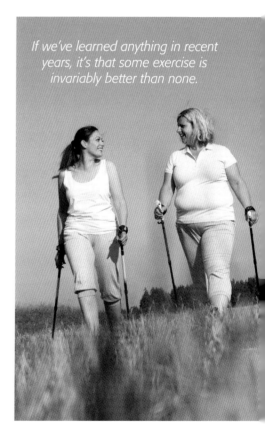

If we've learned anything in recent years, it's that some exercise is invariably better than none.

Exercise and health outcomes

Two recent studies (*Heart,* July 2014; *Mayo Clinic Proceedings,* Sept. 2014) in patients with heart disease came to similar conclusions. The least physically active patients were at the greatest risk for recurrent heart problems and earlier death; the most physically active patients (those performing strenuous physical activity on a daily basis) actually had higher death rates than more moderate exercisers (i.e., those exercising two to four days per week).

Another study of more than 13,000 runners (*Journal of the American College of Cardiology,* Aug. 2014) found that their risk of dying from heart disease was 45 percent lower than non-runners over a 15-year follow-up. Interestingly, maximal survival benefits were observed among those who ran at more moderate distances, speeds and frequencies each week. Even more sobering was the fact that those who ran at an easy pace for as little as five to ten minutes a day had virtually the same survival benefits as those who pushed themselves harder or longer.

Other studies in older adults have now reported a strong statistically significant association between chronic high intensity aerobic exercise and a heightened risk of developing atrial fibrillation (*Circulation,* Aug. 2008)—a heart rhythm irregularity associated with the triggering of strokes. In contrast, moderate intensity physical activity such as walking reduced the risk for atrial fibrillation by about one-third. Collectively, these studies, and other reports, have led to the phrase "cardiac overuse injury," which is increasingly used to describe the potential consequences of the "more exercise is better" strategy.

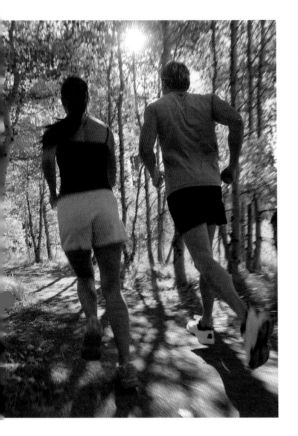

Optimal dosing of exercise?

According to the Physical Activity Guidelines for all Americans, 150 minutes per week of moderate intensity physical activity (e.g., walking) or 75 minutes per week of vigorous physical activity (e.g., jogging or running) are recommended to improve health and well-being. Why half the time for vigorous exercise? The intensity, or associated energy cost of running, is greater than walking. Therefore, running (or walking up a treadmill grade) is more cardioprotective than walking—and you can get equal or greater benefits in less time.

In essence, when it comes to the survival benefit of exercise, intensity and duration are inversely related. According to one widely-cited report (*Lancet,* Oct. 2011), a five-minute run is equal to a 15-minute walk, and a 25-minute run is comparable to a 105-minute walk. On the other hand, for the previously sedentary patient, suddenly embarking on a vigorous or high intensity exercise program (i.e., running) may be downright dangerous.

Ease into running

Most experts now strongly recommend a transitional exercise phase—walk before running. Gradually increase your walking pace, from 2 to 3 to 3.5 to 4 miles per hour. After two or three months, if you are symptom-free during fast walking, you can start to jog (slowly at first) or start increasing the treadmill grade or incline. This transitional phase will decrease the incidence of injury, gradually raise the fitness level, and minimize transient spikes in relative risk, which can occur when going from a habitually sedentary lifestyle to unaccustomed high intensity physical activity.

Take-home messages

If we've learned anything in recent years, it's that some exercise is invariably better than none. A landmark study (*Lancet,* Oct. 2011) found that persons who walked just 15 minutes a day had a 14 percent reduction in death rates over an average follow-up of eight years, as compared with their completely sedentary counterparts. In fact, the primary health beneficiaries of an exercise program are those at the bottom of the fitness chain, that is, those in the least fit, least active cohort. Simply making the transition from poor fitness to below average can reduce your overall risk for premature death by up to 40 percent.

If one embraces the current mantra, "exercise is medicine," when it comes to good health and longevity, it appears that overdosing is possible.

Snow Removal: A Potentially Hazardous Winter Workout

Barry A. Franklin, Ph.D.

During the winter months, an increased incidence of heart attack and sudden death has been reported after heavy snowfalls: "At least 8 people died Wednesday in the Detroit area after snow-related exertion. In Wayne County alone, 17 heart attack deaths were attributed to exertion since the snow began Tuesday. Most of the victims were older men clearing their driveways and walks" (*The Detroit Free Press, January 16, 1992; section A:1*).

In response to these alarming reports, we initiated a series of studies at Beaumont Hospital to clarify the physical demands and risks of snow removal. During the first experiment, we monitored heart rate, blood pressure, and oxygen consumption (to assess total body energy expenditure) in 10 healthy, inactive men while clearing a 4-inch high tract of heavy wet snow for 10 minutes (*Journal of the American Medical Association, March 1995*).

The heart rate and blood pressure of most of our subjects catapulted to dangerously high levels—comparable to or higher than the maximum values achieved by the same subjects during exhaustive treadmill exercise testing! Energy expenditure during shoveling was nearly 6 times that at rest, equivalent to the energy cost of playing singles tennis. Moreover, the average subject lifted and threw nearly a ton of snow (12 shovels/minute x 16 pounds/shovel x 10 minutes = 1920 pounds)—equivalent to the weight of a mid-size automobile.

A trigger for heart attacks? In a second study, we reported on 20 heart attack victims who were admitted to our hospital's emergency center over a 12-day period of cold temperatures and blizzard conditions, 5 of whom (all men, aged 55 to 77 years) were engaged in snow removal (*American Journal of Cardiology, June 2001*). All of the men had a history of heart problems or coronary risk factors, including a sedentary lifestyle, and 4 of the 5 were classified as obese. Interestingly, 2 of the 5 patients had been using an automated snow thrower, rather than shoveling.

Sudden death after snow removal? In a third study, we reviewed death records from the medical examiners' offices of 3 counties in the weeks before, during, and after 2 heavy snowfalls that occurred in the greater metropolitan Detroit area. Of the 271 people who experienced sudden cardiac death, 36 (33 men, 3 women) were engaged in snow removal (*American Journal of Cardiology, October 2003*). Four of the individuals were using an automated snow removal device (i.e., electric snow thrower) at the time of their death.

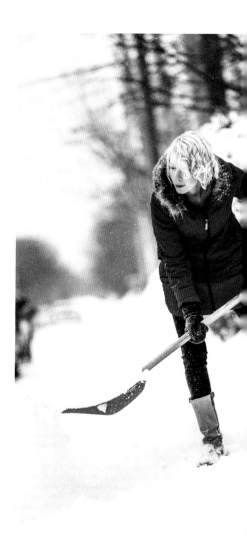

Individuals at risk? Those who are over 45 years of age who have a history of heart problems, symptoms suggestive of a cardiac problem (exertional chest pain/pressure, palpitations, dizziness) or major coronary risk factors (cigarette smoking, high blood pressure, elevated blood cholesterol, diabetes, and sedentary lifestyle) are at increased risk of cardiovascular complications during manual or automated snow removal.

Finally, as a reminder of the potentially threatening cardiac demands of snow removal, paste a copy of this label to your snow shovel or electric snow thrower:

WARNING:
USE OF THIS INSTRUMENT FOR SNOW REMOVAL MAY BE HAZARDOUS TO YOUR HEALTH!

EXERCISE CAUTIOUSLY IN THE COLD

Cross-country skiing and snowshoeing may be hazardous for persons with known or suspected heart disease. Both sports rely heavily on the upper extremities, which can increase blood pressure and put added stress on the heart. As the altitude increases, these activities can increase the heart rate and blood pressure to potentially dangerous levels. The bottom line: Heart attacks and even fatal heart rhythm abnormalities may result.

(*AHA's Heart Insight Magazine,* Feb. 2011)

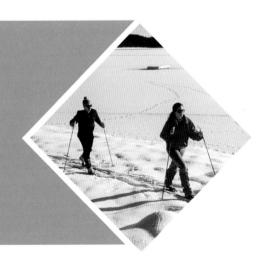

Cardiovascular Benefits of Yoga

Justin Trivax, M.D.

Current recommendations regarding the prevention of heart disease advise individuals to integrate "structured exercise," specifically moderate intensity aerobic activity, into one's routine five days a week, complemented by strength training two days a week. Although there is no mention of regular yoga practice in these recommendations, there is increasing evidence that yoga is not only beneficial for prevention, retardation, and reversal of heart disease, but is also important for spiritual healing and well-being.

Your blood pressure is elevated. You blame it on chronic stress and the bag of chips you finished in the waiting room. Your doctor wants to treat you with medication. What should you do? Practice yoga. Although many physicians have become accustomed to prescribing multiple antihypertensive medications, in a randomized controlled trial of middle-aged adults, daily yoga practice was as effective as medical therapy in controlling high blood pressure (*Indian Journal of Physiology and Pharmacology,* April 2000). Yoga effectively reduces blood pressure by reducing excitatory hormones such as adrenaline, noradrenaline and aldosterone. It also improves the functioning of specialized receptors that control blood pressure.

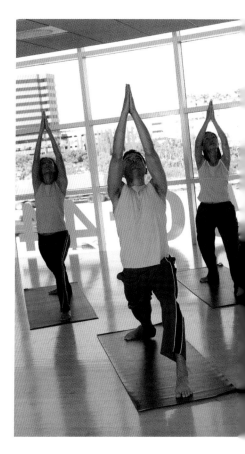

Your doctor notes that your cholesterol level has increased, you are borderline diabetic, and you've gained 30 pounds in the past two years? Now what? Practice yoga. Modern-day yoga has become more rigorous, recruiting large muscle groups and substantially increasing caloric expenditure. Yoga lowers cholesterol levels, decreases body weight and fat stores, and improves the body's ability to transport sugar to working muscles. A 17 percent decrease in LDL-cholesterol was reported in patients with moderately elevated cholesterol who participated in daily yoga for three months (*Acta Physiologica Scandinavica Suppl,* 1997). In a study of over 100 patients with diabetes, improvements of blood glucose and reductions in oral diabetes medication were noted in those who completed a 40-day yoga class (*Diabetes Research Clinical Practice,* Jan. 1993).

Maybe you were experiencing exertional chest pain and you had an abnormal stress test. A subsequent cardiac catheterization showed moderate blockage in your coronary arteries. You don't want stents and you don't want bypass surgery. Time for yoga? Some studies suggest that it may complement conventional medical therapy. In addition to treatment with certain medications (cholesterol medications [statins], aspirin, and blood pressure drugs), patients with documented coronary disease who participated in a one-year yoga intervention several times per week used less nitroglycerin for angina, demonstrated improved cardiorespiratory fitness, required much less need for revascularization with stents or bypass, and actually exhibited more coronary plaque regression and less plaque progression when compared with a sedentary group (*Journal Association of Physicians India,* July 2000).

You had a heart attack 10 or 20 years ago? What's done is done, but now only one-third of the pumping capacity of your heart remains and you often feel short of breath. What can you do? Practice yoga (in addition to remaining on standard medical therapy, of course). Nineteen patients with advanced heart failure were studied to determine the effect of yoga on their health. Ten were randomly given standard medical therapy. The other nine were given standard medical therapy complemented by a yoga intervention. After eight weeks, the yoga patients showed greater improvements in levels of inflammatory markers, exercise capacity and quality of life (*Journal of Cardiac Failure,* June 2008). It has been postulated that yoga improves heart failure symptoms by reducing sympathetic drive, similar to beta-blocker therapy, and through improved breathing techniques.

The popularity of yoga continues to rise. What was once considered to be a system of physical and mental disciplines may now become central in the treatment of patients seeking alternatives or complements to traditional medical therapy. As we continue to learn more about the advantages of yoga, perhaps we can all benefit from less drugs and more downward dog.

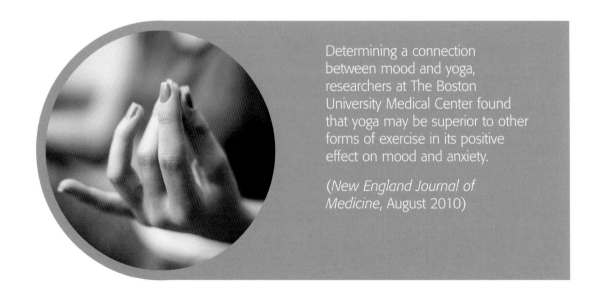

Determining a connection between mood and yoga, researchers at The Boston University Medical Center found that yoga may be superior to other forms of exercise in its positive effect on mood and anxiety.

(*New England Journal of Medicine,* August 2010)

Tai Chi: A Highly Therapeutic, Slow-Motion, Exercise Alternative

Cindy Haskin-Popp, M.S.

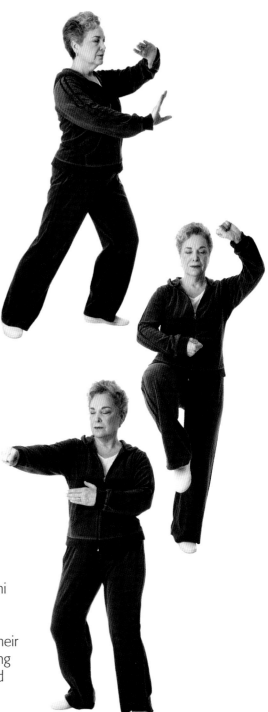

Tai chi, an ancient martial art practiced by the Chinese for more than 3,000 years, has recently gained popularity in Western culture as the scientific evidence in support of its immense health benefits continues to mount. This exercise art form, often described as "meditation in motion" by its proponents, combines slow, fluid movements with deep breathing and mental imagery to optimize overall health and well-being. Tai chi's positive effects on health include improvements in balance and stability, flexibility, muscular strength and endurance, aerobic capacity and psychological well-being (*Evidence-Based Complementary Alternative Medicine,* Sept. 2013; *BMC Geriatrics,* Oct. 2013).

These health benefits can be enjoyed by all, regardless of age, gender, chronic disease, fitness and skill level because of the non-competitive and progressive nature and multiple styles of tai chi. In fact, increasing research supports the safety and effectiveness of tai chi for a wide variety of chronic health conditions, such as cardiovascular and pulmonary diseases, breast cancer, neurologic and metabolic disorders, rheumatoid diseases, and orthopedic limitations (*Evidence-Based Complementary Alternative Medicine,* Sept. 2013).

The tai chi forms, including varied movements and positions, can be modified to meet the needs and goals of the individual (e.g., performed in a chair or in a pool as opposed to standing or practiced on land). This adaptability makes tai chi an attractive exercise alternative for previously sedentary or frail older adults who need to engage in activities for fall prevention. In July 2011, the American College of Sports Medicine released a position statement that recommended tai chi as an adjunct exercise for adults because of its positive effects on balance, motor control, agility and proprioception (i.e., the ability to sense where your body is in space)—all of which are variables associated with fall prevention.

One widely-cited study compared a 15-week program of simplified tai chi forms with a conventional balance training program in community dwelling adults, aged 70 years and older (*Journal of the American Geriatrics Society,* May 1996). After four months, participants in the tai chi class had reduced their risk of multiple falls by almost half of those participating in the balance training group. Furthermore, after the study's completion, the tai chi subjects reported increased ability to prevent falls by using more effective body mechanics in their environment—an indication of enhanced functional fitness.

Individuals with sufficient functional fitness are able to perform activities of daily living safely and independently without undue fatigue. Tai chi provides functional fitness training and, as a result, complements a conventional aerobic and strength building exercise program (*Medicine & Science in Sports & Medicine,* July 2011).

Functional fitness activities train multiple muscle groups throughout the body to work together as a unit, rather than isolating and exercising a muscle group independently. In other words, functional fitness activities like tai chi train the movement pattern, programming it in the brain, thus enhancing the mind-body connection. This training of the neuromotor system translates into improved coordination and stability while at rest and during movement.

In addition to its health benefits, tai chi has many other attributes that make it an appealing activity. It doesn't require expensive equipment, adjunctive devices or special clothes to perform. It can be practiced in most places, such as the comfort of your own home, a fitness center or a hotel room. It is not weather-dependent (an ideal activity for Michiganders who want to be active year-round). And, it can be performed independently or in a group.

There are many resources available to the individual interested in learning tai chi that run the spectrum from self-taught methods using the wide variety of DVDs found on the market to classes offered to the community.

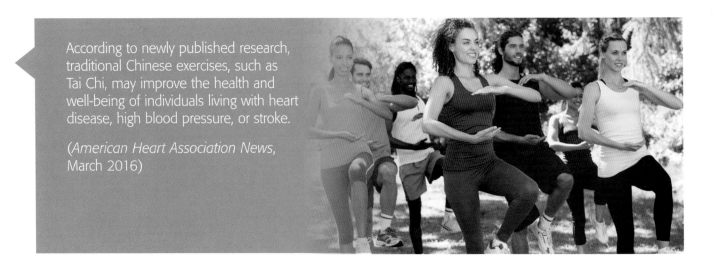

According to newly published research, traditional Chinese exercises, such as Tai Chi, may improve the health and well-being of individuals living with heart disease, high blood pressure, or stroke.

(*American Heart Association News,* March 2016)

Heel Pain? An Exercise Impediment

Barry A. Franklin, Ph.D.

Heel pain is commonly attributed to inflammation of the fibrous tissue that is attached to the heel bone and runs along the bottom of your foot. This condition is called plantar fasciitis. Pain is most intense when first standing. Most people experience their most intense pain in the morning, immediately after waking, when trying to take their first steps. Common causes of plantar fasciitis include a sudden increase in the amount of weight-bearing activities (e.g., walking, running) you do, or repeated trauma to the plantar fascia. Treatments may include: daily stretches (see figures); change in shoe type; custom orthotics; anti-inflammatory medications; rest; night splints; corticosteroid injections; and, ice or cold therapy. However, if you have diabetes, neuropathy, or cardiovascular problems, talk with your physician before initiating these therapies. A good podiatrist can be especially helpful in this regard.

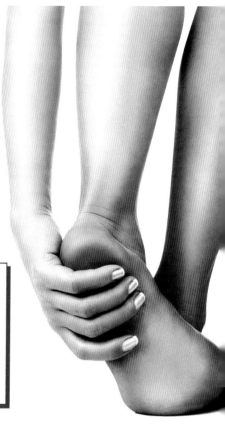

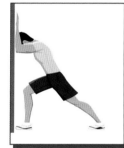 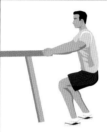 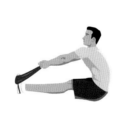 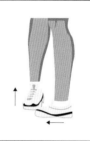

Maintaining Your Exercise Motivation: Practical Suggestions

Lisa Schornak, M.S.

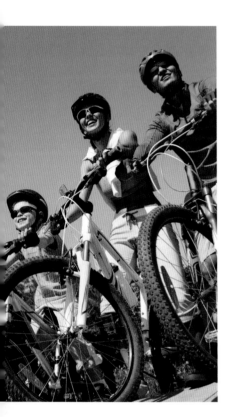

There are numerous ways to increase your motivation to exercise but here are a few practical ones that are highly effective for most people. Think about why you are exercising. Do you need to make it part of a healthy lifestyle? Is it to lose weight and get in shape? Could it be to control modifiable risk factors, including chronic stress?

Be realistic and set reasonable goals. Remember why your exercise program is so important. Only look towards your next workout. If you look down the road too far you may stumble. Keep track of your progress. Whether it is time accumulated, pounds or inches lost, or miles covered, document (record) your achievements. Reward your efforts; not with ice cream, but with a movie, a new workout item or a trip to the spa.

Remember, as Ralph Marsten so aptly put it, "What you do today can improve all your tomorrows." Make exercise part of your daily routine. Could you ever imagine not buckling your seat belt when you get in your car or not brushing your teeth for a few days? Next time someone asks you to join them for a walk at lunchtime or after work for a new exercise class, just say "yes."

Recognize that regular exercise helps control stress. It allows time for quiet contemplation. Exercise, like a brisk walk, gives you time to plan the day ahead and organize your thoughts. Regular exercise can also help reduce body weight, fat stores and blood sugar values. Physically fit people live longer, demonstrate lower resting heart rates and blood pressures and often enjoy a better night's sleep.

Make exercise convenient and fun. Remember how good you feel after your workout. Regular exercise improves self-confidence and relieves stress. Try to vary your exercise routine. Taking a Spin or Zumba class might be just the motivation you need. Involve the entire family by taking a bike ride or playing tennis at your local park. Think: move more, sit less. Join a volleyball or wallyball league. Sometimes just having a partner who is counting on you to be there is enough motivation to get you moving again.

Perhaps Dr. Joseph Alpert, editor of *The American Journal of Medicine*, summed it up best by his answer to a question that he often gets. "Patients often ask me how often they should exercise. My response? You only have to exercise on the days that you eat."

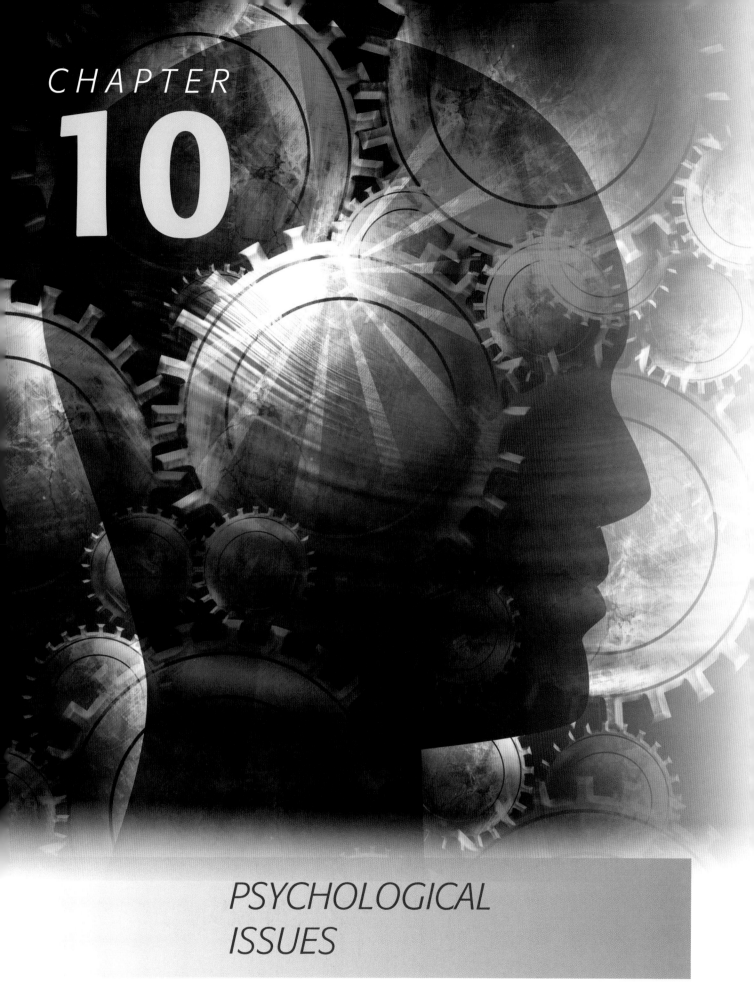

10

PSYCHOLOGICAL ISSUES

Impact of Psychosocial Risk Factors on the Heart

Barry A. Franklin, Ph.D.

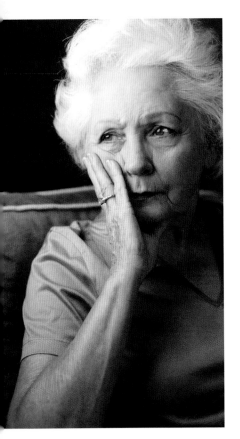

To combat cardiovascular disease, physicians and allied health care professionals often focus on modifying conventional risk factors such as cigarette smoking, high blood pressure, elevated blood cholesterol and diabetes. However, a review of published research demonstrated that only 75 percent to 90 percent of the causes of coronary artery disease are explained by these conventional risk factors, either alone or in combination *(American Journal of Cardiology,* Feb. 2009). An escalating body of research now provides strong evidence that at least some of the remaining incidence (10 percent to 25 percent) may be attributed to the adverse effects of psychosocial stressors.

Emerging psychosocial risk factors

The importance of psychosocial variables in the development, clinical manifestations, and prognosis of patients with heart disease has received increased attention in recent years. Consider these sobering reports (*The Physician and Sportsmedicine,* Oct. 2009):

- According to one widely cited study, persons who demonstrated a Type-A behavior pattern (hard-driving, competitive, impatient, persistent sense of time urgency), were twice as likely to develop coronary heart disease as compared with their more mellow Type-B counterparts. However, other studies suggest that only some components of the Type-A behavior pattern (like hostility) are more closely linked to the development of heart disease.

- Researchers at Harvard reported that the risk of experiencing a heart attack in the two hours following an 'angry confrontation' increased two to three fold.

- In several studies, patients who met the criteria for depression were at least three to five times more likely to die during the first year following their heart attack than were nondepressed patients.

- According to the World Health Organization, when depression occurs in conjunction with other chronic diseases, including angina pectoris (chest pain), arthritis, asthma and diabetes, it produces significantly greater decrements in overall health than the medical condition alone.

- Acute emotional stress/distress has been implicated in the occurrence of fatal cardiovascular events in persons with underlying heart disease. A review of the county coroner's records from the time surrounding the massive Northridge, Cal. earthquake on January 17, 1994, revealed that the associated emotional stress triggered a disproportionate number of sudden deaths, from a daily average of less than five in the preceding week to 24 on the day of the earthquake.

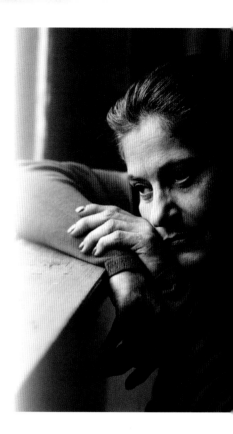

- Researchers in Germany reported that the stress associated with viewing an exciting World Cup soccer match more than doubled the risk of an acute cardiovascular event (heart attack, stroke, etc.).
- Research has now shown that anxiety worsens the prognosis in cardiac patients, and chronic job strain is an independent predictor of recurrent coronary events in patients who have had a recent heart attack.
- One study that examined the prognostic importance of social resources among medically treated individuals with heart disease found that unmarried patients with no confidant had a five-year survival of only 50 percent compared with 82 percent for those who had either a spouse, confidant, or both.

Adverse responses → cardiovascular disease

Psychological risk factors have been implicated as precursors of initial and recurrent coronary events, as well as targets for counseling and behavioral interventions. These risk factors are believed to worsen or exacerbate the development of cardiovascular disease by two mechanisms: encouraging unhealthy behaviors such as cigarette smoking, sedentary living, eating foods that are high in calories and/or fat, and increasing the non-compliance to prescribed cardioprotective medications; and eliciting physiological responses that may lead to insufficient oxygen delivery to the heart muscle, threatening heart rhythms, more vulnerable plaque, and the potential for blood clotting.

Implications for screening and counseling

Unfortunately, the influence of psychosocial risk factors in cardiovascular disease remains under-recognized compared with conventional risk factors. Psychosocial risk factors contribute independently to cardiovascular events, presumably by encouraging unhealthy behaviors and causing adverse changes in nervous, hormone, blood clotting and inflammatory systems. Recognizing this relationship offers an important target for cardiovascular education, counseling and behavioral interventions, even after controlling for major risk factors. This focus should serve to maximize the potential for cardiovascular risk reduction by addressing at least a portion of the 10 percent to 25 percent incidence of heart disease that is unexplained.

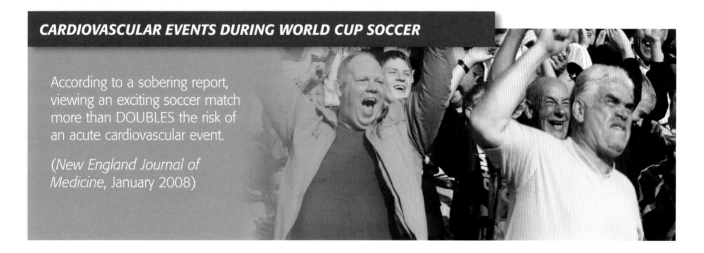

CARDIOVASCULAR EVENTS DURING WORLD CUP SOCCER

According to a sobering report, viewing an exciting soccer match more than DOUBLES the risk of an acute cardiovascular event.

(*New England Journal of Medicine*, January 2008)

My Heart Is Healing, but I'm Not Feeling Like My Old Self

Daniel Stettner, Ph.D.

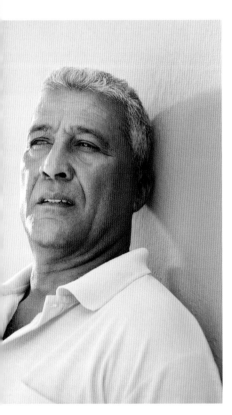

Having had a heart attack or cardiac surgery may also have created major psychological distress for you and your family. Many cardiac patients come 'face-to-face' with fears of dying or death. Cardiac events can affect your overall physical and psychological well-being. Thus, it's common for people who have come through such experiences to feel depressed. Depression or major life traumas have been reported to precede heart attacks in up to 50 percent of all cases. In other studies, depressed patients were at least 3 to 5 times more likely to die during the first year following a heart attack than were nondepressed patients. Although the link between clinical depression and increased cardiac mortality remains unclear, it appears that depressed patients are less likely to take prescribed medications and adhere to recommended behavior and lifestyle changes intended to reduce the risk of recurrent cardiovascular events.

Depression is where people feel very sad and empty; moreover, some may experience these feelings for long periods of time. Self-confidence and self-esteem are typically very low. It is common to feel hopeless and helpless with depression. Depression is much more intense than sadness alone or just feeling upset or 'blue.' It usually interferes with how you live your daily life. For many cardiac patients, depression manifests as fear, anger, anxiety, loss of control, and worry that the heart problems will happen again. It is also common to 'bottle up' these concerns, and not want to talk about them, thinking and hoping that the feelings will just go away.

How do you know if depression is a problem for you? The following screening test, adapted from the Harvard Department of Psychiatry National Depression Screening Day Scale, commonly called the HANDS™ questionnaire, is designed to help identify individuals who are likely to be suffering from a depressive disorder that may require treatment.

It is very important that you talk openly and often about what you've been through. As you may already have discovered, there may be limits to how long your family and friends will be willing to listen to you. They may not understand how important it is for you to share your concerns and worries. That is why support groups, an exercise-based cardiac rehabilitation program, professionals (including clergy) and others who are good listeners are so important in your recovery. When you talk and share your thoughts and feelings, it helps you feel much better. The combination of such assistance and your own personal health rehabilitation may resolve the depression.

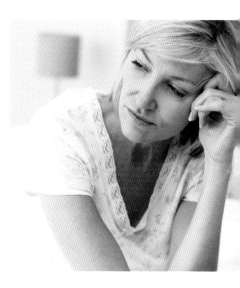

In some cases, special anti-depression medicines, in addition to talking, can also be very helpful. Others emphasize the salutary effects of regular exercise, social support, or both, in dealing with depression. Remember, you are not alone on this journey of treating the manifestations of cardiovascular disease. According to clinical psychologist Dr. Judith Schwartzman, "Depression can be thought of as an extreme and prolonged response to stress." Yet, it can be overcome. Effectively dealing with depression can be a vital part of your personal health recovery.

DEPRESSION SCREENING TEST			
1.	I feel sad most of the time	Yes ____	No ____
2.	I don't enjoy the things I used to do	Yes ____	No ____
3.	I sleep too little or too much	Yes ____	No ____
4.	I don't feel like eating or eat too much	Yes ____	No ____
5.	I can't make decisions	Yes ____	No ____
6.	I have difficulty concentrating	Yes ____	No ____
7.	I feel hopeless	Yes ____	No ____
8.	I feel worthless	Yes ____	No ____
9.	I get tired for no reason	Yes ____	No ____
10.	I think about suicide*	Yes ____	No ____

Scoring:

If you answered "yes" to 4 or more of these questions, and you have felt this way every day for 2 weeks or more, you may be suffering from clinical depression and should consult a healthcare professional for a complete evaluation.

*If you answered "yes" to question #10, seek help immediately, regardless of your answer to any of the other questions.

Beyond Medications: The Healing Power of Inner Peace

Kavitha Chinnaiyan, M.D.

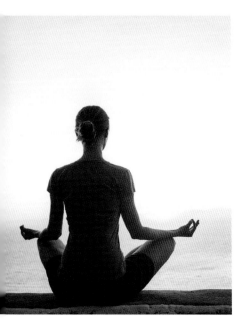

Technological advances and powerful new medications have changed the management of heart disease over the last two decades. Greater insights into disease mechanisms are continually reshaping the landscape of cardiovascular medicine. Importantly, the medical community is beginning to understand the power of the mind and its influence on not only disease causation, but also on the perception of disease. Depression, anxiety, stress and other psychosocial factors are not only risk factors for developing heart disease, but can be triggered by heart attacks, percutaneous or surgical procedures, congestive heart failure or other diagnoses. This observation is not unique to heart disease; any chronic illness can result in psychological disorders resulting in exponential suffering. These disorders result from the perceived loss of quality of life or functional status, fear of having another event and fear of death. These conditions in turn affect recovery of function, quality of life and long-term survival. Worry and anxiety negatively impact the ability to make positive changes in diet, physical activity and unhealthy behaviors such as smoking, further perpetuating the disease process.

Suffering is the result of becoming identified with the perceived cause of distress or pain. Reflecting and ruminating over loss of health or quality of life arise from reliving the past, while worry and fear of future cardiac events result from projecting into the future. Although medications can help with psychological stressors, effective strategies that result in mindfulness during daily activities are found to be increasingly beneficial.

Mindfulness is heightened self-awareness that supports non-judgmental observation of passing emotional states, bodily sensations and thought forms, resulting in mental stillness and inner peace. The ability to focus on immediate experience without reference to the past or future is the goal of yoga and other esoteric practices. In addition to improved sleep and greater relaxation, mindfulness results in greater acceptance of the disease state and life situations, openness to ongoing experience, curiosity and forgiveness.

Quieting of the mind's incessant commentary results in lowered blood pressure and inflammatory markers via the autonomic nervous system. Cultivation of inner peace via mindfulness is associated with greater self-care related to chronic illness and increased motivation to make impactful lifestyle changes. Present moment awareness results in the ability to choose diet and activity without being driven by habit or conditioning.

Meditation is the most effective method for cultivating inner silence. A twice-daily practice of breath awareness is simple and transformative, impacting all facets of life including health, well-being and relationships. In the context of inner peace, suffering becomes optional in the presence of bodily pain and distress.

As important as technological advances and discovery of novel therapies are, they are incomplete without integration of mental and psychological processes that accompany chronic illnesses. Prescribing meditation instead of or as a complement to medications might have far-reaching beneficial effects on the management of heart disease.

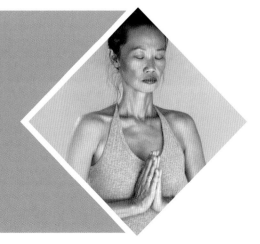

Studies find that a selected mind-body intervention (transcendental meditation) significantly reduced risk for mortality, myocardial infarction, and stroke in coronary heart disease patients.

(*Circulation: Cardiovascular Quality and Outcomes*, September 2016)

Yoga and Meditation for Heart Disease?

Kavitha Chinnaiyan, M.D.

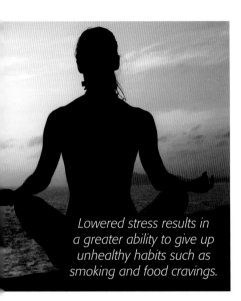

Lowered stress results in a greater ability to give up unhealthy habits such as smoking and food cravings.

Heart disease continues to be the number one killer in the United States and has rapidly become one of the major killers in most developing nations. Nevertheless, cardiovascular disease is largely a disease of "lifestyle" and therefore is preventable. Although genetic factors contribute to its development, a widely cited review of published research concluded that 75 to 90 percent of coronary artery disease incidence is explained by "lifestyle" risk factors, either alone or in combination. Thus, focusing on major cardiovascular risk factors (i.e., high blood pressure, elevated blood cholesterol, cigarette smoking, overweight/obesity, sedentary lifestyle, diabetes) and aggressive modification of them can save lives as demonstrated in numerous studies over the last few decades.

Psychosocial factors such as depression, anxiety, anger and social isolation also appear to play a role in the development of heart disease. It has become increasingly apparent that 10 to 25 percent of the "unexplained" heart disease may be partially attributed to psychosocial risk factors, demonstrating the power of the mind-body connection and lending credibility to the ancient wisdom that we are more than our bodies. Accordingly, identification and alleviation of these conditions may not only decrease the incidence of heart disease and its ramifications, but also promote overall well-being. This is where yoga and meditation come in.

Yoga is often viewed primarily as a popular fitness activity designed to improve strength, vitality and flexibility through challenging exercises. In reality, these exercises comprise just one component of yoga. Derived from the Sanskrit root, (yuj = union) yoga is a comprehensive science that strives for union or joining of the mind, body and spirit in awareness. The central and dominant practice of yoga is meditation, which is the systematic process of allowing the mind to become still for specific periods of time each day. By incorporating meditation, the main benefits of yoga can increasingly be experienced "off the mat" in how one handles the everyday stresses in life, as one cultivates the ability to experience deep contentment, peace and joy even amidst chaos. There are far-reaching benefits that come from a still mind as gleaned over the last few decades. Hundreds of studies have examined the effects of yoga and meditation on heart disease, repeatedly demonstrating significant improvements in not only conventional risk factors, but also in symptoms of heart disease, reduced need for cardioprotective medications and in the decreased rate of progression of atherosclerosis, the systemic process that leads to heart attacks and strokes.

In another study (*Circulation,* Nov. 2012), 201 African American patients with known coronary heart disease were randomized to a meditation-based program versus standard health education. Patients that meditated regularly cut their risk for death, heart attack and strokes by nearly half over a follow-up period of 5.4 years! How does this happen? Magnetic resonance imaging studies of long-term meditators show clear differences in the areas of the brain that "light up" compared to non-meditators—these areas correspond to parts of the brain involved in processing emotions, thoughts and most importantly, hormonal activity (for example, the pituitary gland). Moreover, meditation results in substantial lowering of stress hormones such as cortisol that plays pivotal roles in causing high blood pressure, high cholesterol and diabetes. Indirectly, lowered stress results in a greater ability to give up unhealthy habits such as smoking and food cravings.

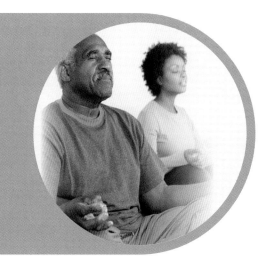

What was once a practice for a centered few has become mainstream American. In fact, at the present time, more than 15 million U.S. adults practice yoga. Not surprisingly, research exists supporting its physical benefits, including the reduction of both heart rate and blood pressure.

(*Monitor on Psychology—American Psychological Association*, November 2009)

Using Stress Management to Aid in Smoking Cessation

Kirk Hendrickson, M.S.

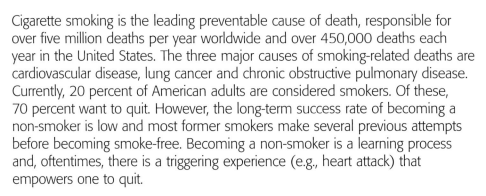

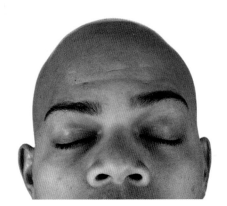

Cigarette smoking is the leading preventable cause of death, responsible for over five million deaths per year worldwide and over 450,000 deaths each year in the United States. The three major causes of smoking-related deaths are cardiovascular disease, lung cancer and chronic obstructive pulmonary disease. Currently, 20 percent of American adults are considered smokers. Of these, 70 percent want to quit. However, the long-term success rate of becoming a non-smoker is low and most former smokers make several previous attempts before becoming smoke-free. Becoming a non-smoker is a learning process and, oftentimes, there is a triggering experience (e.g., heart attack) that empowers one to quit.

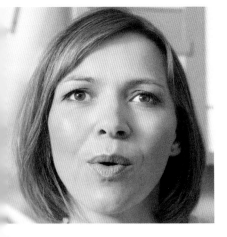

The smoking habit is strongly connected to many facets of the smoker's life. Smoking is also physically and emotionally addicting, making it very difficult to quit. A behavioral therapy program and the use of pharmacologic agents, such as nicotine replacement therapy like Zyban or Chantix, can enhance the likelihood of becoming an ex-smoker. An individual's personal readiness to change is also important in the quitting process.

Emotional stress is a part of every day life, but learning how to manage stress is crucial in achieving a balanced and healthy life. Increased stress has been associated with an increased frequency of smoking. Moreover, emotions like stress or anger are reported by smokers as the number one smoking trigger, as well as a trigger for former smokers to return to the smoking habit. Intuitively, it seems that learning effective stress management techniques can help to achieve smoking cessation.

When stress occurs, a smoker's learned response is to reach for a cigarette to relax. However, the nicotine in cigarettes is actually a stimulant that transiently raises the heart rate and blood pressure. Simultaneously, carbon monoxide decreases the oxygen carrying capacity of the blood. This "relaxing" response is merely a comfortable and familiar behavior that the smoker has learned. Additionally, the nicotine and other chemicals in the cigarettes are feeding the addiction. Thus, these responses actually increase stress on the body.

A proven technique for relaxing is known as diaphragmatic breathing, involving deep breathing from the diaphragm instead of the chest. The diaphragm is a muscle located just below the ribs. Breathing from the diaphragm involves slow deep breaths where the abdomen expands, moving air in and out of the lungs. Take slow, deep breaths; pause for a moment with your lips together and exhale all the air slowly, as if you were blowing up a balloon. Breathing from the diaphragm promotes relaxation in the body, as opposed to the shallow, rapid, chest breathing that occurs when you are anxious. This deep breathing technique and other therapies, such as yoga or tai chi, elicit what is known as the relaxation response.

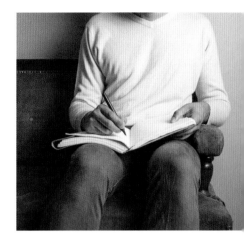

Other stress management techniques include progressive muscle relaxation, which involves tensing and relaxing groups of muscles from head to toe. Tension is maintained for seven to 10 seconds followed by relaxation for 15 to 20 seconds before moving to another group of muscles. Even short bouts of walking (as little as five to 10 minutes), especially if repeated throughout the day, can help with stress management, improve health and replace the habit of smoking. Combining deep breathing and guided imagery or visualization has also proven useful. Moreover, active problem solving techniques and journaling can assist in favorably modifying the stressors of daily life.

All of these techniques should be regularly practiced to replace unhealthy, longstanding stress responses. Since quitting smoking and the symptoms of nicotine withdrawal (including irritability, insomnia, fatigue, headache, inability to concentrate) may provide additional stress on a smoker, it is best to develop an improved response to stressors before establishing a quit date. Additionally, smokers should get plenty of rest, exercise regularly, drink water to fight urges, eat a healthy balanced diet and take a multivitamin. Taking steps to relax and pamper oneself by reading a good book, indulging in a hot bath, or getting a massage are also important. The symptoms of nicotine withdrawal are temporary and last over a couple of weeks but can be overcome. Keys to success include a positive attitude, self-talk and a good support system.

Controlling stress is a critical component in the toolbox used in smoking cessation. Having a strong desire to become a non-smoker, confidence in managing stress, along with a behavioral therapy program and medications to tame urges and decrease the symptoms of nicotine withdrawal will ultimately increase the likelihood of becoming smoke-free. Persistence is the key to success. This goal is well worth the effort in improving health and quality of life.

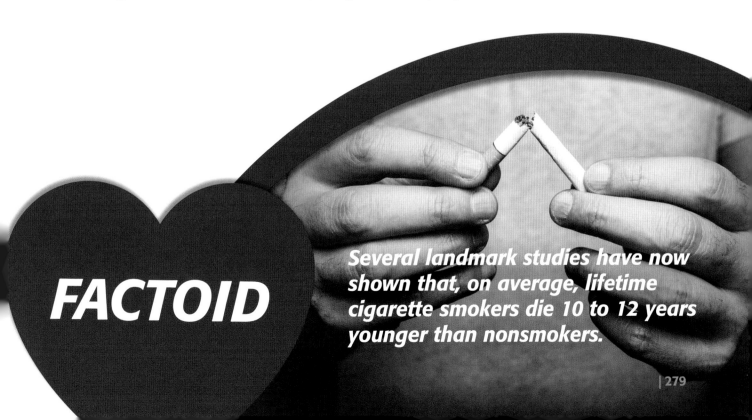

FACTOID

Several landmark studies have now shown that, on average, lifetime cigarette smokers die 10 to 12 years younger than nonsmokers.

Can Pets Influence Our Response to Stress?

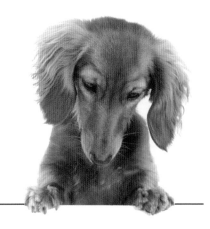

Angela Fern, M.S.

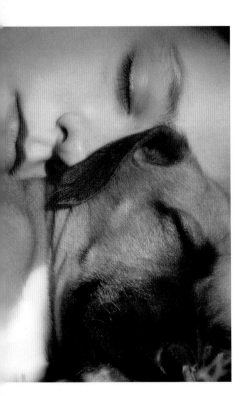

Pets are increasingly used for advertising products on television and in magazines. We see animals in movies and Internet clips. Many businesses now allow their employees to bring their pets to work on selected days each year. Since 78.2 million dogs and 86.4 million cats 'have homes' in the United States, it is apparent that Americans are smitten with their pets. I've often wondered, "Do our pets help us deal with stress?"

Although the term "stress" is understood by young and old alike, the meaning is relative. Stressors, which are triggers for stress, are not the same for every person. Our individual reaction to a stressor can make all the difference in our body's response to it. All people, regardless of circumstance, experience stress, either eustress (good stress) or distress (bad stress) including the hassles of day-to-day living. It is one of the risk factors for coronary artery disease that is considered "modifiable," which means that a positive change in our behavior can influence it. Unfortunately, chronic stress can have serious consequences. For example, takotsubo cardiomyopathy ("broken heart syndrome") is a condition that causes heart attack-like signs and symptoms that is believed to be precipitated by stressful life events.

There are three stages of stress, which are collectively known as the General Adaptation Syndrome. Stage I is the alarm phase involving the "fight or flight" response, where hormones such as adrenaline and cortisol are released. In this stage, increases in heart rate, blood pressure, and breathing occur. Traffic congestion, hassles at work, or family arguments are examples of typical stressors. The second stage is known as resistance, in which we may experience stressful responses over time. The last stage is termed exhaustion because long term stress responses are believed to negatively affect our health, such as increasing risks for chronic disease, digestive problems, weight gain, depression and sleep disorders.

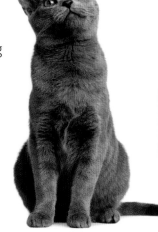

Stress management is an important coping tool for everyone. As individuals, we respond to stress and subsequently, stress relief, differently. While people may disagree on which method is the best to deal with stress, it is vital that common stressors are recognized and handled. At the positive end of the spectrum is eustress, for example, planning a wedding or hosting family for the holidays, which usually ends well. However, the timeline to the finale can be wrought with many stressors. Distress can come in the form of a job loss, the death of a loved one, or as post traumatic stress disorder. The stress response can be severe and lasting and may contribute to chronic illness.

Pets, in addition to other factors, can play a role in reducing stress. There are many interventions to achieve stress management, which include "psychosocial support, regular exercise, stress reduction training, sense of humor, optimism, altruism, faith, and pet ownership" (*Current Atherosclerosis Reports,* Mar. 2006). Additionally, the web site, WebMD, lists several suggestions for ways to relax the body and mind, which include regular physical activity, breathing exercises, gardening, writing and playing with or caring for pets.

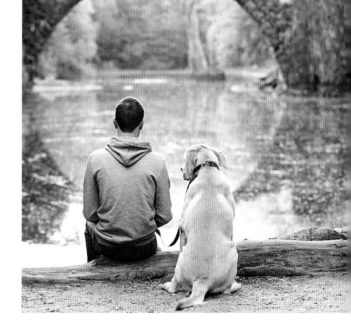

In one study that examined cardiovascular reactivity, when pets (dogs or cats) were present, their owners had lower heart rates and blood pressure at rest, during mental arithmetic (where they also made the least amount of mistakes) and during hand submersion in ice water than when their spouses or friends were present. It was concluded that "pets can buffer reactivity to acute stress as well as diminish perceptions of stress" (*Psychosomatic Medicine,* Sept.-Oct. 2002). In another study that also tested mental stress in subjects performing mental arithmetic, all participants were taking the blood pressure drug, lisinopril. Subjects that also owned pets (dogs or cats) had significantly lower heart rate and blood pressure responses to mental stress than those taking the drug alone (*Hypertension,* Oct. 2001). In conclusion, research suggests that pets can help us feel better and relax. So the next time you feel stressed, spend some quality time with your favorite pet to reduce the associated demands on your heart.

Optimistic Heart Patients Live Longer

Barry A. Franklin, Ph.D.

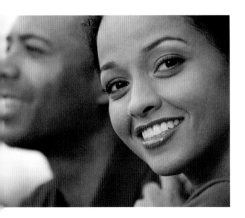

Today, increasing numbers of heart patients are entering their 70s, 80s, and 90s, often outliving their counterparts without heart disease. In our experience, these tend to be patients who take care of themselves and perhaps equally important, develop the mind-set necessary to deal with the challenges of heart disease.

Today, there is considerable evidence in the psychosocial literature to suggest that we get what we expect and attract what we fear. Invariably, those heart patients who not only survive but thrive believe they can achieve longevity and a high quality of life. A classic example is my good friend and esteemed colleague, Joe Piscatella, who had triple vessel coronary artery bypass surgery at the age of 32. He's now 71 years of age.

Several years ago, researchers at Duke University Medical Center tracked the health outcomes of 2,818 patients who had just undergone coronary angiography, a procedure used to confirm their underlying heart disease. At the time, all were given a brief questionnaire to assess how much or how little optimism they felt about their long-term prognosis (*Archives of Internal Medicine,* Feb. 2011).

Over the next 15 years, 1,637 of the study patients had died, and about half of the deaths were related to heart disease. The researchers found that favorable expectations were a strong predictor of overall survival. Patients who scored low on optimism tests were 30 percent more likely to die during the follow-up period, even after the researchers controlled for potential confounding variables, including age, gender, heart disease severity, other medical conditions, and depression. These findings add to a compelling body of scientific evidence that supporting optimistic expectations may be associated with significant survival benefits.

The authors suggested two possible reasons why optimism may lead to better cardiovascular outcomes. First, the optimistic patient may be more likely to heed the doctor's advice, take prescribed medications and adopt long-term lifestyle changes, compared with a pessimistic patient. Second, optimism may help buffer the health consequences associated with chronic stress and anxiety.

I vividly remember counseling a new patient in our cardiac rehab program. Bill, a 48-year-old truck driver in good physical condition, had recently experienced a mild heart attack. His face was racked with anxiety and depression—he clearly thought his life was over and that he was on "borrowed time."

I reviewed his medical records and found that his ejection fraction after the heart attack, a key index of heart function and survival, was still within the normal range. His fitness from a post-heart attack exercise stress test was "high" for a healthy man his age. Thus, two key prognostic indicators were in his favor. "If you take care of yourself, you've probably got many, many years ahead of you," I told him.

Heart patients often assume the worst. We've got to do a better job in promoting hope and optimism. By doing so, especially when it's truly justified, we may be helping them greatly—perhaps more than we'll ever know.

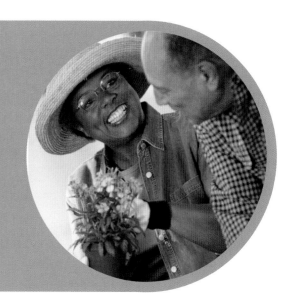

CARDIAC PATIENTS WITH POSITIVE ATTITUDES LIKELY TO EXERCISE, LIVE LONGER

Researchers used a questionnaire to assess the moods of 607 heart patients in a Denmark hospital. Five years later the investigators found that the most positive patients exercised more and had a 42 percent reduced risk of dying (from any cause). Importantly, exercise acted as a mediator in the relationship between well-being and reduced mortality.

(*Circulation: Cardiovascular Quality and Outcomes,* Sept. 2013)

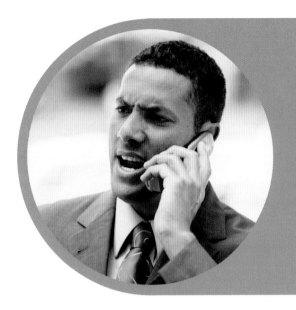

OUTBURSTS OF ANGER AND THE RISK OF A HEART ATTACK

In an analysis of nearly 3,900 patients who were interviewed during their hospitalization for a confirmed heart attack or acute myocardial infarction (AMI), the risk of experiencing AMI was more than two-fold greater after outbursts of anger compared with at other times. Moreover, greater intensities of anger were associated with greater relative risks of cardiac events triggered by anger. Compared with nonusers, regular beta-blocker users had a lower susceptibility to heart attacks triggered by episodes of anger.

(*American Journal of Cardiology*, Aug. 2013)

SOCIAL SUPPORT AND HEALTH OUTCOMES AFTER A HEART ATTACK

A widely-cited study found that among patients 55 years of age or younger who survived heart attacks, those with low perceived social support had poorer mental health status, quality of life, and more depressive symptoms 12 months after their cardiac event. These findings, which held for both men and women, have implications for subsequent interventions for such patients, including support groups and/ or exercise-based cardiac rehabilitation.

(*Journal of the American Heart Association,* Sept. 2014)

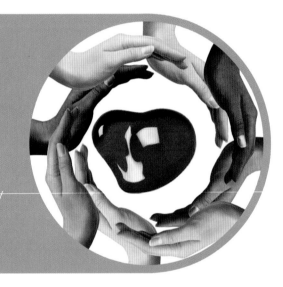

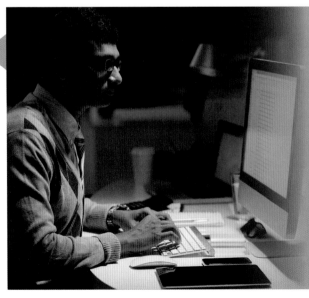

WARNING: WORKAHOLISM MAY BE HAZARDOUS TO YOUR HEART HEALTH

According to one study, people who routinely work 11 or more hours per day had a 60 percent higher risk for heart-related problems, including fatal heart attacks and anginal chest pain, as compared with people who maintained a conventional eight-hour work day. Why? People who often work long hours tend to be type A personalities—aggressive, overcommitted and competitive. Researchers believe that these characteristics can lead to unhealthy lifestyles and high stress levels (*European Heart Journal,* July 2010).

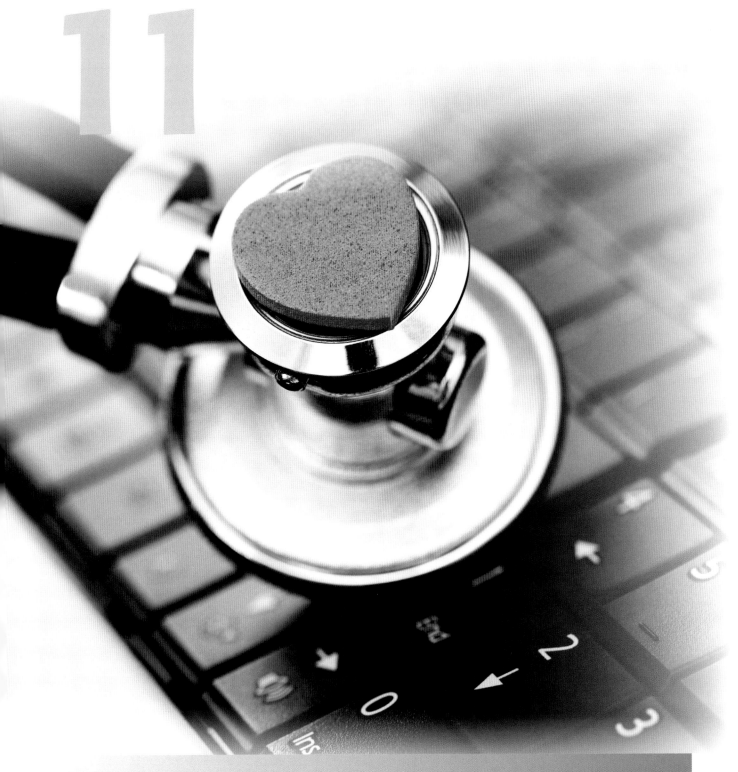

CHAPTER
11

RELATED CARDIOVASCULAR ISSUES/TREATMENTS

Pulmonary Hypertension: The Other High Blood Pressure

Samuel Allen, DO
Jacqueline Brewer, RN

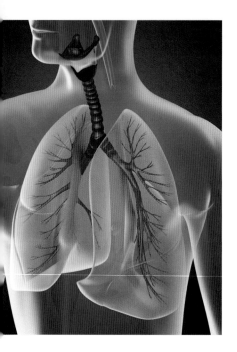

High blood pressure within the lungs is known as pulmonary hypertension, or PH. This form of high blood pressure, which is unlike systemic high blood pressure (commonly called "high blood pressure"), is caused when the small blood vessels within the lungs become thicker and cause the opening inside the vessel to narrow. Therefore, these vessels cannot carry as much blood to deliver oxygen to the body. This affects not only the lungs but also the heart. Over time, this high pressure puts strain on the heart causing the right side of the heart to fail.

Symptoms of PH are often confused with other respiratory or lung conditions and therefore commonly misdiagnosed, or diagnosed at a later time. These symptoms include breathlessness, swollen ankles and legs, chest pain, dizziness, fainting, and fatigue. These symptoms can occur during activity or simply at rest. With PH, "the worse you feel, the sicker you probably are."

A diagnosis occurs through the process of exclusion, or the ruling out of other diseases. Many tests are conducted including but not limited to an ultrasound of the heart, blood testing, a lung scan, chest x-ray, six-minute walk test, a sleep study, pulmonary function testing, and ultimately a right heart catheterization. The right heart catheterization is considered the "gold standard" test for diagnosing PH since it is the only test to precisely measure the pressure within the vessels.

PH can be classified into 5 different groups. When PH is triggered from another disease, it is called secondary. Treatment for secondary PH involves treating the underlying disease only to decrease the pressure within the vessels. When PH is the result of an unknown cause we call it "primary PH," and it is known as pulmonary arterial hypertension, or PAH. PAH is what we refer to as an "orphan disease," due to the fact that this is an extremely rare disease, reported to have an incidence of 15 cases per 1 million people. PAH affects women more than men by a factor of 2.5. Treatment for PAH has expanded considerably in the last 3 years. There are now 14 FDA-approved therapies ranging from oral, inhaled, intravenous, and subcutaneous medications. There are also many clinical trials that are available to those diagnosed with PAH.

Varicose Veins:
The Blue Epidemic

Amr Abbas, M.D.

Varicose veins are the most common cardiovascular disease manifestation, exceeding the incidence of heart disease, peripheral artery disease and stroke combined. The condition affects both men and women; however, it is more frequently found in women. Normally, veins have one-way valves that direct the flow of blood from the feet upward, toward the heart, and from the skin inward, preventing it from leaking backward due to gravity. If these valves become defective, blood may leak backward causing swelling at the ankle, spider and varicose veins and, in advanced stages, skin discoloration and ulcers in the leg. This is known as venous insufficiency.

People who are overweight, work in occupations that require prolonged standing, including physicians, nurses, police officers and teachers, as well as individuals with a family history of varicose veins, are more likely to develop this condition.

Treatment is initially directed at wearing compression stockings and decreasing the intake of dietary salt. If this approach fails, leaking veins can be collapsed with a long tube that is advanced through them with laser or radiofrequency energy. The procedure is known as endovenous ablation, requires only local anesthesia, takes 30 to 45 minutes and is relatively pain-free. The large varicose veins are then either removed through very small incisions or injected with a chemical substance to collapse them.

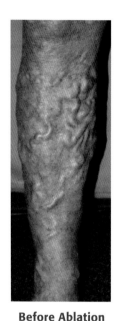

Before Ablation   **After Ablation**

Normal Vein   **Varicose Vein**

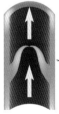 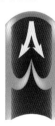 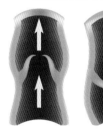

Valve   Valve
Open   Closed   Leaky Valve

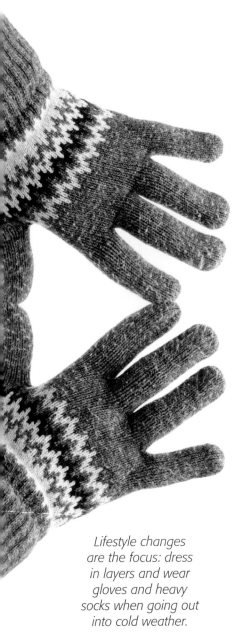

Lifestyle changes are the focus: dress in layers and wear gloves and heavy socks when going out into cold weather.

Raynaud's Disease: Tis the Season

Terry Bowers, M.D.

Definition and symptoms

Do you suffer from painful discoloration of your fingers or toes in cold weather? You're not alone; approximately 3 to 5 percent of people in cold climates experience symptoms of Raynaud's disease. It is more than just having cold hands or feet, but it's not frostbite. Women are affected more often than men (approximately 75 percent of the cases), typically between the ages of 15 and 40. The disorder is characterized by episodic spasms called vasospastic attacks that cause the small arteries in the fingers or toes to constrict and limit blood flow to that digit.

The symptoms range from discoloration to tingling, numbness or severe pain. An attack affects just one or two fingers or toes, with different attacks not necessarily affecting the same digits. The duration of the symptoms is variable but can persist until the hand or foot is warmed. A person with Raynaud's can experience three phases of skin color change: whiteness when blood flow is interrupted, blueness because the fingers/toes are not getting enough oxygen-rich blood or redness when blood flow returns.

Causes and diagnosis

Raynaud's disease is caused by an overactive response of the small blood vessels in your fingers or toes to cold or emotional stress. It is not associated with an underlying disease process such as lupus or scleroderma. If you have severe small vessel vasospasm due to inflammatory diseases such as lupus, atherosclerotic vascular disease, trauma, or connective tissue disease then you have a secondary condition called Raynaud's phenomenon. However, most people with Raynaud's disease do not have an underlying disease. The diagnosis therefore is made on clinical grounds. All the testing performed is to rule out an underlying disease. There is no lab test that can be done to establish primary Raynaud's disease.

Treatment

The goal of treatment is to reduce the severity and frequency of attacks. Lifestyle changes are the focus: dress in layers and wear gloves and heavy socks when going out into cold weather. Small heating pouches that can be placed in pockets, mittens and boots can give added protection. Avoid holding cold drinks, frozen foods or touching cold metals. Hats are particularly important to avoid chilling because a great deal of body heat is lost through an exposed scalp. It is important to avoid cigarette smoking or secondhand smoke as these increase vascular vasoconstriction. Also practice good skin care by keeping your hands/feet moisturized. If conservative measures fail there are medications that can be used to dilate blood vessels and decrease the attacks, including calcium channel blockers, alpha blockers and vasodilators.

You should see your doctor if you are concerned about the attacks, or if you develop sores or ulcers on your fingers or toes. If attacks always affect the same finger or toe on only one side then secondary Raynaud's is more likely and should be evaluated by your doctor.

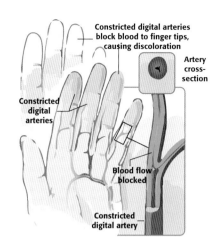

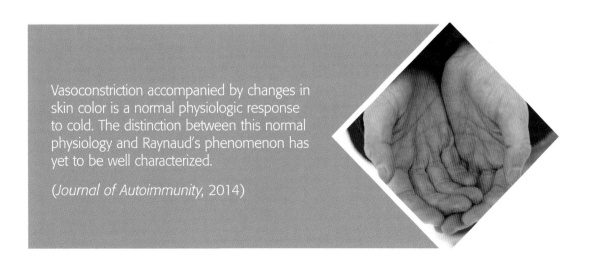

Vasoconstriction accompanied by changes in skin color is a normal physiologic response to cold. The distinction between this normal physiology and Raynaud's phenomenon has yet to be well characterized.

(*Journal of Autoimmunity*, 2014)

Venous Thromboembolism: A Clot in the Vein That Can Be Deadly

Terry Bowers, M.D.

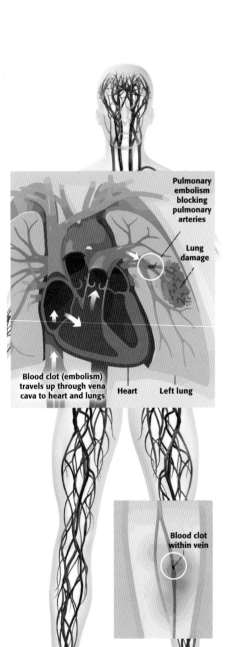

Pulmonary embolism blocking pulmonary arteries

Lung damage

Blood clot (embolism) travels up through vena cava to heart and lungs

Heart

Left lung

Blood clot within vein

We all know people that seemed to be healthy, developed leg pain or swelling and then died suddenly. The medical terminology for this condition is deep venous thrombosis (DVT), which causes leg swelling and pain due to a clot in the leg vein. If the clot breaks away and travels in the venous system to the lung where it lodges in the pulmonary artery it is called a pulmonary embolism (PE), which is a common, lethal disorder that affects hospitalized and non-hospitalized patients. Venous thromboembolism (DVT and/or PE) results from a combination of hereditary and acquired risk factors. The risk for this disorder is increased in people with cancer, infection, severe acute medical illness, immobilization, a prior history of venous clotting, smokers, the elderly (over 75 years), and patients after orthopedic and major surgery.

Venous thromboembolism is the third most common cardiovascular disorder after heart attack and stroke. It is believed that there are approximately 1 million cases in the U.S. each year, accounting for an estimated 300,000 deaths per year.

PE is also the third most common cause of hospital-related death, yet is the most common preventable cause of hospital-related death. The key to prevention is diligent attention to those patients at risk with anticoagulation therapy and leg compression devices, which can reduce the occurrence of this killer by as much as 70 percent.

Although prevention is the best treatment, early detection is essential in patients who develop venous clotting to keep it from migrating to the lung. If suspected, an ultrasound of the leg veins should be done as soon as possible to identify the clot. This is a simple test to perform that does not cause any discomfort. Once a clot travels to the lung, patients develop shortness of breath, cough (occasionally with blood), high heart rates and experience chest pain that worsens with breathing. Unfortunately, it can also cause sudden collapse and death. If PE is suspected, a computed tomographic scan of the chest is performed to evaluate the lung arteries for a blood clot.

Treatment is focused on blood thinners (anticoagulants) that keep the clots from progressing and allow the body to dissolve the clot. In extreme cases we can give blood clot dissolving medications called thrombolytics. There is now a new oral form of anticoagulation called Xarelto that has greatly simplified treatment of patients with these disorders. Numerous medical centers are actively involved in research efforts to improve outcomes of patients with venous thromboembolism.

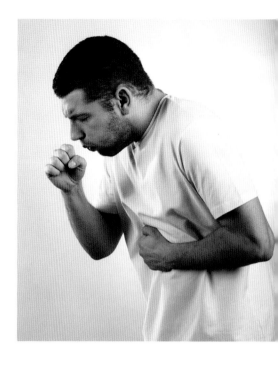

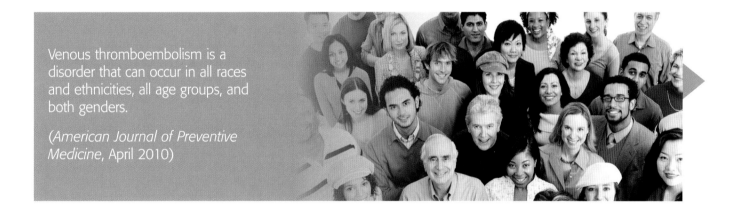

Venous thromboembolism is a disorder that can occur in all races and ethnicities, all age groups, and both genders.

(*American Journal of Preventive Medicine*, April 2010)

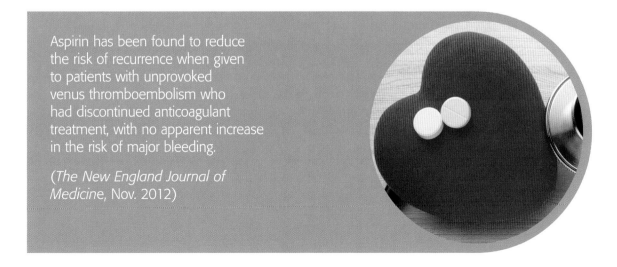

Aspirin has been found to reduce the risk of recurrence when given to patients with unprovoked venus thromboembolism who had discontinued anticoagulant treatment, with no apparent increase in the risk of major bleeding.

(*The New England Journal of Medicine*, Nov. 2012)

Novel Clot Extraction Techniques for Pulmonary Embolism

Terry Bowers, M.D.

Extensive pulmonary emboli in both left and right lungs

Clots that develop in the legs can break loose and flow to the lung arteries where they obstruct flow. These clots are called pulmonary emboli (PE) and are very common, occurring in more than 500,000 people per year. There are many acquired and congenital risk factors that are known to increase the risk of PE. The clinical manifestations of PE are dependent upon how much of the lung is affected and how the right side of the heart responds. Consequences range from sudden death to those patients that have no symptoms. The treatment in those that are very sick is to eliminate the clot. Strategies to do so include anticoagulants that keep further clotting from occurring, followed by infusion of clot dissolving medications or mechanical removal of the clot with catheters or surgery. Clot dissolving medications called thrombolytics are proven to be effective in the sickest patients. Unfortunately, thrombolytics expose the patients to major bleeding, including a small but real risk of bleeding into the brain. Surgery for PE is reserved for those patients that don't have other options because it requires open heart surgery. Thus, there is a gap between what we know about PE and what we currently have to treat patients.

Currently, clinicians are actively working on techniques to remove clots from the lungs in sick patients with PE without having to use clot dissolving medications. Intuitively, the lower the dose necessary, the lower the major bleeding risk. Our multidisciplinary team derives expertise from interventional cardiology and radiology, vascular and cardiothoracic surgery, pulmonary medicine, and hematology. The system approach is used to ideally enhance outcomes by improving survival, decreasing long term complications of the clot and to reduce the risk of therapy-related bleeding. Our goal is to develop a systematic approach that allows the physician to easily, rapidly and safely remove the entire clot from the pulmonary artery in a single setting with a cost effective strategy. There are three promising new devices that are being studied in patients with PE to achieve that goal: the Angiovac system, Indigo system and the FlowTriever system.

The Angiovac system uses a large bore catheter with a balloon expanded opening that aggressively vacuums the clots from large veins in the body and filters them from the blood. We have used this system to remove extensive amounts of clot from the inferior vena cava in several patients who had no other viable option. New developments in this system now make it possible to use it to remove clots from the lung arteries.

Another device is called the FlowTriever, which has an oversized catheter that can be tracked from the neck vein or the groin vein up to the lung artery. A self-expanding cage is maneuvered into the large clot, the cage retracts and the clot is suctioned out simultaneously.

The third device is called the Indigo system, which uses a smaller catheter that is easy to track up to the affected lung branches. The Indigo catheter has a simple suction system and a clot separator that breaks the clot into pieces, allowing it to be suctioned out without clogging the catheter. This simple system may be highly effective in selected patients with PE.

More research is necessary to identify the most effective and safest strategy to remove the pulmonary artery clots that can lead to low blood pressures and even death due to right heart failure. These new devices offer promise to achieve clot removal with a low risk of bleeding.

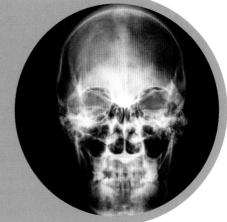

On average, a stroke occurs every 40 seconds in the United States, resulting in someone dying from a stroke every four minutes, which speaks to the need to develop more effective drugs, cures, and procedures to treat stroke.

(*Science Daily*, February 2013)

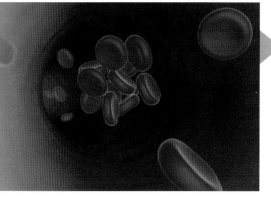

The optimal initial treatment for a clot-caused (ischemic) stroke remains intravenous delivery of the clot-busting medication tissue plasminogen activator (tpa). When given within a few hours of stroke symptoms, tpa can dissolve the clot and reestablish blood flow to the brain, limiting stroke disability.

(*American Heart Association Focused Update*, June 2015)

Patent Foramen Ovale: A Common Finding but a Rare Problem

George S. Hanzel, M.D.

Patent foramen ovale

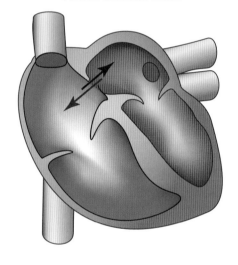

As medical imaging continues to improve, we frequently find "abnormalities" that just a generation ago would have gone undetected. Fortunately, these "abnormalities" are often really normal variants that infrequently cause harm. One such "abnormality" is a hole in the heart called a patent foramen ovale (PFO).

Prior to birth, everyone has a hole in the wall that separates the two upper chambers of the heart, the right and left atrium. In most people the hole closes shortly after birth. However, the hole does not completely seal in 20 to 25 percent of people. This flap is called a PFO. The PFO is frequently discovered incidentally when a patient undergoes an echocardiogram (an ultrasound of the heart) for other reasons.

For the vast majority of people, PFOs pose no clinical consequence and do not require any treatment or follow-up testing. For these persons reassurance is the best medicine. However, in a very small percentage of patients, PFOs can lead to stroke. A clot in a vein can break off and travel to the heart and through the PFO from the right atrium to the left atrium, and ultimately to the brain, causing a stroke. After one has a stroke due to a PFO the risk of having a recurrent stroke increases significantly.

The best treatment for patients with a PFO related stroke is controversial. Traditionally, patients have been treated with blood thinners, such as aspirin or warfarin. There are now minimally invasive techniques available to close PFOs. A small catheter, or tube, is inserted into the vein in the groin and advanced into the heart. The catheter is used to place a patch to cover and close the PFO.

Believe it or not, PFOs are also associated with migraine headaches. The lungs inactivate many chemicals in the bloodstream. Blood that travels through a PFO can carry chemicals that provoke migraines. It is thought that closure of the PFO might improve migraines.

Aneurysms: A Bubble in the Vascular System?

O. William Brown, M.D.

An aneurysm is a ballooning of an artery. It can occur anywhere in the body and most commonly involves the main artery called the aorta. The aorta carries blood from the heart and travels down the middle of the body. When it gets to the belly button, the aorta splits with one branch going to each leg. Like balloons, when an aneurysm gets too big it can pop or rupture. If the aorta ruptures, it can be fatal. Therefore, it is important to detect and treat aneurysms before they rupture. The likelihood of a successful recovery following an elective operation to repair an aortic aneurysm is approximately 98 percent. However, if an aneurysm is not treated until it ruptures, the chance of survival is 50 percent at best.

The best ways to diagnose an aortic aneurysm are with an ultrasound of the abdomen, a physical examination, or both. People who suddenly feel a large pulse in their abdomen should make an appointment to see their physician. People over the age of 65, or people who have a family history of aortic aneurysm, should undergo an ultrasound of the abdomen.

Symptoms associated with aortic aneurysms depend upon the location of the aneurysm. People who have aneurysms of the thoracic aorta (portion of the aorta in the chest) may develop chest pain, upper back pain or shortness of breath. People with aneurysms of the abdominal aorta may develop severe lower back pain or abdominal pain.

Aneurysms of the aorta that are larger than 5 centimeters (2 inches) usually require treatment. In the past, treatment required a large incision in the chest or abdomen and the replacement of the aneurismal segment with an artificial artery. Today, we can treat most aneurysms with stent grafts. These grafts are placed in the aorta through small incisions in each groin. Most people can go home the next day and resume full activity within one week.

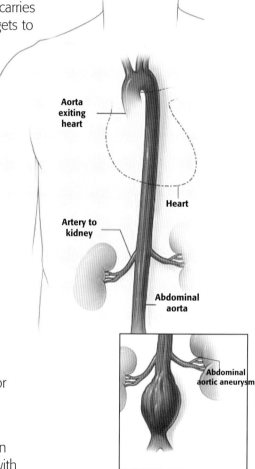

Aorta exiting heart

Heart

Artery to kidney

Abdominal aorta

Abdominal aortic aneurysm

Aortic Dissection: A Trigger for Sudden Cardiac Death

Jeffrey Altshuler, M.D.

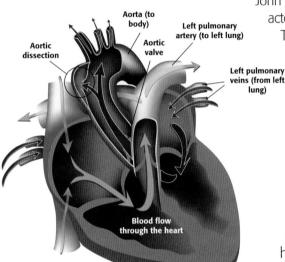

Aorta (to body)

Aortic dissection

Aortic valve

Left pulmonary artery (to left lung)

Left pulmonary veins (from left lung)

Blood flow through the heart

John Ritter, the son of famous country/western star Tex Ritter, was an American actor, comedian and voice-over artist. He was best known for playing Jack Tripper on the hit ABC sitcom Three's Company, for which he won an Emmy and a Golden Globe Award in 1984. Ritter died at the age of 54 from an aortic dissection on Sept. 11, 2003—ironically on 9/11.

Of all the events that can cause sudden cardiac death, one of the most overlooked is an aortic dissection. While not truly a "heart" problem, it is just as dire both in the short term and during a patient's lifetime.

The aorta is the main blood vessel that carries blood from the heart to branch arteries throughout the body. It is shaped like a candy cane as it passes through the chest. The first part called the ascending aorta feeds the coronary arteries, which provide oxygenated blood to the heart muscle. The aorta then curves, which is called the arch, giving off the subclavian arteries to arms and carotids to the brain before becoming the descending aorta passing through the chest into the abdomen.

Like all arteries the aorta is composed of three layers. A dissection occurs where there is a tear in the inner layer called the intima, allowing blood into the middle layer, peeling the layers apart. While this can happen anywhere in the aorta, the most common spots are in the ascending aorta just beyond the coronary arteries, in the descending aorta just past the left subclavian artery or, less commonly, in the arch. Once a dissection occurs, the tear can propagate forwards or backwards, which can block any of the branches of the aorta in the chest, abdomen or legs.

The most common symptoms of a dissection are sudden severe chest or back pain, often described as being hit by an axe. If the dissection blocks major arteries there may also be symptoms related to lack of blood flow in the organs supplied by those arteries.

Seeking immediate medical care is imperative as this is truly a life threatening situation. Without treatment, 1 percent of people with dissections will die each hour and 90 percent will die within two weeks.

Treatment depends on the location of the dissection. If the ascending aorta is involved, immediate surgery is undertaken to replace that portion of the aorta. If the ascending aorta is spared and the dissection is limited to the distal aorta, the initial treatment involves blood pressure control and intensive care unit monitoring. Once the acute event has been treated, patients with dissections must be monitored for the remainder of their lives for adverse aortic changes. They can live a normal life; however, they must monitor their blood pressure closely and avoid vigorous or high intensity activities, which may involve straining.

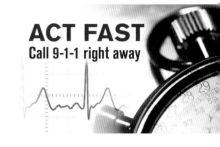

People who are at higher risk for aortic dissections include those who are hypertensive (particularly untreated), and those with a bicuspid aortic valve or a family history of dissection at a young age. Nevertheless, more than 70 percent of dissections are in hypertensive individuals.

In addition, there are several genetic disorders of the connective tissue, including Marfans Syndrome, Loeys-Dietz syndrome and Ehlers-Danlos syndrome that are associated with a high risk of dissection. People with aortic aneurysms (particularly if they are large) are at increased risk of experiencing aortic dissection; however, dissections can and do occur in normal sized aortas.

Currently, there are no screening tests to determine if a person is at risk for aortic dissection. However, if there is a family history of dissection, aneurysm, sudden cardiac death or the genetic conditions previously mentioned, an echocardiogram or computed tomographic scanning may be helpful. If you, or a friend or loved one experiences the excruciating symptoms associated with aortic dissection, remember the actor John Ritter, and dial 911.

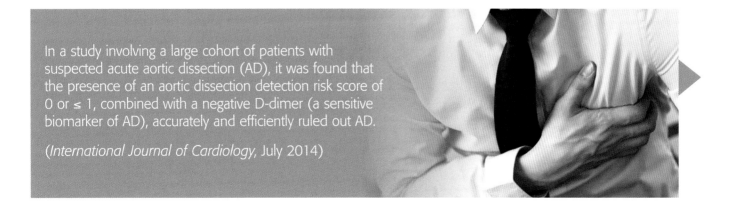

In a study involving a large cohort of patients with suspected acute aortic dissection (AD), it was found that the presence of an aortic dissection detection risk score of 0 or ≤ 1, combined with a negative D-dimer (a sensitive biomarker of AD), accurately and efficiently ruled out AD.

(*International Journal of Cardiology*, July 2014)

Cardio-Oncology: New Issues Created by Treatment and Survival

Terry R. Bowers, M.D.

Research is currently ongoing to determine if patients with a weakened heart muscle that need a specific cancer treatment can safely receive that therapy if used in conjunction with selected cardioprotective agents.

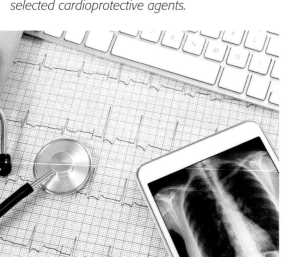

As modern-day patients increasingly survive previously fatal cancers, these survivors often develop and ultimately die from some sort of heart disease. The ultimate goal for patients with cancer is to prolong survival, maintain a good quality of life, and limit the cardiotoxic effects of therapy. It is clear that emerging chemotherapeutics, although effective, have an undeniable cardiovascular risk.

The toxicity of therapy comes in three forms: radiation that leads to premature coronary disease, pericardial disease and valvular heart disease; chemotherapeutics that target the heart muscle, potentially leading to congestive heart failure and cardiac arrest; and, direct effects of chemotherapeutics on the vascular system, leading to hypertension and thromboembolism, clots that can result in stroke and pulmonary embolism.

The reason for the adverse effects is that the heart and vascular tissue have a high rate of metabolism, similar to cancer cells, which is the target of the chemotherapeutics. Some of the adverse effects are immediate, but most occur long after cancer treatment is completed, oftentimes two to 10 years later.

Oncologists have recognized this risk and increasingly have consulted cardiologists to care for these patients since they are surviving to the point that the adverse effects are manifested.

Collaboration between oncologists and cardiologists is necessary in this growing arena; however, there are no current guidelines available to gauge risk assessment and tailor therapy for cancer patients at risk for cardiovascular disease. Patient education about the potential cardiotoxicity and symptoms attributable to the development of heart disease is an important first step. Baseline cardiac evaluations with electrocardiograms and echocardiograms in patients receiving potentially cardiotoxic chemotherapy is essential.

Repeat studies are performed once signs/symptoms develop or at intervals that are not yet defined in the absence of these harbingers. In addition, there are exciting current research initiatives to identify echocardiographic changes and abnormal blood tests that appear before the heart muscle weakens, allowing the oncologist to modify the therapy before irreversible damage occurs. Once these adverse effects are noted, we need to develop and implement best practice treatment strategies that are currently not available. Cardio-oncology research is now focusing on identifying specific types of heart muscle weakening that occur with chemotherapeutics, using magnetic resonance imaging and echocardiography to identify them.

The next step is to determine whether patients at risk can be treated with cardiac medications before or during their cancer treatments that will help protect their heart and vascular system. Prevention of cardiotoxicity is of the utmost importance. Cardiac medications called angiotensin receptor blockers, angiotensin-converting enzyme inhibitors, and beta-blockers have been shown to prevent a decline in heart function if used early in those adversely affected. Research is currently ongoing to determine if patients with a weakened heart muscle that need a specific cancer treatment can safely receive that therapy if used in conjunction with selected cardioprotective agents.

Lastly, new cancer treatments are developing rapidly. Cardiology researchers should be involved early in their development to better understand their cardiovascular effects and potentially minimize adverse outcomes. The strategy of cardiology consultation for cancer patients that have developed cardiac decompensation is now evolving into a collaboration between cardiologists and oncologists to prevent, screen, detect and treat these patients proactively. Cardio-oncology is an emerging area that will translate to better outcomes for our patients.

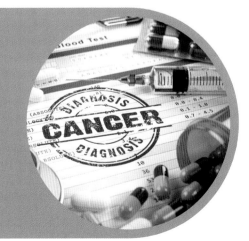

According to the American Heart Association, cardiovascular disease, which includes heart disease as well as strokes and diseases of the blood vessels, claims more lives than the next five leading causes of death combined, including cancer.

(*Journal of The National Cancer Institute*, July 2005)

Countering Brain Injury With Therapeutic Hypothermia

William Devlin, M.D.

Clinicians have long known the potential benefits of altered body temperature in treating certain medical emergencies. The greatest benefit comes from cooling to lower temperatures. Recently, there has been a heightened interest in the use of therapeutic hypothermia for the treatment of patients who experience cardiac arrest (i.e., abrupt cessation of heartbeat). The idea behind this is that lowering body temperature can preserve brain function in such patients, reducing the likelihood of brain injury.

For many years, emergency rooms have had to warm up people who suffered drowning in cold water because they found that when body temperature drops, individuals can go into a hibernation state. The old adage is "never pronounce a cold body." Patients who were thought to be dead or to have little chance of survival without brain damage have survived and demonstrated miraculous recoveries.

Although we are not exactly sure how therapeutic hypothermia works, it is clear that there can be significant benefits when it is applied. The most important aspect about resuscitating an individual who experiences a potentially lethal heart rhythm is to provide immediate cardiopulmonary support: cardiopulmonary resuscitation or CPR. It is still recommended that everyone be familiar with basic life support techniques to help increase the chance of someone surviving a cardiac arrest. Classes in basic life support are available through the American Heart Association, Red Cross and your local hospital. Activating advanced life support by calling 911 is also critically important.

The idea behind therapeutic hypothermia is that lowering body temperature can preserve brain function in such patients, reducing the likelihood of brain injury.

Individuals who experience a cardiac arrest either outside the hospital or even while in a medical facility are considered for therapeutic hypothermia. It can be administered in several ways, either through cooling pads outside the body or through a catheter that is inserted into a central vein. The cooling protocol generally runs for 24 hours and then the patient is allowed to rewarm slowly. This can often be a stressful situation for family members, but is being widely used as an attempt to preserve brain function and activity.

Hopefully you and your families will never have to go through an experience like this. Fortunately, an increasing number of hospitals have the capability of using therapeutic hypothermia to potentially counter brain injury in patients who are successfully resuscitated from a cardiac arrest.

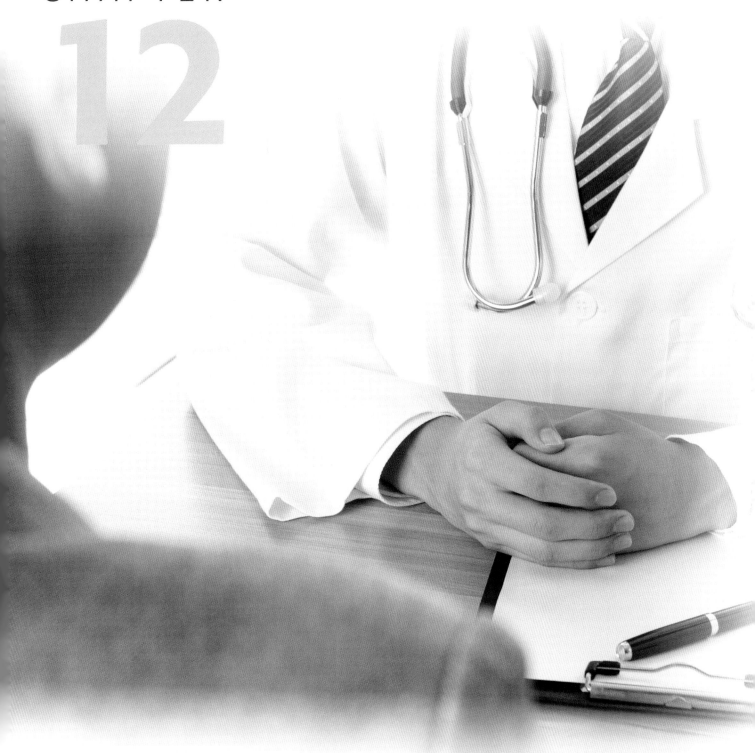

CHAPTER
12

ASK THE
CARDIOLOGIST
Robert N. Levin, M.D.

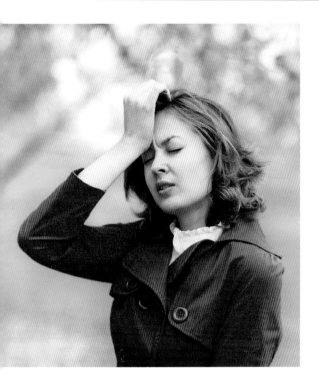

Question: One of my co-workers recently received some very upsetting news by phone, leading her to develop chest pain and what seemed like a heart attack. At the hospital, she was told that she had "Broken Heart Syndrome," and her heart pump function returned to normal several days later. Is this possible?

Answer: Yes. "Broken Heart Syndrome," also known as Takotsubo cardiomyopathy (named after a round-bottomed narrow-necked Japanese ceramic fishing pot used for trapping octopus) or "apical ballooning syndrome," is a temporary severe decrease in heart wall motion in the absence of coronary artery blockage. The patient develops chest pain and an increase in cardiac enzymes, and the heart takes on a peculiar "ballooning" configuration, hence the name of the disorder. The syndrome is thought to be mediated by adrenaline metabolites, a chemical known as neuropeptide Y, and possibly brain natriuretic peptide. The disorder occurs most commonly in post-menopausal women, who develop chest pain and electrocardiographic abnormalities and elevated heart enzymes suggestive of a heart attack, but without sustaining permanent heart damage. Episodes are usually preceded by extreme psychological or emotional stress. Treatment includes monitoring (usually in the Coronary Care Unit) and supportive care. The prognosis is favorable, and the heart pump function usually returns to normal within days to several weeks. The underlying mechanisms are incompletely understood, and it is unclear which medications may benefit patients with this syndrome. Treatment may include beta blockers or angiotensin converting enzyme inhibitor drugs, as well as blood thinners during the early phase of the disorder when ballooning of the heart muscle occurs.

Note: All of the questions (Q) and answers (A) included in this chapter were provided by Robert N. Levin, M.D.

Question: Should I worry if my blood pressure briefly spikes to 180/100 millimeters of mercury and then returns to normal?

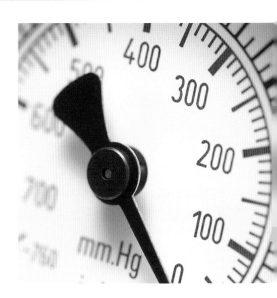

Answer: This is a situation that merits a check-up and a discussion with your doctor. Even if your blood pressure is normal 90 percent of the time, complications of high blood pressure can occur as a result of intermittent "spikes." Such blood pressure spikes can be a normal response to periods of emotional stress, or may represent the phenomenon known as "white coat hypertension." This condition is precipitated by an encounter with a health care worker wearing a white lab coat (my colleagues who do not don white coats tell me that they still frequently see blood pressure "spikes" during office visits). Alternatively, these blood pressure spikes could be a "marker" for the future development of sustained high blood pressure.

"Target organs" affected by either temporary or sustained hypertension include the retina, brain (risk of stroke), heart (risk of heart attack) and kidneys.

One easy way to check for blood pressure spikes is to have a 24-hour blood pressure monitor, which is a device that you wear for a day and return to your doctor. Your doctor will review your average blood pressure over a prolonged period of time and determine whether you require treatment. The challenge of starting patients on medications for intermittent blood pressure spikes is that the physician runs the risk of lowering the blood pressure too much when spikes are not occurring, and this can make you feel dizzy, tired or even pass out. Because of these issues, we often need to exercise a "trial-and-error" approach with medications.

Question: My niece recently passed out while playing basketball at school. She was told she experienced "sudden death." She was resuscitated and was found to have long QT syndrome. What is this and how is it treated?

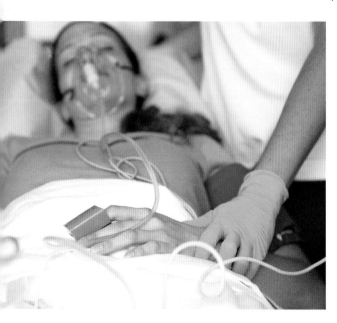

Answer: Sudden death in an apparently healthy young person can be due to various cardiac causes, one of which is the long QT syndrome. This syndrome is characterized by an abnormal prolongation of one of the electrical intervals routinely measured on an electrocardiogram; the QT interval is the equivalent of a battery being recharged—it represents recovery or recharging of a heart muscle cell after it fires. Prolongation of this recharging period makes the heart muscle cells more vulnerable to electrical discharges, which can trigger potentially deadly heart rhythms that cause individuals to lose consciousness. Death is usually due to ventricular fibrillation. Physical and emotional stress are common triggers of passing out or sudden death in the long QT interval syndrome.

There are many causes of long QT intervals, including, ironically, some rhythm stabilizing medications and metabolic disorders such as low magnesium, low potassium or low blood calcium. Many cases are due to hereditary prolonged QT syndrome, which is due to various genetic mutations.

Hereditary long QT is usually a condition of the young. Fainting and sudden death are less likely in patients greater than 40 years of age. Family members of individuals with long QT interval should be screened, with at least an electrocardiogram performed. All individuals with QT prolongation should be screened for acquired causes such as low potassium, low calcium, underactive thyroid or medication-related causes.

Genetic testing for the common types of long QT syndrome is now available commercially, and can identify a gene mutation in 50 to 75 percent of individuals in whom the diagnosis seems to be warranted. Treatment options for symptomatic patients with long QT syndrome include beta-blockers, such as nadolol or atenolol. A physician may tailor the treatment to the type of QT interval involved. Implantable defibrillators are being used more often in patients at high risk for sudden death, including those with symptoms before puberty, those with very long QT intervals and those who repeatedly lose consciousness due to electrical rhythm problems despite beta-blocker therapy. However, this treatment remains somewhat controversial. Restriction of patients' participation in athletic activities is usually advised as passing out or sudden death is often adrenaline-mediated.

Question: I was told by my cardiologist that I have a leaky mitral valve, but I have no symptoms whatsoever. Is this a condition that requires surgery?

Answer: Mitral regurgitation is a backward leakage of the heart valve that separates the upper chamber (atrium) from the lower chamber (ventricle) on the left side of the heart. When the left ventricle contracts, it normally pumps blood into the aorta, which is the main conduit leading out of the heart. In mitral regurgitation, some of the blood moves forcefully into the aorta when the ventricle contracts, but some of the blood also leaks backward into the left atrium. Treatment of leaky valves (as opposed to narrowed valves) is an art, in that there are no precise fixed values one can use to assess whether the patient needs surgery. Over time, your cardiologist will monitor your symptoms (shortness of breath or fatigue), pumping ability of the heart (known as ejection fraction) and the size of the main pumping chamber (left ventricle) of the heart. With aging, the left ventricle tends to enlarge and the pumping activity tends to decrease after many years of mitral valve leakage.

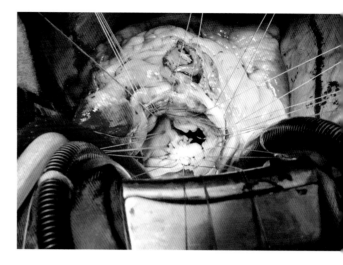

An exception to this approach would be an acute form of mitral regurgitation, which sometimes occurs with valve infection, heart attack or with rupture of one of the chords tethering the valve leaflets in place; this often requires urgent surgery.

Question: I recently had an implantable cardioverter/defibrillator (ICD) implanted by my cardiologist after I had loss of consciousness due to a serious heart rhythm irregularity. The device shocked my heart while I was exercising, and my cardiologist started me on a drug called amiodarone. Why do I need to take medications if I already have an ICD?

Answer: An implantable cardioverter defibrillator (ICD) is a pacemaker-like device that is implanted under the skin on the chest, and shocks or "defibrillates" the heart in order to restore a normal rhythm. The analogy that I use for my patients is to consider an ICD as a "fire extinguisher," in that the device will not activate unless there is a "fire." What many patients don't realize is that the ICD is really not doing anything other than monitoring your heartbeat, unless a dangerous rhythm problem arises, in which case it will shock your heart back into a normal rhythm. Approximately 36 percent of patients who have ICDs implanted never require a shock; however, if a patient does develop a recurrent electrical rhythm problem that causes the device to repeatedly fire, your cardiologist may opt to start you on a rhythm-stabilizing medication (e.g., amiodarone) to prevent recurrence of the rhythm problem, so that you hopefully will not require another "shock" by your ICD (an unpleasant experience).

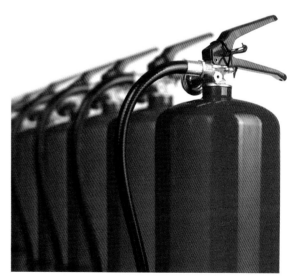

Question: I'm a 40-year-old woman and have experienced recent dizzy spells when I get up from a lying down position. My heartbeat speeds up when I have these spells. My doctor said I have "POTS." What is this and how is it treated?

Answer: "POTS" is an acronym for "postural orthostatic tachycardia syndrome." The disorder is not new, but has had many different names over the last 150 years. POTS is a condition characterized by dizziness or near fainting when standing up from a lying down position, with an accompanying increase in the pulse rate by more than 30 beats per minute. The faintness or lightheadedness is usually relieved by lying down again. The condition is more common in women than in men, and usually occurs between the ages of 15 and 50. Some women report an increase in POTS episodes just before their menstrual periods. It is normally not a serious condition.

POTS can also occur with pregnancy, viral illness, trauma, major surgery, irritable bowl syndrome, or mitral valve prolapse. The cause of POTS is not well understood. Some researchers have suggested a possible "imbalance" between the sympathetic nervous system (which governs the "thermostat" that controls heart rate and heartbeat reactions to stress) and it's parasympathetic counterpart (which does the opposite). In most cases, POTS spontaneously improves and may completely subside over time.

Treatment for POTS is aimed at relieving low blood volume or regulating potential underlying circulatory problems. One approach is to add extra salt to the diet; it is usually recommended that patients with the disorder avoid heavy meals, alcohol, extreme heat, and dehydration. Some physicians suggest a drug called fludrocortisone combined with elastic stockings. Others prescribe drugs such as clonidine or midodrine. It is usually recommended that patients drink 16 ounces (two glassfuls) of water before getting up from a lying down position. Other clinicians advise beta-blocker drugs or certain antidepressants. Currently, no single therapy has been found to be universally effective for treating people with POTS.

Question: I've had atrial fibrillation (AF) for many years and I take Coumadin without any problems. I have no symptoms and I'm able to regularly play golf. I have a friend who had an ablation procedure to get rid of his AF. Am I a candidate for this procedure?

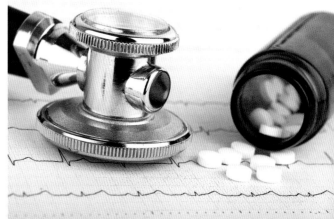

Answer: Atrial fibrillation, known as AF, is a condition characterized by erratic, irregular beating activity of the left atrium (upper chamber) of the heart. There are several issues to consider in treating AF, including controlling the heart rate (i.e., giving drugs that prevent the heart from beating too fast) and preventing clots from forming in the heart; the latter problem is usually addressed with drugs such as warfarin (Coumadin) or dabigatran (Pradaxa). On some occasions, your cardiologist may attempt to "convert" AF to a normal heart rhythm with medications or with a controlled electric shock (cardioversion).

In patients who do not tolerate AF (i.e., have cardiac symptoms despite appropriate medical therapy), ablation is an option. There are both surgical and catheter-based procedures to abolish, or "ablate," AF. A surgeon or cardiologist delivers a radiofrequency stimulus to the left atrium or to the pulmonary veins, which in many cases results in return to a normal heart rhythm. In the "robotic maze" procedure, the surgeon performs the ablation procedure through a small incision in the chest. However, most patients who have these procedures still need to take blood-thinning medications for some period of time, sometimes permanently.

Check with your cardiologist regarding the varied treatment approaches to AF. If you are tolerating your AF and are able to take blood-thinners and rate control medicines without any problems, there is probably no pressing need for you to pursue the option of ablation.

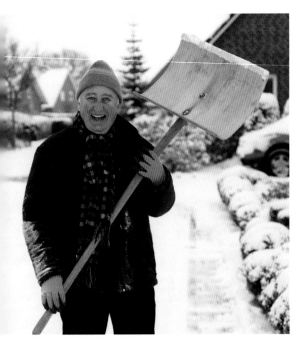

Question: I recently had a stent implanted in one of the arteries in my heart. Do I need to take antibiotics when I have dental work done? Also, a friend told me that I cannot have a magnetic resonance imaging (MRI) scan after receiving a stent.

Answer: When the dentist works on your teeth, even for a simple cleaning, there is a temporary period of time during which bacteria enter the bloodstream, which can cause an infection of some implanted devices and certain abnormal heart valves. Reports of coronary stent infections are exceedingly rare, and we therefore do not advocate taking prophylactic antibiotics after a coronary stent implant.

In the early days of stent implants (more than a decade ago), there was a great deal of uncertainty regarding the effect of MRI scans on metallic stents. It was presumed that the magnetic field could potentially cause stents to migrate, or "move," if exposed to a strong magnetic field. Current evidence supports that MRI scans are perfectly safe with coronary stents, even with "freshly" implanted stents.

Question: I was diagnosed with coronary artery disease about one year ago, at which time my cardiologist placed stents in two of my heart arteries. I have felt fine since then. Is it safe for me to shovel snow? Is a snow blower safer?

Answer: Snow shoveling can be a significant hazard to individuals with coronary artery disease, even if your heart problem has been "treated" by angioplasty or bypass surgery. Every year, we see a significant increase in cardiac events after major blizzards. Shoveling snow usually requires considerable effort because it involves lifting a heavy weight in cold weather. It also constitutes an "abrupt" type of isometric work, especially in deconditioned or sedentary individuals. For persons with coronary artery disease, blood flow may be insufficient to meet this demand, resulting in chest pain, abnormal heart rhythms, heart attack, or even death. Using a snow blower is less taxing than manual shoveling, but the risk remains. Several studies published by Beaumont cardiologists and rehab staff have investigated the hazards of shoveling snow. In one of these reports, of five patients who suffered a heart attack during snow removal, two were using an automated snow blower. We recommend that patients with heart disease refrain from snow removal in any form.

Question: In the past two winters, I have noticed that my fingers turn purple and somewhat painful in cold weather. My doctor recently diagnosed me with Raynaud's Syndrome and prescribed nifedipine. What is Raynaud's Syndrome?

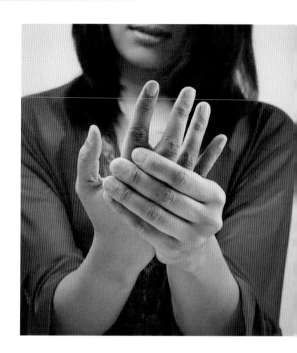

Answer: Raynaud's Syndrome is a condition that causes fingers or toes to become pale, cold, or numb. Sometimes the fingers can even turn red, white, and blue! This happens because the smallest arteries that bring blood to the fingers or toes can develop spasm when exposed to cold or stress. Smoking, cold climate, and certain health conditions (such as autoimmune disorders) may trigger or exacerbate the condition. Although most people have never heard of Raynaud's Syndrome, it is surprisingly common, affecting 10-20% of the population. Many patients can cope with symptoms simply by keeping warm, controlling stress, exercising, stopping smoking, and wearing gloves in cold weather. If these measures are not successful, your physician may prescribe a medication for the condition, usually a calcium channel blocker such a nifedipine or amlodipine.

Question: I've heard that alcohol can have beneficial effects on the heart. Is this true, and how much is beneficial?

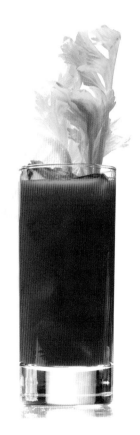

Answer: This is a complex question, and the answer is that it's partially true. Studies have shown that moderate alcohol intake can be beneficial to the heart, likely by increasing the body's own clot-busting (endogenous) tissue plasminogen activator, increasing "good" or high-density lipoprotein (HDL) cholesterol, and possibly by inhibiting clumping of platelets, which are clotting elements in the blood. Unfortunately, most medical trials that have studied alcohol have measured it in "grams," rather than ounces or shots. It is quite difficult to assess how many grams constitute an ounce of alcohol, let alone the confounding factor that beer and hard alcohol have very different alcohol contents. Basically, moderate alcohol intake can be defined as two one-ounce "hard alcohol drinks for an average-build male (roughly equivalent to two shots of 80-proof spirits, two 12-ounce bottles of beer, or 6-8 ounces of wine) and half this amount for an average-size female. For patients who do not already consume alcoholic beverages, we generally do not advocate that they start drinking for heart health. The American Heart Association recommends that if alcoholic beverages are consumed, they should be limited to no more than 2 drinks per day for men and 1 drink per day for women, and ideally should be consumed with meals (Circulation, July 2006). Alcohol intake that exceeds the "moderate" range can have serious cardiac (and other medical/social) consequences, including heart rhythm irregularities, cardiac muscle weakness, high blood pressure, and liver and pancreatic disease. Plato, quoting from the inscription in the temple at Delphi, suggested "nothing in excess." This is a worthwhile recommendation to keep in mind!

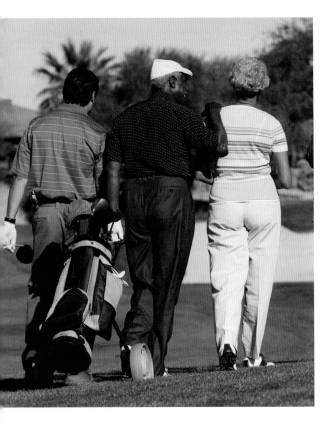

Question: Does my weekly round of golf count as exercise for my heart?

Answer: I would strongly support your golf activities in that there are numerous associated health benefits. Studies demonstrate that golf is a moderate intensity activity. How much exercise you derive from golf depends on a number of factors. You get much more exercise if you walk 18 holes, especially if you use a pull cart or carry your own bag. You burn more calories on a hilly course than on one with a flat terrain. Although the walking in golf is not continuous, you use considerable energy traversing the 3 to 4 miles of an average golf course. If you are very fit, walking a golf course is not likely to replace vigorous exercise training; however, if you are sedentary and deconditioned, golf can help you to improve your fitness. Recognize that you need to exercise regularly and that one round of golf a week would be inadequate. Some golf courses require that golfers use a motorized cart, and this may diminish health benefits. In these circumstances, try to add some exercise by parking the cart away from your ball and walking to it. You can also usually trade off using the cart with your partner, so one of you can get in some additional exercise.

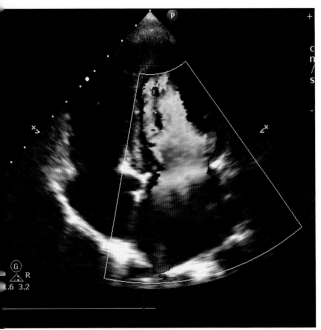

Question: I'm 72 years old and have been told by my doctor that I have a heart murmur due to aortic valve thickening. Is this a serious problem?

Answer: Aortic valve thickening, also known as aortic sclerosis, is considered a normal part of the aging process. It is often accompanied by a mild heart murmur and is generally confirmed by an echocardiogram (ultrasound exam of the heart). Aortic sclerosis is present in as many as 40% of individuals older than 75 years of age.

Although aortic sclerosis is a relatively benign condition, some patients will go on to develop narrowing of the aortic valve opening, known as aortic stenosis. Approximately 16% of patients with aortic sclerosis will develop more significant narrowing of the valve, with approximately 2.5% developing severe aortic stenosis.

Patients with aortic sclerosis should be followed closely. Studies have shown mixed results as to whether aggressive cholesterol-lowering therapy might retard the valve narrowing process, in that the valve looks much like an atherosclerotic plaque under the microscope. Research examining antibiotics for this disease has been disappointing.

Question: My doctor said I have hypertrophic cardiomyopathy, and advised that I avoid vigorous exercise. What is hypertrophic cardiomyopathy?

Answer: Hypertrophic cardiomyopathy (HCM), the most common cause of sudden death in athletes, is characterized by a reduced left ventricle cavity (main pumping chamber of the heart) and a thickened heart muscle. The enlarged heart muscle cells result in extra-forceful contractions. Problems that can occur with HCM are related to increased stiffness of the thickened heart muscle, making the left ventricular chamber cavity difficult to fill, and electrical rhythm disturbances caused by the "super-sized" heart muscle cells. Vigorous physical activity makes it difficult for the main pumping chamber to fill, and also predisposes the patient to sudden death by virtue of heart rhythm irregularities. Most of the symptoms (especially shortness of breath) of HCM can be alleviated by medications; however, if the heart muscle is particularly thick or if the patient experiences fainting spells, they may benefit from an implantable defibrillator.

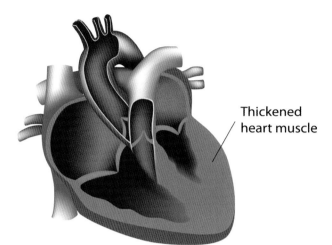

Thickened heart muscle

Few disorders have inspired as much controversy as HCM in regard to potential treatment modalities. Some cardiologists have advocated dual-chamber pacemakers, whereas others have used catheter-delivered alcohol to create a "controlled" heart attack to intentionally shrink the size of the overgrown muscle. Still others have performed myotomy/myectomy procedures (which literally slice out segments of the thickened heart muscle) to treat the condition. To date, the only feasible "nonpharmacologic" treatment of HCM is an implantable defibrillator in high-risk patients (i.e., patients who are adolescent and/or have passed out, adults who have had "sudden death," and patients with certain documented electrical rhythm problems). Although beta-blockers are commonly prescribed for this disorder, other drugs may also be used, such as calcium channel blockers or Norpace.

Most patients with HCM are advised to avoid vigorous exercise, which can trigger threatening heart rhythms, fainting, or even sudden cardiac death. Abnormal heart rhythms may, in some instances, be effectively treated with yet another drug – amiodarone. Clearly, there is a genetic component to this structural cardiovascular abnormality, and promising studies exploring the genetic origin of HCM and the potential for gene therapy represent exciting developments in the field of cardiology.

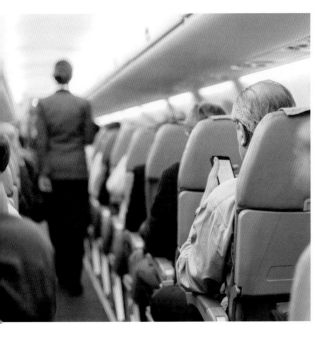

Question: I noticed that my legs swell whenever I take a long airplane trip. What causes this?

Answer: Many people experience mild leg swelling (edema) during and immediately after air travel. The swelling is due to several factors, including low cabin pressure in the aircraft, stagnant collection of blood in the leg veins (stasis), and dehydration due to cabin atmosphere. These factors can create the "perfect storm" for development of clots in the legs, which in turn can cause a serious or even life-threatening condition whereby these clots travel to the lungs. This scenario has been exacerbated in recent years by a phenomenon known as "coach class syndrome," in that the airlines have shortened the "pitch" between seats, leading to cramping and crowding (not to mention the larger passengers), which can make deep vein blood clots more likely to form. The best way to reduce the likelihood of this problem is to stay well-hydrated during the flight, avoid alcohol and caffeine (both of which can worsen dehydration), "pump" (contract and release) your feet and calves during the flight, and get up to move around the cabin as often as possible, ideally every hour.

Question: I have a friend who takes a special antioxidant vitamin packet every day. Would this help my heart?

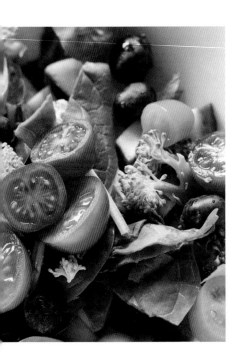

Answer: There have been very few controlled trials that have appropriately evaluated these products, which are expensive. There is a huge, multibillion-dollar vitamin industry that would like you to pay dearly to "reverse the aging process." I counsel my patients to increase their consumption of foods that are naturally high in antioxidants. Such "heart-healthy" foods include:

Beans	Oranges	Spinach	Walnuts
Blueberries	Pumpkin	Tea	Yogurt
Broccoli	Salmon	Tomatoes	
Oats	Soy	Turkey	

You should also incorporate a regular exercise program into your cardioprotective routine for maximum antioxidant benefit and to improve fitness and blood vessel tone. A healthy diet and regular aerobic exercise will ultimately lower your risk of heart attack and stroke.

Question: Should I be taking vitamin D to enhance my heart health?

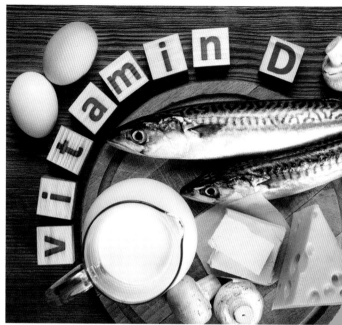

Answer: Several years ago, researchers reviewed the relationship between vitamin D deficiency and cardiovascular disease (Journal of the American College of Cardiology, December 2008). The authors emphasized that vitamin D deficiency seems to predispose people to develop high blood pressure, diabetes, metabolic syndrome, heart muscle thickening, and inflammation of the blood vessels. A study of male health professionals demonstrated a two-fold increase in heart attack risk in those who were deficient in vitamin D (Archives of Internal Medicine, June 2008). The Framingham Offspring Study showed similar findings.

Low 25-hydroxy vitamin D levels (20 ng/ml or less) are found in 27% to 57% of the United States population. The desirable concentration is at least 30 ng/ml, but less than 150 ng/ml. The average American adult consumes about 230 International Units (IU) of vitamin D daily. The recommended "adequate" intake of vitamin D is 200-600 IU, though many experts suggest taking 800-2000 IU daily.

The most potent source of vitamin D is sunlight, with 5 to 10 minutes per day of sun exposure stimulating the skin to produce 3,000 IU of vitamin D. Of course, those who live in the northern part of the globe tend to get significantly less sun exposure than those who live closer to the equator.

People are more likely to be vitamin D deficient if they are dark-skinned, elderly, obese, or a smoker. Factors that can decrease vitamin D concentrations include medications (e.g., seizure medication, steroids, antiviral medication), kidney or liver disease, sunscreen use, or institutionalization.

Muscle pain and weakness are generally the first symptoms of vitamin D deficiency. Good natural sources of vitamin D are cod liver oil, salmon, tuna, fortified milk and orange juice. Clearly, large randomized clinical trials are needed to clarify the relationship between vitamin D deficiency and cardiovascular disease. I would advise that you talk with your physician regarding adequate intake of vitamin D. He/she may want to obtain a vitamin D blood level prior to advising vitamin supplementation.

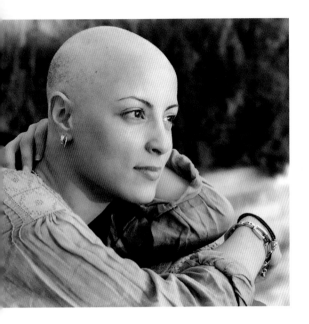

Question: I have breast cancer, and I am currently on chemotherapy including a drug called doxorubicin. My oncologist referred me to a cardiologist to monitor my heart function. What type of tests will my cardiologist do?

Answer: Doxorubicin is a member of a class of drugs called anthracyclines, which are commonly used to treat various forms of cancer. The anthracyclines (and also taxanes and trastuzumab) can cause oxidative damage to the energy components of the heart muscle cells, and can potentially weaken the heart muscle, a process known as cardiotoxicity. The risk of damage to the heart is proportional to the cumulative amount of drug given, so your cardiologist and oncologist will be tracking how much of the drug you have received over time. There is an 18 percent chance of developing cardiotoxicity on these drugs, and 2 to 4 percent of patients develop severe congestive heart failure.

For many years now, the gold standard to assess heart function has been to evaluate the left ventricular ejection fraction, which is a measure of how well the heart contracts. This is typically measured by performing serial echocardiograms (sometimes after each cycle of chemotherapy), or sometimes MUGA (nuclear) scans. Recently, however, we have discovered that there are more sensitive and perhaps more reliable methods for assessing the potential for heart muscle damage in patients on chemotherapy. These include a longitudinal strain index, which can be measured during an echocardiogram in some ultrasound labs. The longitudinal strain index measures the strain on the heart muscle, much like you would measure the tension in a spring.

Another recent and exciting development is measurement of certain biomarkers, including troponin I, NT-pro-BNP, myeloperoxidase (MPO), GDF-15, and galectin-3. These are measured by blood tests performed at baseline (before chemotherapy) and after three months of chemotherapy. Of these, it seems that troponin I and MPO might be the most reliable and predictive of development of heart muscle damage. Nevertheless, the left ventricular ejection fraction remains an important and useful index of heart pump function.

The goal in performing these tests is to determine if you are approaching an irreversible or advanced level of heart muscle damage, prior to the damage actually occurring. If this occurs, your cardiologist might prescribe certain cardioprotective medications, such as beta blockers and angiotensin-converting enzyme inhibitors to help prevent further damage. Alternatively, your oncologist may decide to change your chemotherapy regimen.

It is important that your cardiologist and oncologist communicate regularly regarding these issues.

Question: My internist referred me to a cardiologist because of resistant hypertension. What is resistant hypertension and how is it treated?

Answer: Resistant hypertension is defined as elevated blood pressure that is uncontrolled on three different blood pressure medications, or appropriately controlled on four or more medications. This problem has become much more prevalent in the United States in the past several decades. The prevalence of resistant, or refractory, hypertension was 7 percent in the late 1980s, and is now 20 percent. The problem is more common in African Americans, patients with chronic kidney disease and patients with diabetes. It is slightly more common in women and in older people. Resistant hypertension substantially increases the risk for chronic kidney disease, stroke, heart attack, and overall mortality. Many patients with resistant hypertension have an excess of a body hormone called aldosterone, which can be measured with a simple blood test. They may also have increased activity of the sympathetic nervous system. Obesity and obstructive sleep apnea can also contribute to a nonresponse to blood pressure medicines, as does excessive salt intake. Treating sleep apnea with a mask that keeps the airway open during sleep (continuous positive airway pressure—CPAP) often decreases the blood pressure, as does treating aldosterone excess with a drug such as spironolactone.

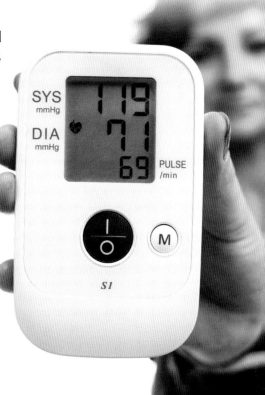

Some patients have a syndrome known as pseudo-resistant hypertension, which may include the patient not taking their prescribed medications properly, inadequate dosing of the medication, or taking drugs (such as nonsteroidal anti-inflammatory agents) that can interfere with the action of the antihypertensive drugs.

To determine if your blood pressure is truly resistant or refractory, your physician may ask you to check your home blood pressure readings and compare them to the office blood pressure. If there is a disparity between these readings, your physician may arrange an ambulatory blood pressure monitor to better determine your true blood pressure levels.

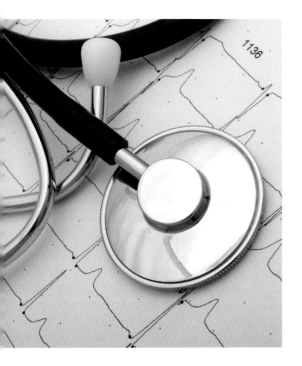

Question: Recently, my cardiologist evaluated me and obtained an electrocardiogram and echocardiogram during my office visit. She said that I have congestive heart failure, but that my heart pump function on the ultrasound test is normal. How is this possible?

Answer: Congestive heart failure (CHF) is an inability of the main or lower pumping chambers of the heart (the ventricles) to fill and pump properly, causing a back-up of blood from the heart into the lungs. This effectively results in congestion of the lungs, liver, abdomen and lower extremities.

There are various types of CHF other than the "garden variety" caused by inability of the heart to contract properly. One example would be a heart valve disorder, such as a narrowing or leakage of a heart valve, which can cause back-up of blood from the upper chambers of the heart (the atria) into the lungs, resulting in shortness of breath and diagnosis of CHF. Some heart rhythm irregularities can also cause abnormal increases in the pressures in the heart, without impairing the pump activity.

Very commonly, especially with advancing age, we see "heart failure with preserved systolic function," or "diastolic" CHF, meaning the walls of the main pumping chambers of your heart are stiff, making it difficult for the main pumping chambers to fill between beats; however, the walls squeeze in a normal fashion when the heart contracts. The analogy I use with my patients is to imagine a balloon which, in place of thin latex walls, is composed of half inch tire rubber; when you exhale and blow into the balloon to try to inflate it, it takes a great deal of effort to fill (inflate), though it empties appropriately when you release the stem.

Treatments of diastolic CHF can be challenging. One of the main approaches is to attempt to control blood pressure in patients who have longstanding high blood pressure with thickened heart walls. Other options include diuretics or water pills, and sometimes calcium channel blockers which may allow the stiff walls to "relax" and for the chambers to fill more easily. Spironolactone (Aldactone) has been used by some cardiologists, though recent research shows this drug to be less promising than initially thought. Another drug alternative for this disorder is candesartan, an angiotensin receptor blocker, which tends to decrease the risk of hospitalization but otherwise showed no benefit. Additional research is needed to determine the optimal therapy for this condition.

Question: When I went for my last check-up, my doctor did an electrocardiogram and said I have a "right bundle branch block." What is this and how is it treated?

Answer: The electrical system of the heart consists of two groups or bundles of electrical fibers, much like small freeways consisting of miniature electric wires. One group is on the left side of the main pumping chamber (left ventricle) and is known as the "left bundle branch" system. The other is on the right side of the septum (muscular "wall" dividing the two heart chambers) and is designated as the "right bundle branch."

In patients who have a right bundle branch block, the electrical impulses travel through the "city streets" of the electrical system of the heart, rather than using the main "freeways," or bundle branches. This means the electrical impulses eventually travel through the heart muscle, but it takes longer, causing a "conduction delay" on the electrocardiogram.

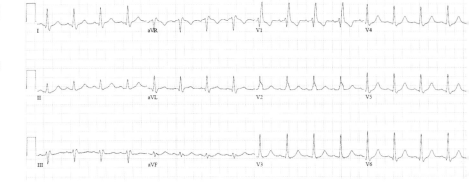

Five percent of apparently healthy adults have a right bundle branch block, and it often does not reflect anything wrong with the heart. In some instances, however, the right bundle branch block can be caused by an underlying coronary artery blockage, which may be discovered during a stress test, heart catheterization, or coronary computed tomography angiogram. In other instances, it can be caused by structural abnormalities of the heart, such as congenital heart disease, heart muscle disorders, or even a clot in the lungs. Your physician may recommend an echocardiogram and possibly a chemical stress test to identify these disorders.

Question: I have congestive heart failure, and have read that I should be taking an angiotensin converting enzyme (ACE) inhibitor drug along with my Coreg. I have moderate kidney disease, am not on dialysis, and my cardiologist put me on Isordil and hydralazine, but did not prescribe an ACE inhibitor. Will I still benefit from this combination of drugs?

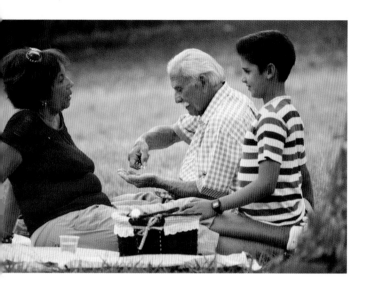

Answer: Congestive heart failure (CHF) is a decreased ability of the heart to pump sufficient blood to your body, resulting in backup of blood from the heart into the lungs and associated shortness of breath. Standard therapy for CHF typically includes a diuretic, such as furosemide (Lasix) or bumetanide (Bumex), a beta blocker (such as metoprolol or carvedilol), an ACE inhibitor drug (such as enalapril, also known as Vasotec) and sometimes an additional water pill such as Aldactone (spironolactone). A failing heart is "load-dependent," meaning there is disruption of the filling pressure of the heart (preload) and of the resistance against which the heart beats (afterload). One of the mainstays of treating CHF is to attempt to reduce the filling pressures in the heart, meaning to decrease both preload and afterload. Although ACE inhibitors can achieve this goal, they can also be problematic in some patients with kidney dysfunction, as they are metabolized by the kidney and may sometimes result in an elevated blood potassium.

The combination of a nitrate drug, such as isosorbide, which reduces preload, and a drug such as hydralazine, which reduces afterload (resistance to outflow from the heart), can achieve essentially the same results (including mortality reduction) as an ACE inhibitor, without having any adverse effects on the kidney. The only downside to this combination is that compliance is not always optimal in that each drug must be taken several times daily.

I'd suggest you discuss with your cardiologist the goals of therapy in your particular case, and the pros and cons of different drug regimens.

Question: My cardiologist diagnosed me with pericarditis and prescribed colchicine. I used to take this medication for my gout. Why did my doctor prescribe this medication?

Answer: Pericarditis is an inflammation or infection of the sac that encases the heart (the pericardium). It usually affects young and middle-aged individuals. There are many possible causes of pericarditis, including viruses (especially Coxsackie viruses), bacterial infections, tuberculosis, kidney disease, autoimmune diseases (such as lupus, rheumatoid arthritis, scleroderma, and Sjogren syndrome), tumors, trauma, and certain medications (such as hydralazine or procainamide). In Western Europe and North America, 80 to 90 percent of cases are labeled "idiopathic," meaning a definitive cause is not identified.

The most common presentation of patients with pericarditis is chest pain, often described as a "sharp" pain that becomes worse when taking a deep breath and is often improved by sitting up and leaning forward.

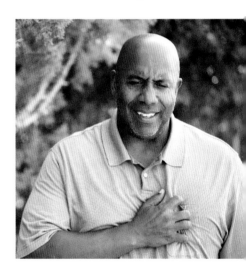

The most common presentation of patients with pericarditis is chest pain, often described as a "sharp" pain that becomes worse when taking a deep breath and is often improved by sitting up and leaning forward. Your health provider diagnoses pericarditis by physical examination, including listening for a crunching sound known as a "friction rub." Additional diagnostic studies may include an electrocardiogram, and sometimes an echocardiogram or computed tomography (CT) scan. The echocardiogram or CT scan may reveal fluid in the pericardial sac.

The mainstay of treating pericarditis that is idiopathic or viral in origin is NSAIDS, or non-steroidal anti-inflammatory drugs, which include aspirin, and drugs such as ibuprofen or indomethacin. Steroids were previously used quite often for pericarditis, especially for recurrent cases or cases not responding to aspirin or NSAIDS. However, it is currently felt that steroids should be restricted to patients who do not tolerate NSAIDS or who have contraindications to their use, and only after failure of first line therapy with NSAIDS and colchicine.

Recent evidence supports using colchicine in addition to NSAIDS for treating pericarditis; this drug has been shown to improve remission rates in one week, and to reduce recurrence rates, especially when compared with NSAIDS alone. Colchicine is an anti-inflammatory drug which has been used for many years to treat gout. It works by preventing granulocytes, which are a certain type of white blood cell, from having an inflammatory effect. Colchicine has been shown to decrease the risk of treatment failure and to prevent recurrence of pericarditis. It is generally given for three months for acute pericarditis cases, and for six months for recurrent cases. The most common side effect is gastrointestinal upset, especially diarrhea, which occurs in 7 to 10 percent of people who take colchicine.

In patients who do not respond to colchicine and NSAIDS, your physician may prescribe drugs that more strongly block the immune system, such as azathioprine, intravenous immunoglobulin, or anakinra injections (interleukin receptor blockers). These are newer approaches and may result in additional side effects. Additional studies are needed to confirm the efficacy of these newer drugs.

You should have a discussion with your health provider regarding the duration of your therapy with NSAIDS and colchicine. Most patients require only one to two weeks of therapy.

Question: My nephew had aortic valve regurgitation and had to have his aortic valve replaced. I, too, have aortic regurgitation, but my cardiologist is not replacing my valve. He is following me by performing echocardiograms every year. Why is he not fixing my valve?

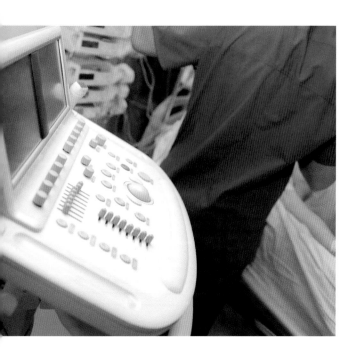

Answer: Aortic regurgitation is a condition characterized by backward leakage of blood into the left ventricle of the heart during the relaxation (diastolic) phase of the cardiac cycle, usually due to a defective aortic valve. Several conditions can cause this, including calcification and stiffening of the valve (often coincides with the aging process), rheumatic inflammation of the valve, valve infection or a congenitally abnormal valve. Over time, the left ventricle, or main pumping chamber of the heart, compensates for this extra (leaking) blood volume in two ways: it enlarges to accommodate the extra (regurgitant) blood volume or it starts to show signs of decreased pumping ability (ejection fraction).

Replacing or repairing regurgitant valves (as opposed to stenotic or narrowed valves) constitutes an "art" in that there is often a fairly long latent period until the patient becomes symptomatic and the valve needs to be replaced. Your cardiologist will likely advise that your valve be replaced when you start to show signs (on cardiac ultrasound) of enlargement of the left ventricle, a decrease in the heart's ejection fraction or with associated symptoms (usually shortness of breath).

In recent years, cardiologists have embraced a somewhat lower threshold to fix leaking heart valves, in that the morbidity and mortality of the procedure is far lower than it was in the past.

Question: I have been taking metoprolol for the past two years, which was prescribed by my cardiologist for episodes of paroxysmal supraventricular tachycardia (sudden rapid heart rate), along with mild elevation of my blood pressure. If I work out on my elliptical machine within a few hours of taking my metoprolol, I can only get my heart rate to 116 beats per minute (bpm). If 24 hours have passed since taking my pill, I can get my heart rate up to 140 bpm. Is my exercise doing any good for me if I can't adequately increase my heart rate?

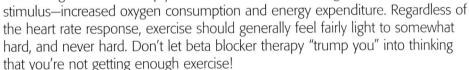

Answer: Metoprolol is a beta-blocker and works by slowing the heart, especially during exercise. As long as the metoprolol is in your system, you may not be able to achieve your prescribed target heart rate; however, you are still benefiting from the exercise. If you use the same workload, you are still doing the same amount of work but at a lower heart rate. A common misconception is that the rise in heart rate during exercise is what causes the body to become aerobically fit. But the increased heart rate during exercise is simply a marker for the real training stimulus—increased oxygen consumption and energy expenditure. Regardless of the heart rate response, exercise should generally feel fairly light to somewhat hard, and never hard. Don't let beta blocker therapy "trump you" into thinking that you're not getting enough exercise!

Question: I recently had a drug coated stent placed in my right coronary artery. Why do I still have to take Plavix if my stent has a drug coating to prevent blockage?

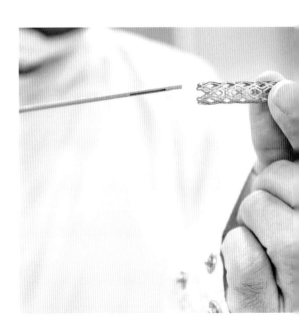

Answer: There are two things that we are concerned about after implanting a stent in a coronary artery. One is development of a clot in the stent, which is a result of blood being exposed to stainless steel and can occur in the first few hours to first several months. A clotted stent almost always causes a heart attack, and this type of heart attack can be quite serious. Plavix (clopidogrel), Effient (prasugrel) and Brilinta (ticagrelor) are drugs used (in addition to aspirin) to minimize the chance of this occurring. The second issue is somewhat less ominous and is known as "restenosis," or renarrowing within the stent. This is due to development of scar tissue inside the stent. Although this may be more innocuous than a clot, it can sometimes cause clinical problems. It does not involve clot formation. The purpose of the drug coating on the stent is to minimize the possibility of scar tissue formation. Patients with drug coated stents are advised to continue the combination of Plavix and aspirin (to prevent clots) for a minimum of one year.

Question: I am on warfarin (Coumadin) for atrial fibrillation due to a leaking mitral valve. I saw an advertisement for Pradaxa on TV. Can I take Pradaxa in place of warfarin?

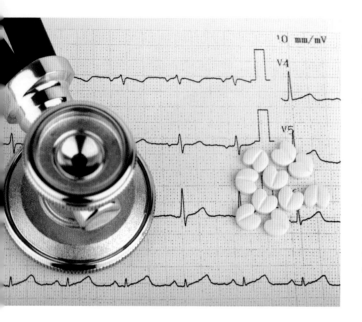

Answer: Although several new agents have been approved and are being investigated as "replacements" for warfarin, there are still some potential pitfalls with the new drugs. The new class of drugs works by blocking a clotting protein known as factor X. The problem with these drugs is that they are approved only for nonvalvular atrial fibrillation, meaning they are not FDA approved for atrial fibrillation due to valvular heart disease. A positive finding was that all of these drugs had a lower rate of hemorrhagic (bleeding) stroke compared to warfarin. The initial studies with dabigatran (Pradaxa) showed efficacy similar to warfarin, with some excess heart attacks. One potential drawback to these drugs is the inability to reverse them if there is a bleeding problem. Other drugs in this class include rivaroxaban (Xarelto), which has been studied in both heart attacks and in nonvalvular atrial fibrillation and is FDA approved. An even more promising agent was recently approved, and this drug is called apixaban (Eliquis). In a large study known as the ARISTOTLE trial, apixaban was found to be superior to warfarin in preventing stroke or embolism (clot which travels to the brain), caused less bleeding and resulted in a lower mortality rate.

At this point, anti-X or anti-Xa agents are not a viable alternative for patients with mechanical (metallic) heart valves; these patients should remain on warfarin. I'd suggest you have a discussion with your cardiologist regarding the optimal blood thinner in your situation.

Question: My doctor said that I have congestive heart failure due to cardiomyopathy. What is cardiomyopathy and how is it treated?

Answer: Cardiomyopathy is any type of heart muscle disorder. In the United States, the most common type of cardiomyopathy is heart muscle weakness due to plaque buildup in the coronary arteries that supply blood to the heart. Another form of cardiomyopathy is dilated cardiomyopathy, meaning the heart is enlarged and weakened, usually due to factors other than coronary artery blockage. Some of these are idiopathic, meaning we do not know the cause. Others are due to a virus that may have infiltrated the heart muscle in the past and caused heart muscle weakening; about 20 to 30 percent of these will reverse and the heart pump function will return to normal. Some are due to toxin exposure, with multiple agents including alcohol, cocaine and occupational chemicals. Less common forms of cardiomyopathy include hypertrophic cardiomyopathy, which causes an asymmetric overgrowth of heart muscle cells with an inordinately strong increase in heart muscle pumping action; restrictive cardiomyopathy, which is a stiffening of the heart muscle resulting in abnormal filling of the main pumping chamber; and, infiltrative cardiomyopathy, caused by abnormal protein deposition in diseases such as amyloidosis and sarcoidosis. Less common causes of cardiomyopathy include thyroid disease, peripartum state (pregnancy) and muscular dystrophy.

In the United States, the most common type of cardiomyopathy is heart muscle weakness due to plaque build-up in the coronary arteries that supply blood to the heart.

Your cardiologist will likely perform some tests to determine which type of cardiomyopathy you have, usually including a physical examination, chest X-ray and echocardiogram. He or she may also wish in some cases to perform cardiac catheterization, and in others to obtain a magnetic resonance imaging scan or even a (catheter-based) biopsy of the heart muscle.

The treatment depends on the type of cardiomyopathy, and is generally tailored to the individual patient. Common drugs to treat congestive heart failure due to the weak pump type of cardiomyopathy include water pills (such as furosemide), beta blockers (such as metoprolol or carvedilol) and ACE-inhibitors (such as lisinopril). In some cases, if the heart pump function is severely impaired, the patient may require an implantable defibrillator to shock any potential life-threatening rhythm disturbance that might occur; one form of implantable defibrillator can even resynchronize the heart muscle and actually make it pump more efficiently.

Question: My LDL cholesterol is elevated, and I have had adverse effects to three different statins over the past two years. Are there drugs to lower LDL other than statins?

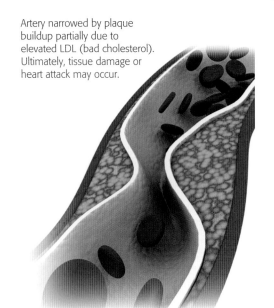

Artery narrowed by plaque buildup partially due to elevated LDL (bad cholesterol). Ultimately, tissue damage or heart attack may occur.

Answer: Elevated LDL, or bad cholesterol, is a key risk factor for heart attack and stroke. There is a promising new class of non-statin drugs that appear to be very effective at lowering LDL. The drugs are known as PCSK9 inhibitors, and are given once or twice monthly in the form of an injection, much like insulin shots. These are bioengineered antibodies that block PCSK9, a protein that interferes with the body's ability to clear LDL cholesterol, a different mechanism from how statins work. About 10 percent of patients on statins (approximately 5 million patients) suffer muscle pain or other side effects that prevent them from taking these drugs.

The anti-PCSK9 drugs include Amgen's evolocumab, alirocumab from Sanofi and Regeneron, and bococizumab from Pfizer. One of the more recent studies with evolocumab, called "DESCARTES," evaluated 901 patients and found a 57 percent reduction in LDL compared to placebo (*New England Journal of Medicine,* May 2014). Adverse events included upper respiratory tract infection, flu and back pain.

What is not known is whether the profound additional reduction in LDL will translate into meaningful decreases in heart attacks, strokes, and other complications of cardiovascular disease.

Question: My wife booked us for a vacation in Colorado in approximately two months. I have coronary artery disease and have had three stents placed in the past. Will the high altitude in Colorado be a problem?

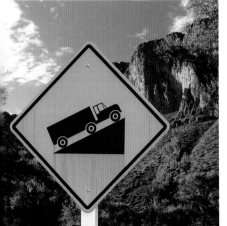

Answer: If all you have is coronary artery disease and placement of previous stents, with generally preserved heart pump function, you will not likely have a problem at high altitude. High altitude is sometimes associated with pulmonary hypertension, or elevated pressures in the lungs. The relatively low pressure of oxygen in air at high altitude causes the lung vessels to constrict, which in turn elevates pulmonary pressures. At sea level, oxygen pressure is about 150 mmHg. At high altitude (3,000 to 5,500 meters) the oxygen pressure decreases to 80 to 100 mmHg. At extremely high altitude (5,500 to 8,840 meters), the oxygen pressure in the atmosphere decreases to 40 to 80 mmHg. In most patients with "routine" coronary artery disease or heart valve problems, this does not pose a problem, with the provision that one should avoid vigorous or strenuous physical activity at high altitude. Transient dysfunction of the right ventricle (portion of the heart that pumps to the lungs) can occur with strenuous exercise at high altitude. In general, patients with emphysema or with certain forms of complex congenital heart disease tend to have more of a problem at high altitude, as do patients with congestive heart failure that require home oxygen therapy. Discuss your individual situation with your cardiologist or primary care physician.

Question: I have mitral and aortic heart valve thickening problems, and my doctor said that it's due to my systemic lupus. How can lupus affect the heart?

Answer: Systemic lupus erythematosus (known as SLE) is an "autoimmune" (connective tissue) disorder whereby the body makes antibodies to its own cellular hereditary material, called DNA, or deoxyribonucleic acid. This often causes joint pain, rash, and possibly heart, lung, kidney, or brain abnormalities. The disease process can affect virtually all parts of the heart. Pericarditis, or inflammation of the sac around the heart, is the most common cardiac problem in systemic lupus. This may also result in pericardial effusion, which is a collection of fluid in the sac around the heart. Another possible abnormality could be any type of electrical rhythm abnormality of the heart. A third potential complication would be coronary arteritis, which is an inflammation of the walls of the coronary arteries. This is usually treated with high dose steroids. In addition to coronary arteritis, lupus patients can experience coronary artery spasm, coronary clotting, or migration of a clot within the artery. Heart valve involvement is common in patients with systemic lupus. Patients can develop noninfectious vegetations (thickening) of the heart valves, sometimes referred to as "marantic endocarditis" or "Libman-Sacks" endocarditis. Valve thickening is the most common finding on the cardiac ultrasound (echocardiogram), and most frequently involves the mitral valve. Pulmonary artery hypertension, or elevated pressure in the lungs, can also be caused by SLE and can be assessed by echocardiogram with Doppler. Heart valve involvement can also include valve narrowing, ruptured chords attached to the valve, clotting events, or clots in the chamber of the heart, all of which have been reported in patients with SLE. The treatment depends on the type and severity of involvement.

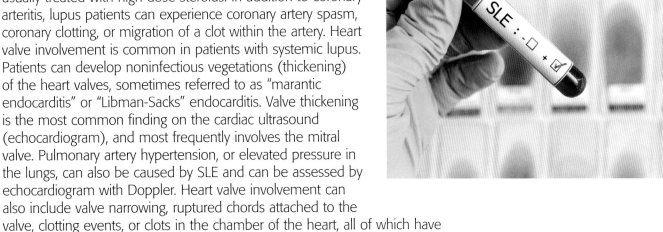

In summary, SLE can affect all parts of the heart, including the pericardium, endocardium (inner lining of the heart chamber), heart muscle cells, heart valves, conduction system, or coronary arteries.

Question: I have been hospitalized several times for congestive heart failure, and am currently taking furosemide, lisinopril, carvedilol and spironolactone. My cardiologist tells me that my medication regimen is "maximized." However, I occasionally need to be hospitalized because of associated heart failure symptoms. I understand that there are new medications that may lessen the need for re-hospitalization and may actually reduce my mortality risk. What are these medications?

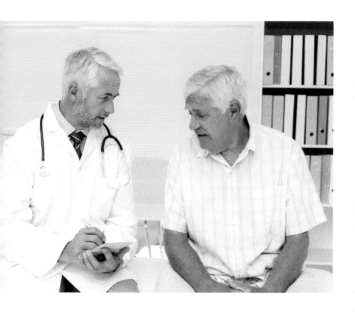

Answer: Congestive heart failure is characterized by an inability of the heart to effectively pump blood to the body organs, resulting in a back-up of blood into the lungs and shortness of breath. As you indicate, your cardiologist has you on optimal medical therapy for heart failure. Typical heart failure therapy includes a diuretic, an angiotensin converting enzyme (ACE) inhibitor, a beta blocker (such as carvedilol), and sometimes spironolactone. Recently, several new medications have been studied and some have now been approved by the Food and Drug Administration for adjunctive treatment of congestive heart failure. One medication, called Entresto, is actually a combination of two drugs, sacubitril and valsartan. Sacubitril blocks a protein known as neprilysin, which causes blood vessels to constrict and the body to retain salt. By blocking neprilysin, we can relax blood vessels and minimize the likelihood of retaining sodium. In this particular drug, sacubitril is combined with valsartan, which is an agent that blocks a hormone called aldosterone, which also causes blood vessel constriction and salt retention. Sacubitril/valsartan was studied in the PARADIGM-HF trial (*European Heart Journal,* Aug. 2015) and patients who received it demonstrated a decreased risk of recurrent hospitalization and death from heart causes. Adverse side effects of the drug included low blood pressure (18 percent), elevated potassium (12 percent), coughing (9 percent), and kidney failure (5 percent). Entresto should not be used in combination with an ACE inhibitor or with a drug known as aliskiren, a renin inhibitor used to treat high blood pressure. It is also not recommended in patients with abnormal liver function or those who are pregnant.

Another new drug that has been approved for treatment of congestive heart failure is called Corlanor (ivabradine). This is a medication that works by affecting your heart's electrical activity in order to slow the heart rate. The value of heart-rate reduction was evaluated in a randomized, placebo controlled trial that included 6,558 adults with congestive heart failure, demonstrating a decreased risk of worsening heart failure, cardiovascular death or repeat hospitalization (*Lancet,* Sept. 2010). Potential side effects include slow heart rate, high blood pressure, atrial fibrillation and visual disturbances. It should not be used in patients with abnormal liver function and/or those who are pacemaker dependent.

Although these new medications appear to have exciting potential, they have not been extensively studied at this point in time, and are fairly costly. You should discuss these with your physician (and your insurance carrier) to see if they may be appropriate for you.

Question: I saw my cardiologist because of shortness of breath, and she informed me that I have mitral stenosis. She prescribed metoprolol. What is mitral stenosis and how is it treated?

Answer: Mitral stenosis is a narrowing of the mitral valve, which is a two-leaflet valve that controls blood flow from the upper chamber (left atrium) to the lower chamber (left ventricle) on the left side of the heart. The mitral valve is so named because it resembles a bishop's mitre. When the mitral valve narrows, a pressure gradient develops across the valve, and the pressure (and size) of the left atrium increases. The increased left atrial pressure is reflected directly via the pulmonary veins to the lungs, causing the shortness of breath that you describe. The higher the patient's heart rate (pulse), the higher the left atrial pressure and the worse the shortness of breath.

The mainstay of treating mitral stenosis is rate control,—i.e., slowing the pulse with medication so that the pressure gradient decreases. This is usually accomplished with drugs such as beta-blockers (such as metoprolol), calcium channel blockers (such as diltiazem or verapamil) or digoxin. In the past, patients with mitral stenosis had to undergo open heart surgery to replace the valve once it became critically narrowed (the degree of valve narrowing can be easily and accurately measured by your cardiologist via echocardiogram and Doppler). The current preferred therapy for mitral stenosis is mitral balloon valvuloplasty, whereby the valve opening is widened via a catheter-mounted balloon guided from a blood vessel near the groin up to the heart. The success rate of mitral valvuloplasty is excellent, with good durability (minimum 10 to 15 years) in most patients, though the procedure is not feasible if the patient also has moderate to significant backward leakage through the valve (mitral regurgitation).

One of the main complications of mitral stenosis is development of an irregular heart rhythm known as atrial fibrillation, occurring as the left atrium enlarges. Patients with mitral stenosis who develop atrial fibrillation usually require blood thinners (such as warfarin), in that the combination of atrial fibrillation and mitral stenosis is very conducive to development of blood clots.

If your shortness of breath does not resolve despite slowing of your pulse with medications, you should discuss with your cardiologist whether open heart surgery or balloon valvuloplasty might be indicated. He or she may wish to monitor your condition via periodic echocardiograms and possibly stress testing.

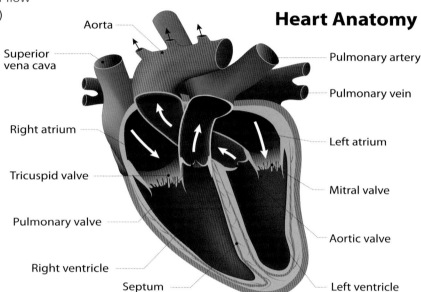

Heart Anatomy

Aorta

Superior vena cava

Right atrium

Tricuspid valve

Pulmonary valve

Right ventricle

Septum

Pulmonary artery

Pulmonary vein

Left atrium

Mitral valve

Aortic valve

Left ventricle

Mitral stenosis is a narrowing of the mitral valve, which is a two-leaflet valve that controls blood flow from the upper chamber (left atrium) to the lower chamber (left ventricle) on the left side of the heart.

Question: My internist referred me to a cardiologist because I feel occasional "skips" and "thuds" in my chest. The cardiologist said I have PVCs. What are PVCs and how are they treated?

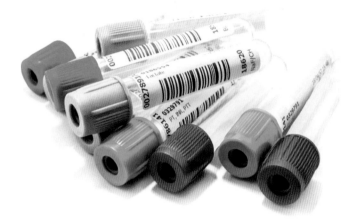

Answer: PVCs (premature ventricular contractions) are extra beats, or "rogue" beats, that arise from the left ventricle (main pumping chamber of the heart) and occur prematurely in the cardiac cycle. In many instances, PVCs are benign and often a cause is not identified.

The first thing that your cardiologist will likely do is obtain a panel of blood tests to check your blood potassium level, magnesium, calcium, and possibly thyroid function. Your cardiologist may obtain an ambulatory 24-hour electrocardiogram monitor or possibly a two- to four-week Event monitor to assess the nature and frequency of your PVCs. You will also likely have an echocardiogram, which is an ultrasound exam of the heart, or other form of cardiac imaging to assess for valve problems and other types of "structural" heart disease. Additionally, you may undergo an exercise stress test, depending on your risk factor profile and/or symptomatology.

Treatment of PVCs depends on the level of symptoms and on the cause. The treatment may consist merely of avoiding alcohol, nicotine, caffeine, chocolate, cola, and tobacco products, all of which can sometimes precipitate or exacerbate PVCs. Your cardiologist might prescribe a beta blocker or other rhythm-stabilizing drug if necessary. If the PVCs are infrequent or not terribly symptomatic, you may not require any therapy at all.

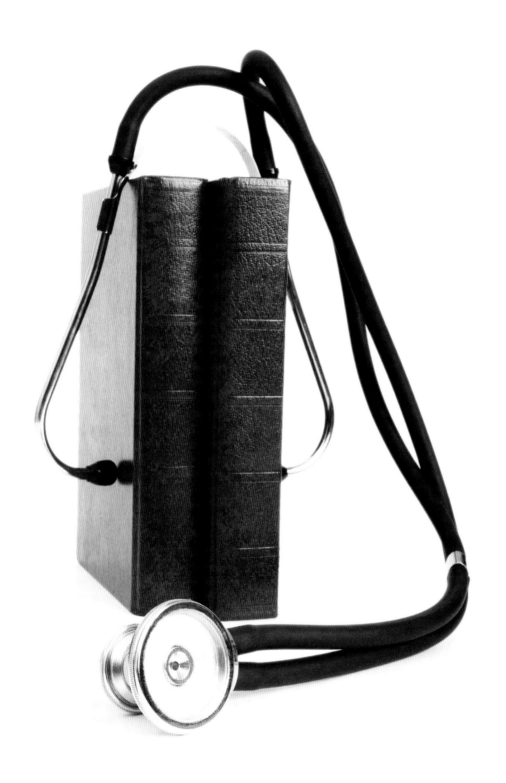

APPENDICES

Appendix A

Beaumont, Royal Oak

Array of Cardiovascular Services

An integral part of Beaumont Health, Beaumont Hospital, Royal Oak is a 1,100-bed hospital that is a major academic, research and referral center with Level I trauma designation. A member of the Children's Hospital Association, it was named Michigan's first Magnet-designated hospital for nursing excellence. The hospital ranks among the top hospitals in the United States for inpatient admissions and for surgical volume.

Beaumont, Royal Oak has also been named the "most preferred hospital" in a five-county area for 21 consecutive years in a consumer survey conducted by the National Research Corporation. In addition, it is the No. 2 hospital in Michigan with nine national medical specialty rankings on the 2016-17 lists of "America's Best Hospitals," compiled by *U.S. News & World Report*. Furthermore, it has also been recognized seven times as a Top Ten Quality Leader by Vizient (formerly the University HealthSystem Consortium). Beaumont is the exclusive clinical teaching site for the Oakland University William Beaumont School of Medicine. For additional information on Beaumont, Royal Oak, visit its website at www.beaumont.edu.

About Beaumont Heart & Vascular Care

Beaumont, Royal Oak is recognized among "America's Top 25 Hospitals" for cardiology and heart surgery by *U.S. News & World Report* for 2016-17. The Beaumont Heart and Vascular Center is a comprehensive, state-of-the-art facility that's dedicated to the prevention, diagnosis, and treatment of heart problems. Beaumont's Ernst Cardiovascular Center offers a collaborative approach to treating and managing the most complex heart and vascular conditions, including atrial fibrillation, heart valve disease, heart failure, and aortic aneurysm and dissection. The center also offers low-cost, preventive heart screening for adults and high school students. Beaumont's Tyner Center for Cardiovascular Interventions at Beaumont, Royal Oak is a 1,600 square-foot, high-tech, "hybrid" operating room/catheterization suite for cardiovascular interventions, blending catheter-based procedures with minimally invasive surgery. Beaumont's Ministrelli Women's Heart Center is the first such entity in Michigan devoted exclusively to the prevention, diagnosis, and research of heart disease in women. Find out more about the various heart and vascular care units at http://www.beaumont.edu/heart/

Heart and Vascular Center: Beaumont's Heart and Vascular Center is dedicated exclusively to the prevention, diagnosis, and treatment of heart disease.

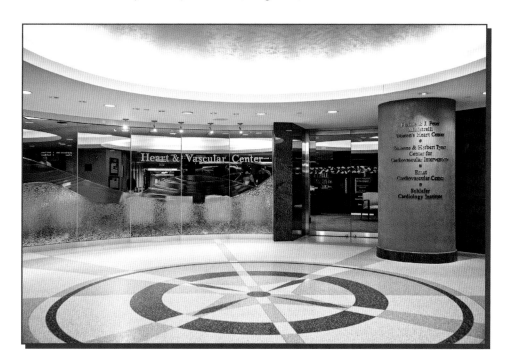

Ernst Cardiovascular Center: The Ernst Cardiovascular Center was created through the generous philanthropy of Max and Debra Ernst. The center is home to multidisciplinary outpatient clinics with a focus on the complex needs of cardiovascular patients.

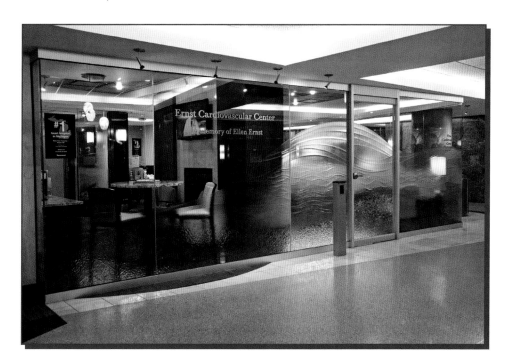

Heart Screening: As part of Beaumont's 7 for $70 heart screening program, the patient undergoes a vascular Doppler of the carotid artery to determine if any blockages exist. This screening consists of a specific series of tests for the diagnosis and prevention of heart and vascular disease.

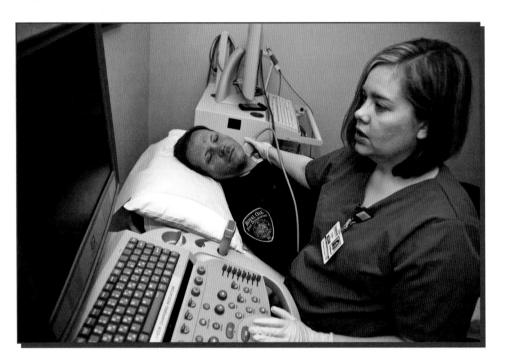

Student Heart Check: To help young people detect their risk for exertion-related cardiac arrest, Beaumont holds free community screenings on an ongoing basis. Many of Beaumont's cardiologists volunteer their time to review the high school students' echocardiograms during the screenings.

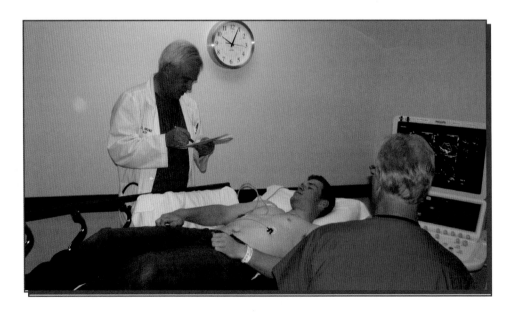

Cardiovascular Performance Clinic: The Cardiovascular Performance Clinic provides athletes or physically active adults with heart screening, training, and counseling services. Blood pressure is monitored while the client undergoes cardiopulmonary exercise testing to determine his fitness level.

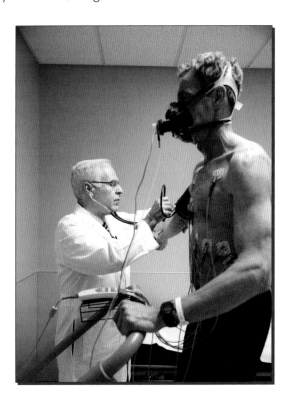

Highly Trained and Skilled Cardiologists: The patient receives follow-up care after receiving alcohol septal ablation treatment, a catheter-based procedure to help patients with hypertrophic cardiomyopathy.

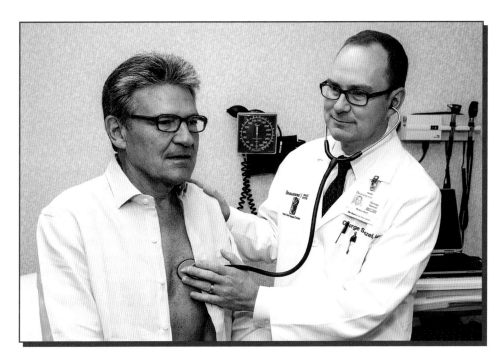

Preventive Cardiology and Cardiac Rehabilitation Center: Beaumont's preventive cardiology/cardiac rehabilitation center provides individually designed, medically supervised exercise and cardiovascular risk factor reduction programs. The center is supervised by trained clinical staff, who are available to answer questions to help patients live a heart-healthy lifestyle. Patients can have peace of mind knowing they have a medically supervised place to exercise after suffering a heart attack or undergoing cardiac surgery or coronary angioplasty.

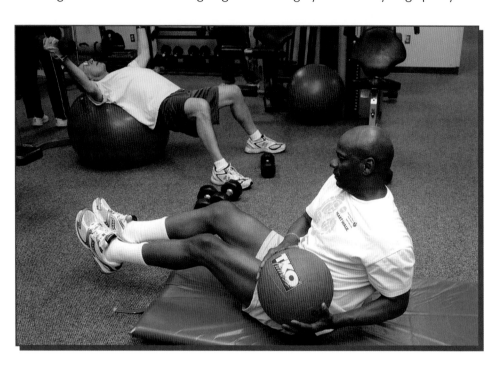

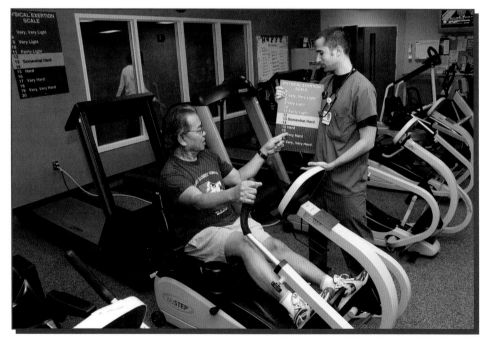

First MitraClip in Michigan: Beaumont cardiologists are leaders in the research and training of innovative procedures for complex structural heart care. Beaumont was the first hospital in Michigan to implant a MitraClip, a commercially approved device that helps high-risk patients with degenerative mitral valve regurgitation or a leaky heart valve. Prior to the procedure, the patient undergoes an echocardiogram.

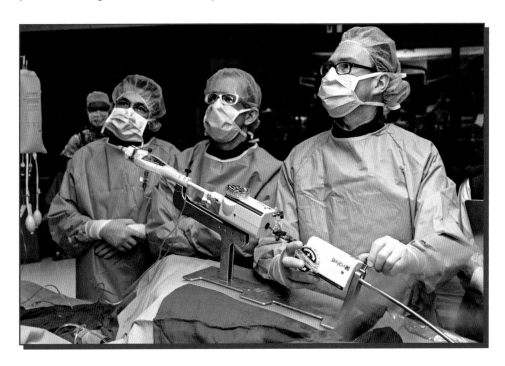

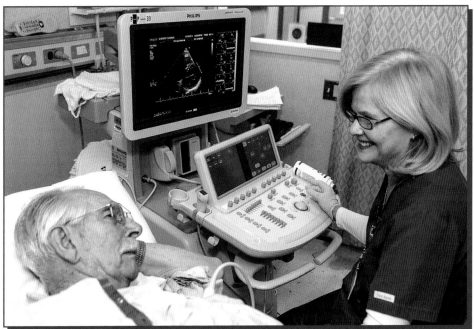

First WATCHMAN Implanted in Midwest: Beaumont cardiologists were the first team in the Midwest to implant a commercially approved WATCHMAN device. The WATCHMAN Left Atrial Appendage Closure Device is a proven alternative to the commonly used blood thinner warfarin for preventing stroke in patients with atrial fibrillation.

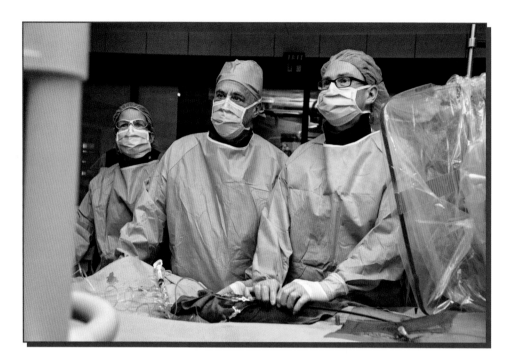

Ministrelli Women's Heart Center: Thanks to a generous donation from Florine and J. Peter Ministrelli, the Ministrelli Women's Heart Center at Beaumont, Royal Oak is the first center in Michigan dedicated to the detection, prevention, and treatment of heart disease in women.

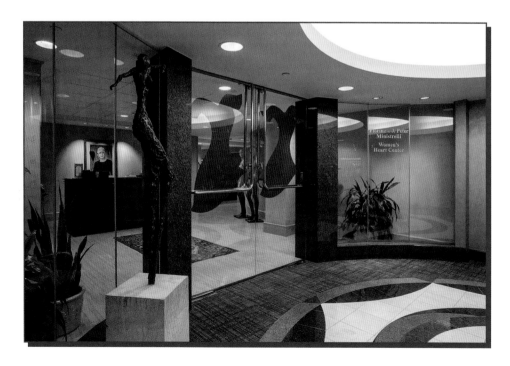

Tyner Center for Cardiovascular Interventions: Beaumont's heart and vascular team are on the cutting edge of research and training. The Tyner Center for Cardiovascular Interventions is a hybrid operating room/cath lab that provides the technology and environment for highly complex structural heart procedures. The facility serves as a major training center for minimally invasive valve replacement and structural heart procedures. Physicians and surgeons from around the world participate in a variety of trainings scheduled in the viewing room annually.

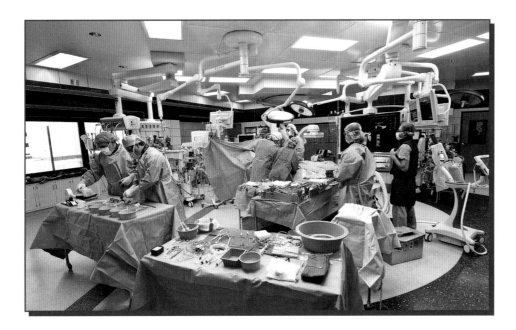

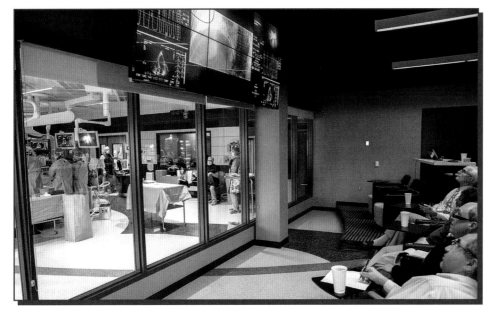

Advanced Clinical Training: Many industry and support teams come to Beaumont annually to be trained in a variety of complex cardiovascular procedures.

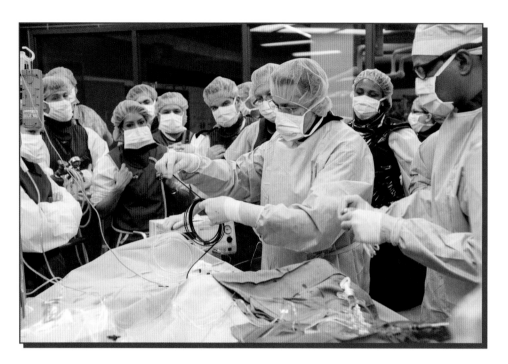

Alcohol Septal Ablation Training: Cardiologists from around the United States regularly participate in trainings, including alcohol septal ablation training, from the cardiovascular experts at Beaumont.

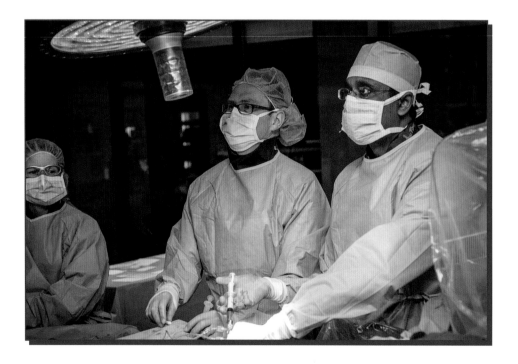

BioSkills Lab: The BioSkills Lab provides hands-on training for physicians and healthcare professionals in the use of new and advanced cardiovascular medical technologies, such as the Impella. Beaumont was the first facility in the United States to use the minimally invasive left ventricular assist device to enhance safety for high-risk cardiac interventions. The BioSkills Lab also includes 16 plug-and-play computer stations for hands-on device manipulation.

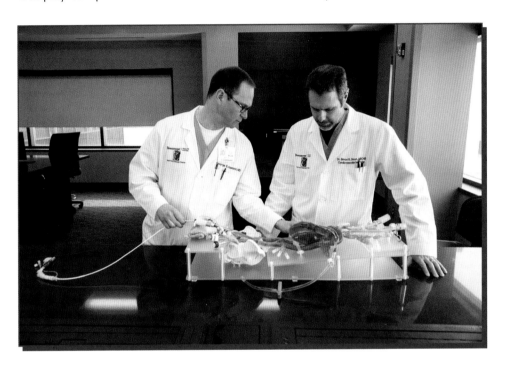

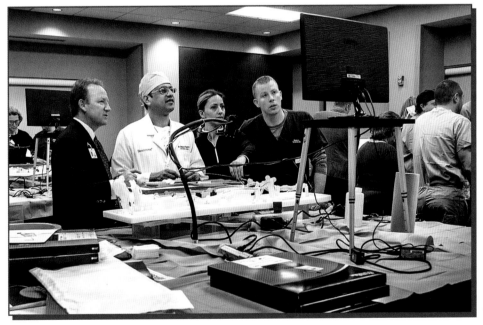

Appendix B

Still More Tips on Heart Health

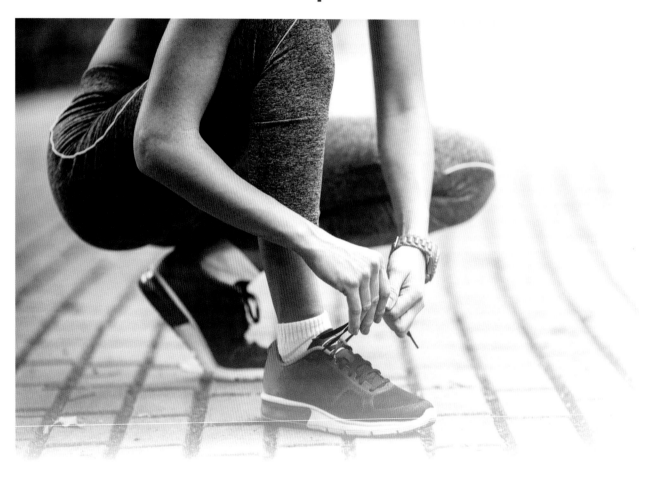

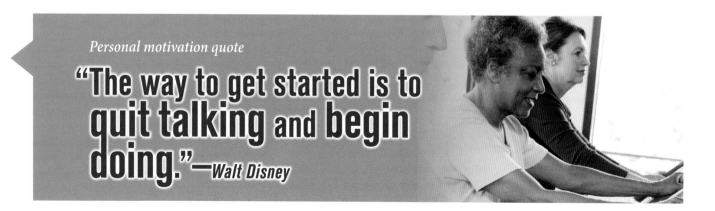

Personal motivation quote

"The way to get started is to **quit talking** and **begin doing.**"—*Walt Disney*

The average Amish man and woman take 20,000 and 15,000 steps per day, respectively. On the other hand, the average American takes just 3,500 steps per day. Interestingly, only about 5 percent of Amish adults are classified as obese.

(*Medicine and Science in Sports and Exercise*, Jan. 2004)

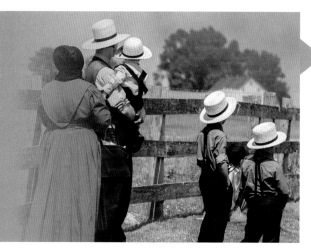

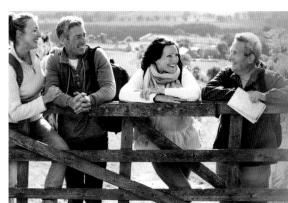

RISK FACTORS AND CARDIOVASCULAR MORTALITY

Physically fit men and women who reach middle-age without any major risk factors (i.e., high blood pressure, diabetes mellitus, elevated blood cholesterol, overweight/obesity, cigarette smoking) have only a 3 to 8 percent likelihood of dying from cardiovascular disease over the next 30 years.

(*Circ Cardiovasc Qual Outcomes*, July 2014)

LIFESTYLE CHOICES AND THE BUILT ENVIRONMENT

Barriers to healthier lifestyle choices often include the built environment. For example, racial/ethnic minority and low-income communities have more convenient access to high-fat, high caloric fast food. In addition, these population subsets are often disadvantaged in access to recreation facilities, positive outdoor surroundings and protection from traffic.

(*American Journal of Preventive Medicine*, Oct. 2004; *Circulation*, Feb. 2012)

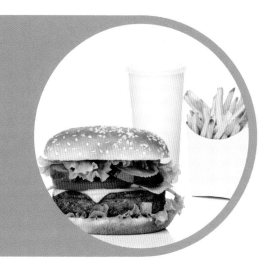

HEART-LUNG FITNESS AND MORTALITY

A measure of aerobic fitness, called metabolic equivalents, or METs, appears to be one of the most powerful predictors of cardiovascular health and longevity. One MET equals the amount of oxygen your body uses at rest. A treadmill test can be used to estimate your MET capacity, the maximum amount of oxygen that you can consume during strenuous exercise. In healthy men and women, each one MET increase in exercise capacity confers a 15 percent reduction in the likelihood of future heart problems. Individuals with a MET capacity of eight or higher had the most favorable health outcomes (*Journal of the American Medical Association*, May 2009).

CARDIAC REHABILITATION: IMPLICATIONS REGARDING PATIENT BENEFIT

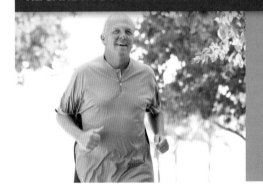

A landmark study clearly demonstrated that cardiac patients with low heart-lung fitness can especially benefit from exercise-based cardiac rehabilitation to improve functional capacity and survival.

(*Mayo Clinic Proceedings*, May 2013)

IMPROVING THE WAY WE REVERSE SUDDEN CARDIAC ARREST

Many out-of-hospital sudden cardiac arrest victims die because bystanders don't perform cardiopulmonary resuscitation (CPR). Studies now report that chest compressions only (Hands Only CPR) for adults by bystander lay rescuers improves survival.

(*New England Journal of Medicine*, July 2010)

TWO STEPS TO SAVE A LIFE:

Call 911

Push hard and fast in the center of the chest

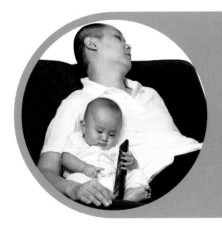

FATHERHOOD ADVERSELY AFFECTS BODY MASS INDEX

In a longitudinal, population-based study that included serial body mass index measurements, men gained an average of 4.4 pounds after becoming first-time dads. In contrast, men who weren't fathers actually lost 1.4 pounds during the 20-year study. The investigators suggested that the new fathers' weight gain may be due to decreases in daily energy expenditure, increases in caloric consumption, or both.

(*American Journal of Men's Health*, July 2015)

CHANGES IN AMBULANCE CALLS AFTER SMOKE-FREE LAW

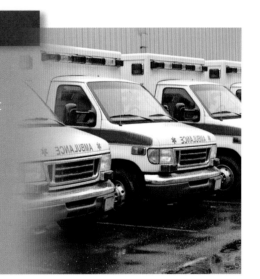

A few years ago, researchers reported that ambulance calls originating from everywhere but casinos dropped by 23 percent when Gilpin County, Colorado implemented a smoke-free law that applied everywhere but casinos. Two years later, when the law was expanded to casinos, ambulance calls from casinos dropped by 19 percent, with no change in calls originating outside casinos. Two implications emerged from the study findings. First, clinicians should advise their patients, especially patients with known or suspected heart disease, to stay away from smoky environments. Second, policy makers should see that all environments, including casinos, are smoke-free. (*Circulation*, Aug. 2013)

SMOKING AND MORTALITY: WOEFULLY UNDERESTIMATED?

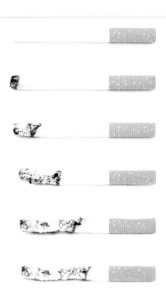

The 2014 Surgeon General's report estimated that cigarette smoking causes more than 480,000 deaths each year in the United States—or about 1 death in every 5. However, according to a recent report, this widely cited number may be an underestimate because it considers deaths only from the 21 diseases that have been formally established as caused by smoking. In the most recent analysis, researchers found that these 21 diseases account for only about 83 percent of the mortality burden from smoking. The addition of diseases currently associated with smoking—but not directly established as caused by smoking—adds an additional 60,000 to 120,000 deaths each year.

(*New England Journal of Medicine*, Feb. 2015)

VERY OBESE ADULTS ALMOST COMPLETELY SEDENTARY

Several years ago, researchers asked 10 morbidly obese adults to wear an activity sensor that kept track of their caloric expenditure, minute-by-minute physical activity, and number of steps per day over three days. The participants spent an average of 23 hours and 52 minutes/day sleeping, sitting, lying down, or performing sedentary activities. These data suggest important links between obesity, low fitness, and cardiovascular disease.

(*Clinical Cardiology,* March 2009).

HOW THEY LIVE LONGER

Long living population subsets in three widely separated areas of the world, including Sardinians, Adventists and Okinawans, share a number of key lifestyle habits. *All don't smoke, put family first, are physically active every day, keep socially engaged, and regularly eat fruits, vegetables and whole grains.*

(*National Geographic,* Nov. 2005)

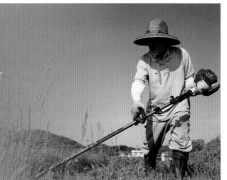

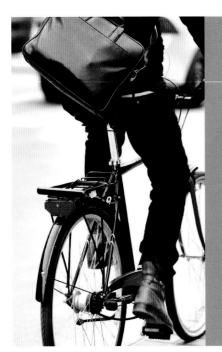

NEW YORK CITY'S LIFE EXPECTANCY IS SKYROCKETING

"If you want to live longer and healthier than the average American, come to New York City," pronounced former Mayor Michael Bloomberg as he released data on the city's life expectancy. Since 1990, when life expectancy in the city trailed the U.S. average by three years, it has lengthened by eight years! How did this come about? To counter the alarming statistics, the city health department introduced a series of initiatives to alter the choices available to its residents. It mandated calorie labels for food sold in chain restaurants and banned trans fats. It prohibited smoking in public places and markedly increased taxes on cigarettes. Finally, it rolled out hundreds of miles of new bicycle lanes and papered subways with information campaigns about the risks of obesity and the benefits of healthier lifestyle choices including regular exercise.

(*Lancet,* June 2012)

THE AMAZING POWER OF ASPIRIN

In March 2009, the U.S. Preventive Health Services Task Force recommended the daily use of aspirin for primary prevention of heart attack and stroke in men and women who haven't been diagnosed with cardiovascular disease. The authors concluded that aspirin is more effective in preventing cardiovascular events in groups of people with traditional risk factors (e.g., elevated blood cholesterol, high blood pressure, cigarette smoking, diabetes, overweight/obese, least active/least fit). Additional evidence shows that aspirin may also play a role in fighting colon cancer, breast cancer, asthma, diabetes and Alzheimer's disease. On the other hand, taking aspirin increases a person's chances of bleeding in the stomach, intestines or brain (called "hemorrhagic stroke").

(Annals of Internal Medicine, March 2009).

ANTIDEPRESSANTS MAY INCREASE RISK FOR ABNORMAL HEART RHYTHMS

Some antidepressant medications such as citalopram (Celexa) and escitalopram (Lexapro) may trigger abnormal heart rhythms and increased cardiac risk. The effect is more likely to occur in patients taking higher doses of these drugs.

(*British Medical Journal,* Jan. 2013)

SNOW SHOVEL-RELATED INJURIES AND MEDICAL EMERGENCIES

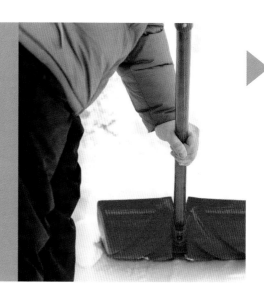

On average, there are an estimated 11,500 snow shovel-related injuries and medical emergencies treated each year in U.S. hospital emergency departments. Cardiac-related visits accounted for an important minority of the cases (7 percent), including all of the reported deaths. Persons with known heart disease, including patients who have undergone previous coronary artery stenting, seem to be at the greatest risk.

(*American Journal of Emergency Medicine,* Jan. 2011; *American Journal of Cardiology,* Aug. 2010)

IS AGE REALLY A NON-MODIFIABLE RISK FACTOR?

Although numerous studies suggest that the aging process promotes heart disease, one review of the scientific data challenged the prevalent notion that age is a non-modifiable risk factor. The authors concluded that age is, to a large extent, simply a reflection of the length of exposure to the burden of risk factors. In an analysis of Framingham data, individuals who attained 50 years of age with optimal risk factors were almost immune to the development of cardiovascular disease.

(*American Journal of Cardiology*, Nov. 2009).

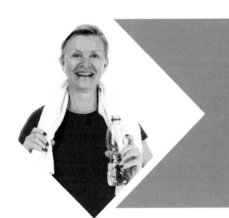

CARDIAC REHABILITATION IN WOMEN

A recent report of nearly 26,000 patients who attended cardiac rehabilitation demonstrated a significantly greater mortality benefit among the women participants than their male counterparts. On the other hand, women were less likely to be referred to and attend cardiac rehabilitation.

(*European Journal of Preventive Cardiology*, Oct. 2015)

SHINGLES INCREASES STROKE RISK

Shingles, a disease characterized by skin eruptions and pain along the involved sensory nerves, increases the risk of having a stroke over the next 12 months. The risk is especially high in individuals with eye-related (ocular) shingles. People who have had shingles should take extra care to reduce stroke risk via lifestyle modification and medication to control blood pressure and cholesterol

(Dr. Daniel T. Lackland, Medical University of South Carolina, Charleston).

WARNING: DEER HUNTING MAY BE HAZARDOUS TO YOUR HEALTH

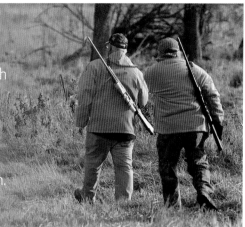

Although gunshot wounds are responsible for hunting fatalities each year, other deaths are commonly attributed to acute cardiovascular events. Several years ago, researchers at Beaumont were the first to report that deer hunting activities can elicit abrupt, sustained, and marked increases in heart rate in middle-aged men. It was concluded that such responses may lead to threatening heart rhythms and the potential for heart attacks or sudden cardiac death.

(*American Journal of Cardiology*, July 2007)

TRIGGERING OF HEART ATTACK BY COCAINE USE

Cocaine has been implicated as a trigger of heart attack in people with and without known heart disease. In the Determinants of Myocardial Infarction Onset Study, the risk of heart attack onset was 24 times over baseline in the 60 minutes after cocaine use!

(*Circulation*, June 1999).

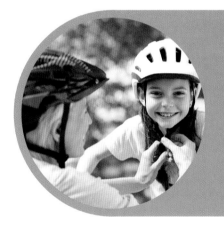

CYCLING ACCIDENTS

Each year, bicycle accidents result in more than 500,000 visits to hospital emergency centers. More than 800 bicyclists die annually, many from head injuries. Most deaths occur between 6 pm and 9 pm, when visibility is diminished. The best defense? Helmets are highly effective in preventing fatal head injuries.

(*Current Sports Medicine Reports*, July/Aug 2012)

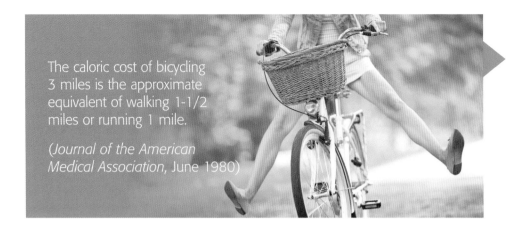

The caloric cost of bicycling 3 miles is the approximate equivalent of walking 1-1/2 miles or running 1 mile.

(*Journal of the American Medical Association*, June 1980)

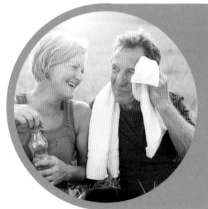

Men who exercise vigorously at least 3 hours a week are 30 percent less likely to suffer from erectile dysfunction (ED) than men who are sedentary.

(*The Medical Post*)

RUNNING REDUCES THE RISK OF DYING FROM HEART DISEASE

A provocative study of runners found that their risk of dying from heart disease was 45 percent lower than non-runners over a 15-year follow-up. Interestingly, the report also showed that individuals who jogged at an easy pace for as little as 5 to 10 minutes a day had virtually the same survival benefits as those who pushed themselves harder or longer.

(*Journal of the American College of Cardiology*, Aug. 2014)

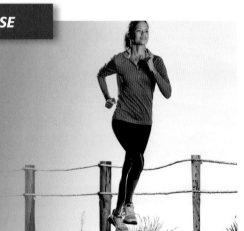

WANT TO LOSE WEIGHT? GET MORE SLEEP

An enlightening study in normal-weight men and women examined changes in appetite-related hormone levels in response to two sleep conditions: short sleep (four hours) and normal sleep (nine hours). The researchers reported that sleep deprivation led to increased levels of hunger-stimulating hormone in men, but not in women. On the other hand, short sleep reduced levels of the satiety (feeling of fullness) hormone in women, but not in men. Take home message: Getting more sleep in both genders may help reduce overeating.

(*Sleep,* Nov. 2012)

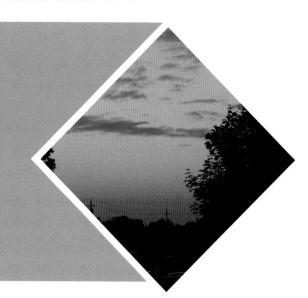

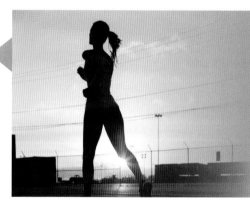

EXERCISE NULLIFIES THE INCREASED DIABETES RISK FROM STATINS

According to a recent report, regular walking or running lowers diabetes, hypertension, and cardiovascular risk in patients with elevated blood cholesterol and should more than compensate for the purported 9 percent increase in diabetes risk from statin use.

(*American Journal of Cardiology,* Nov. 2015)

VIGOROUS PHYSICAL ACTIVITY AND WEIGHT LOSS

According to one sobering report, a 45-minute vigorous exercise bout resulted in a significant elevation in postexercise energy expenditure that persisted for 14 hours. The authors concluded that the nearly 200 calories expended after exercise above resting levels may have implications for weight loss and management. Thus, these findings suggest that the calories expended from vigorous exercise are generally underestimated.

(*Medicine & Science in Sports & Exercise,* Sept. 2011)

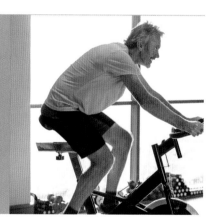

GO FOR A RUN INSTEAD OF A WALK

Because the associated energy cost of running is greater than walking, running (or walking up a grade or incline) is better for the heart than walking. For cardiovascular health, a five-minute run is equal to a 15-minute walk, and a 25-minute run equals a 105-minute walk.

(*Journal of the American College of Cardiology*, Aug. 2014)

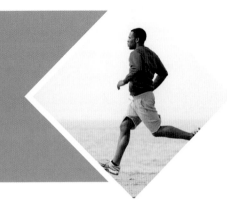

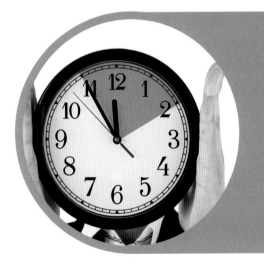

EVEN A LITTLE EXERCISE CAN IMPROVE SURVIVAL IN OLDER ADULTS

A low dose of moderate-to-vigorous physical activity, or about *15 minutes per day*, reduced mortality in older adults by 22 percent. The greatest benefit seemed to accrue among those who went from doing nothing, or only a minimal amount of physical activity, to doing more. These findings should help convince currently inactive older adults that even a little exercise has health and longevity benefits.

(*British Journal of Sports Medicine*, Aug. 2015)

SURVIVAL OF THE FITTEST

Numerous studies have now identified a low level of heart-lung fitness, expressed as metabolic equivalents (METs), as an independent risk factor for all-cause and cardiovascular mortality. The most common way to determine your MET capacity is through a treadmill stress test. An exercise capacity of less than 5 METs indicates a higher mortality group, whereas an exercise capacity of 10 METs or higher identifies individuals with an excellent long-term prognosis. Persons in the low fitness group (less than 5 METs) should be strongly encouraged to improve their exercise tolerance by starting and maintaining a regular, progressive walking program.

(*Mayo Clinic Proceedings*, Sept. 2009).

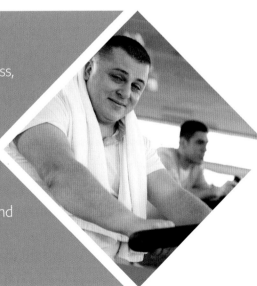

CALORIE COUNTS ON RESTAURANT MENUS ARE OFTEN UNDERESTIMATED

According to a study involving 10 chain restaurants, the actual calories for many popular meals averaged 18 percent higher than the value listed on menus. Self-defense: Because of variations in ingredients and portion sizes, recognize that you may be consuming more calories than are suggested.

(*Journal of the American Dietetic Association,* Jan. 2010).

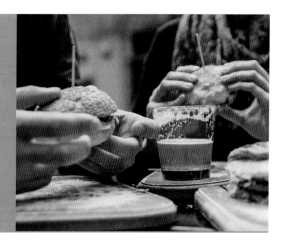

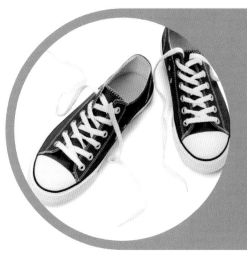

FITNESS TRUMPS BODY WEIGHT IN REDUCING MORTALITY

According to one study, if you maintain or improve your fitness level, even if your body weight remains unchanged or increases, you can reduce your risk of death. In contrast, researchers found no association between changes in body fat or weight and death risk.

(*Circulation,* Dec. 2011)

CALORIC INTAKE FROM FAST FOOD IS DECREASING

During 2007 to 2010, fast food from restaurants such as McDonald's, Burger King and Wendy's accounted for 11 percent of American adults' daily calories. That's lower than it was between 2003 and 2006, when fast food accounted for nearly 13 percent of adults' daily caloric intake.

(*National Center for Health Statistics,* Feb. 2013)

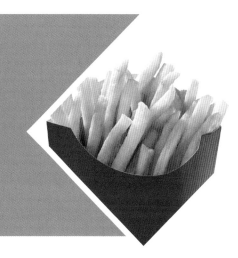

BEANS FOR LOWER BLOOD SUGAR

One review of 41 clinical trials concluded that diabetics who ate one-half cup of beans a day—garbanzo, black, white, pinto or kidney beans—had significantly lower fasting blood glucose, insulin and hemoglobin A1C levels, a marker of long-term glucose control.

(Cyril Kendall, Ph.D., Department of Nutritional Sciences, University of Toronto)

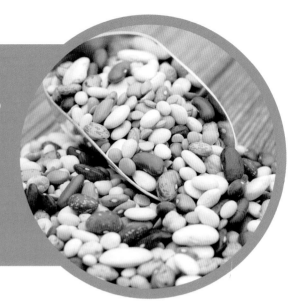

NUTS AND HEART HEALTH

How can you significantly reduce your risk of developing heart disease? By eating a handful of nuts five or more times a week! Even those who eat nuts once a week have less heart disease than those who don't eat any nuts. Tree nuts such as almonds, Brazil nuts, cashews, chestnuts, hazelnuts, macadamias, pecans, pine nuts, pistachios and walnuts are packed full of beneficial nutrients for heart health. (www.nutsforlife.com.au)

WEIGHT-LOSS SECRET?

In a classic report, researchers found that drinking just 500 ml of water transiently increased the metabolic rate (energy expenditure) by 30 percent in men and women. Based on their measurements, they estimated that one could lose more than 5 pounds per year by increasing water ingestion by 1.5 liters per day. It was suggested that this cost-free intervention may serve as a useful adjunctive treatment in overweight and obese individuals to attain an increase in energy expenditure.

(*Journal of Clinical Endocrinology and Metabolism*, Dec. 2003)

RED MEAT CONSUMPTION LINKED TO DIABETES RISK

People who increased their red meat consumption by more than half a serving a day had a 48 percent greater likelihood for developing type 2 diabetes, whereas those who reduced their consumption of red meat by the same amount had a 14 percent lower risk for acquiring this metabolic condition.

(*Journal of the American Medical Association,* July 2013)

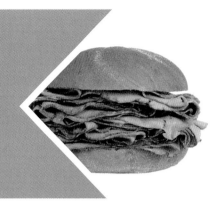

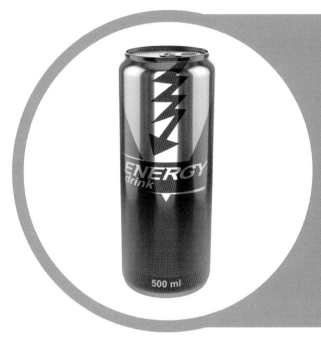

CARDIOVASCULAR EVENTS AFTER INGESTION OF ENERGY DRINKS

Clinical researchers reviewed 17 cases of energy-drink related acute cardiac events. Of the 11 cases related to a serious complication, five reported excessive energy drink consumption, and four reported co-ingestion with alcohol or other drugs. Most of the adverse effects are associated with the high caffeine content of these drinks, approximating 200 to 300 mg in some brands. The investigators suggested that physicians should routinely inquire about energy drink consumption in relevant cases, and that consumers should be advised of the heightened risk of potentially fatal cardiovascular events.

(American Journal of Cardiology, Jan. 2014)

TOMATOES KEEP BLOOD VESSELS HEALTHY

Getting a daily dose (7 milligrams) of the antioxidant lycopene improved the inner or endothelial linings of blood vessels in patients with heart disease. Tomatoes are a good food source of lycopene.

(*PLoS One,* June 2014)

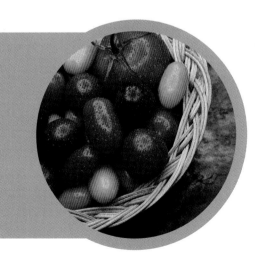

HOLD THE SALT!

An escalating body of scientific evidence now links sodium intake with elevated blood pressure and other adverse cardiovascular outcomes. The American Heart Association recommends that the general population consume no more than 1500 milligrams (mg) of sodium a day because of the harmful effects of sodium—hypertension and increased risk of stroke, heart attack and kidney disease.

(*Circulation*, Jan. 2011)

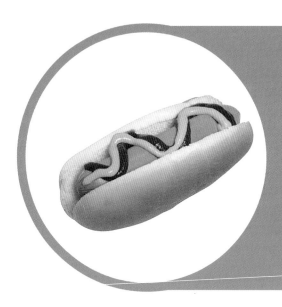

HOW DO YOU MAKE A HOT DOG?

"First you slaughter the animals and cut out all the good parts, the steaks and chops. But you've got a lot of animal left and what are you going to do with it?

The hot dog industry took off when a clever guy invented a machine that works like a kitchen disposal—you dump everything in, eyeballs and all, and grind it up. Voila, the hot dog."

(William Castelli, M.D., former co-director of the Framingham Heart Study).

STRATEGIES TO REDUCE SODIUM INTAKE

Americans average a daily intake of more than 3,400 mg of sodium. This substantially exceeds the maximum intake level (1,500 mg/day) now recommended by the American Heart Association. Dietary sources of sodium are plentiful, are derived largely from processed and restaurant foods, and include many foods not commonly perceived as high sources of sodium. Recent studies also dispel the notion that excess salt intake is due primarily to salt added by the consumer at the table. Such use appears to account for only about 6 percent of sodium consumed.

(National Academy of Sciences, Institute of Medicine, 2012)

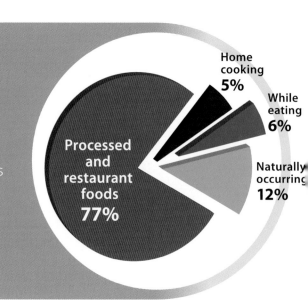

Home cooking 5%

While eating 6%

Naturally occurring 12%

Processed and restaurant foods 77%

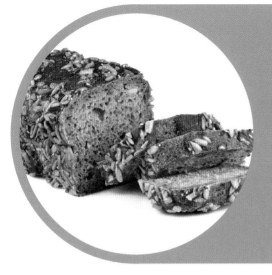

HIGH-FIBER DIET IS LINKED TO LONGER LIFE

People who ate a diet rich in fiber—including whole grains, beans, fruits and vegetables—were 22 percent less likely to die during a 9-year follow-up period than those who ate the least fiber. They were also less likely to die from cardiovascular disease. Why? Researchers believe that fiber has anti-inflammatory properties. It also improves blood cholesterol and its subfractions, triglycerides and glucose levels, reducing the likelihood of disease. The 'take-home message' is: the whiter the bread, the sooner you're dead!

(*Archives of Internal Medicine,* June 2011)

NONCALORIC SWEETENERS MIGHT PROMOTE WEIGHT LOSS

A published statement from the American Heart Association and the American Diabetes Association indicates that there are some data to suggest that noncaloric sweeteners may be used to replace sources of added sugars and that this substitution may result in modest calorie reductions and weight loss.

(*Circulation,* July 2012)

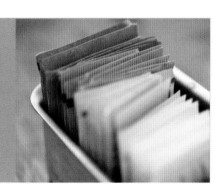

DIETARY FIBER ASSOCIATED WITH DECREASED STROKE RISK

For every 7 grams of fiber consumed daily, the risk for a first-time stroke decreased by 7 percent. This approximates one serving of whole-wheat pasta or two servings of fruits and vegetables each day.

(*Stroke,* May 2013)

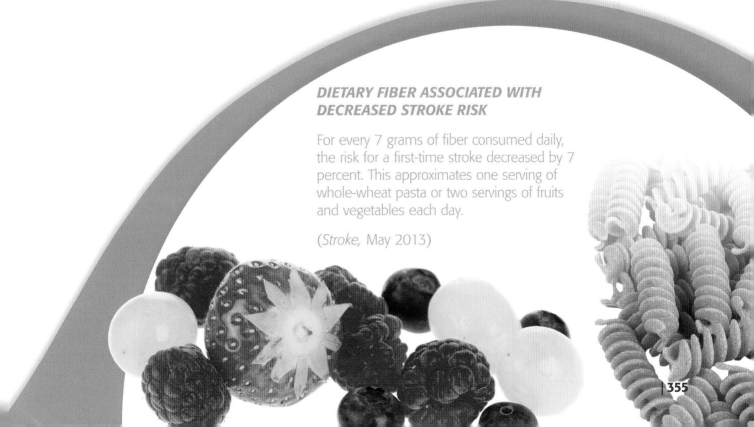

MARATHON RUNNERS AREN'T IMMUNE TO CORONARY ATHEROSCLEROSIS

A provocative study of middle-aged male marathon runners and age-matched sedentary men, all of whom underwent 64-slice CT angiography for a variety of reasons, demonstrated that the runners actually had greater amounts of calcified plaque in their coronary arteries. The researchers suggested that training and racing under demanding conditions, for prolonged periods of time, may actually be injurious to the heart's arteries. For example, distance runners may be leaking calcium into their bloodstream because of repeated trauma to weight-bearing bones .

(*Internal Medicine News,* June 2010)

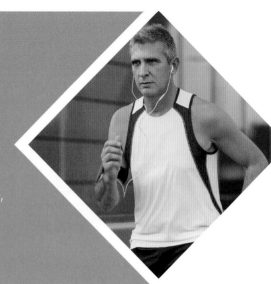

WALKING DURATION ASSOCIATED WITH REDUCED RISK OF STROKE

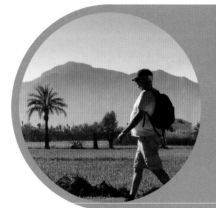

According to a provocative report, time spent walking was associated with a reduced risk of stroke in older men, independent of walking pace or speed. These data suggest that regular walking for extended periods provides an important component of stroke-prevention strategies.

(*Stroke,* Jan. 2014)

HEALTHY FOODS COST MORE

A widely-cited public health study of 11,195 people may help to explain the higher incidence of cardiovascular disease among the poor and less fortunate. People who follow a Mediterranean diet, which emphasizes olive oil, fish and vegetables, spend on average at least $2 a day more than people who consume a conventional American diet.

(*Journal of Epidemiology and Community Health,* Sept. 2009)

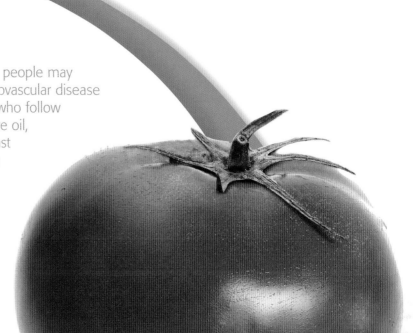

"JUST SAY NO" TO SUGARY DRINKS

Two randomized controlled clinical trials both independently concluded that reducing the consumption of sugar-sweetened beverages reduces weight gain in children and adolescents.

(*New England Journal of Medicine*, Oct. 2012)

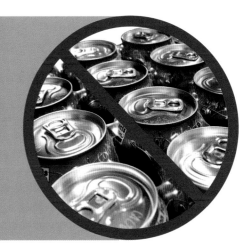

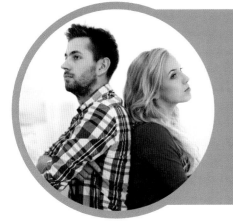

HEART ATTACK, STROKE-PRONE ARTERIES MORE COMMON IN CONFRONTATIONAL PEOPLE

People with confrontational personalities have greater thickening of the neck (carotid) arteries as compared with their more agreeable counterparts, making them more prone to heart attacks and strokes. This held true even after the researchers adjusted for cholesterol levels, blood pressure, smoking status and other risk factors.
(*Hypertension*, Oct. 2010)

SUBOPTIMAL MEDICATION DOSING AFTER ACUTE MYOCARDIAL INFARCTION

Although nearly all patients after a heart attack are discharged on appropriate cardioprotective medications, most patients are prescribed doses substantially below those with proven efficacy in clinical trials. These findings suggest that physician and hospital performance measures may need to better highlight doses of medications to achieve their goal of optimal medical therapy.

(*Journal of the American College of Cardiology*, Nov. 2013)

"Approximately 85 percent of individuals in the U.S. over age 50 have atherosclerotic coronary disease. So for me, the question isn't whether middle-aged and older adults have heart disease—they probably do. It's how to prevent acute cardiac events."

– *Ira M. Grais, M.D.*

DIN: 0123456789
Remain: 0 TAB

TAKE 1 TABLET F
TIMES A DAY AS N

Appendix C

101 Heart-Healthy Facts

1 Physicians and their coronary patients should recognize that exercise-based cardiac rehabilitation, if adhered to, is as beneficial and cost-effective as most contemporary technologies and drug therapies.

2 The most crucial role individuals have in their heart health is as a "self-advocate," accepting the fact that achieving good health is primarily their responsibility.

3 High blood pressure, high cholesterol, and cigarette smoking are key risk factors for heart disease.

4 A heart attack occurs when a coronary artery suddenly becomes blocked or obstructed.

5 To begin the process of healing and recovery from a heart attack, the patient must understand the causes of heart disease and the risk factors that contribute to it.

6 The older a person is, the greater the risk for developing an abnormal heart rhythm known as atrial fibrillation (a-fib).

7 The primary methods to prevent and treat those individuals with metabolic syndrome include lifestyle changes to reduce body weight and fat stores, structured exercise, increased lifestyle physical activity, and the transition to a heart-healthy diet.

8 A number of heart attacks occur without discernable symptoms.

9 The signs that a woman is having angina maybe less obvious than they are for a man; women are more likely to experience nausea, indigestion, or shoulder ache, as opposed to the hallmark chest pain that men often have.

10 Heart attacks have several major warning signs and symptoms, including chest pain or discomfort, upper-body pain or discomfort, shortness of breath, nausea, lightheadedness, and cold sweats.

11 Coronary artery disease and stroke result in three times more deaths in women than all cancers combined.

12 High blood pressure is the second leading modifiable cause of death and disability in the US and contributes to half of all strokes and heart attacks.

13 Patients who have suffered a mini-stroke are twice as likely to suffer a heart attack within the next five years.

14 Angina, which is a symptom of heart disease, often presenting as chest pain, shortness of breath, or both, is caused by inadequate circulation to the heart muscle.

15 A progressive treadmill exercise test is the best way to determine a person's exercise capacity or heart-lung fitness as expressed in metabolic equivalent units.

16 Sudden strenuous exertion may place excessive demands on the heart that cannot be matched immediately by its circulation, leading to electrocardiographic abnormalities, heart rhythm irregularities, or chest pain.

17 Physical activity represents an anti-aging intervention that may be helpful in reducing the impact of age-related diseases.

18 When individuals are diagnosed with atherosclerotic heart disease (i.e., clogged coronary arteries), their cardiologist will commonly recommend medications such as aspirin, cholesterol-lowering statins, beta blockers, angiotensin converting enzyme inhibitors, and nitrates.

19 Salt intake worldwide is at least twice what it should be, with a negative impact on cardiovascular health.

20 Beta-blocker therapy can be useful for preventing recurrent heart attacks and potentially fatal rhythm disturbances in heart attack survivors.

21 Regular exercise can reduce a person's risk of dying from heart disease by up to 50 percent.

22 Common symptoms of congestive heart failure include shortness of breath, activity limitations (fatigue), swelling in the lower extremities, and weight gain due to fluid buildup or retention (edema).

23 Some commonly prescribed medications for congestive heart failure include diuretics, angiotensin converting enzyme (ACE) inhibitors, angiotensin receptor blockers, vasodilators, beta-blockers, cholesterol-lowering statins, and aspirin.

24 At the "heart" of the modern cath lab is sophisticated X-ray imaging equipment which allows the physician to advance thin tubes, called catheters, in real time from the wrist or groin into the heart.

25 As a general rule, it will take a patient about 4-6 weeks to start feeling better after undergoing cardiac bypass surgery.

26 Atrial fibrillation affects 2-3 percent of the population—a percentage that increases as a person ages.

27 The most common cause for myocardial infarction (heart attack) is formation of a blood clot at the site of an inflamed atherosclerotic plaque inside the coronary artery tree.

28 Statins work by blocking an enzyme in the liver called HMG-CoA reductase, which is responsible for converting a cholesterol precursor into true cholesterol.

29 Aquatic exercise has been found to enhance multiple measures of cardiovascular health.

30 Mitral regurgitation is, in essence, an incompetent or "leaky" mitral valve—the one-way valve that separates the left atrium from the left ventricle.

31 Older adults who walk at a three-mile per hour or faster pace tend to outlive those individuals who move at slower speeds.

32 There are 670,000 new cases of congestive heart failure (CHF) diagnosed each year, contributing to 281,000 deaths annually and one million acute CHF hospitalizations.

33 Every heart patient can play an important role in ensuring the best possible outcome from a doctor's visit.

34 Persons with high MET capacities generally live longer and have a lower risk of heart disease than those at the bottom of the fitness/activity continuum—people who are in the least fit, least active subgroup.

35 Traditional Chinese exercises, such as tai chi, may improve the health and well-being of individuals living with heart disease, high blood pressure, or stroke.

36 Atrial fibrillation occurs if the heart emits rapid, disorganized electrical signals from many atrial locations simultaneously rather than from the sinus node alone, causing its two upper chambers (the atria) to fibrillate (contract very fast and irregularly).

37 About one in 10 patients undergoing heart catheterization for suspected angina are found to have total blockage (occlusion) of one of the major arteries that provide blood to the heart muscle.

38 Men and women with stable coronary disease who have no symptoms during routine activities of daily living can generally safely engage in sexual activity.

39 The incidence of chronic disease, such as cardiovascular disease, diabetes, arthritis, and osteoporosis increases with age, with approximately 80 percent of older adults living with one or more of these conditions.

40 Even small amounts of physical activity each week will help reduce heart disease risk, and the benefit escalates as fitness increases, up to a point.

41 Hypertension, diabetes, cardiovascular disease, and tobacco use directly contribute to erectile dysfunction.

42 Aspirin remains a mainstay of therapy for a variety of cardiac disorders, decreasing inflammation in the arteries and preventing the formation of blood clots.

43 The riskiest time of day for heart attacks is between 6 am and noon.

44 An exercise stress test is associated with a very low risk of complications and can help a person's doctor determine whether exertion-related symptoms (e.g., severe shortness of breath, chest pain or pressure) are related to underlying heart disease.

45 Avocados contain monounsaturated fat, fiber, phytosterols, and other nutrients believed to lower the level of cholesterol in the blood.

46 An exercise stress test simultaneously evaluates several variables, which help to build a snapshot of a person's overall cardiovascular health and fitness.

47 Equivalent energy expenditures by moderate-intensity exercise (walking) and vigorous exercise (running) produce similar risk reductions for the development of high blood pressure, elevated cholesterol, and diabetes mellitus.

48 Leg pain that occurs during walking or other types of physical exertion may be due to vascular diseases.

49 Ejection fraction, which is the percentage of blood pumped out of the hearts main pumping chamber, the left ventricle, with each heartbeat, is a key indicator of the contractility of a functioning heart.

50 A person with congestive heart failure, which can occur when the left ventricle has been weakened or damaged, may have an ejection fraction of less than 35 percent.

51 An abnormal electrocardiogram (ECG) test result may suggest the likelihood of underlying heart disease, especially a major blockage of one or more coronary arteries.

52 Shorter people are more likely to develop heart disease.

53 Strenuous physical activity, especially when sudden or unaccustomed in habitually sedentary individuals, may transiently increase the risk for acute myocardial infarction and/or sudden cardiac death.

54 Considerable evidence suggests that chemical stressors, including illicit drugs, can increase the risk of acute myocardial infarctions in persons with and without underlying heart disease.

55 Transcendental meditation, a mind-body intervention, may significantly reduce risk for mortality, myocardial infarction, and stroke in coronary patients.

56 Improvement of environmental air quality is a highly effective way to reduce the population incidence of acute cardiac events.

57 People who routinely get less than five hours of sleep per night have a higher risk of developing heart disease.

58 A cardiac MRI, which creates detailed pictures of the heart using a specialized camera, can be used to diagnose a number of heart conditions.

59 Death rates due to heart disease are the highest in the South and lowest in the West.

60 A coronary artery calcium test identifies signs of plaque in the heart's vasculature, which is a significant risk factor for heart attack.

61 Among older patients with heart disease who undergo cardiac rehabilitation, death rates are approximately 20-35 percent lower than among those who don't participate.

62 On average, a regular endurance exercise program will decrease a person's heart rate by more than three million beats a year.

63 Risk assessment for coronary artery disease is recommended as the first step in the diagnosis and treatment of this deadly medical condition.

64 Heart disease should not be considered a "man's disease," given that cardiovascular mortality is higher in women than men.

65 Approximately one out of three adults in the United States has high blood pressure (hypertension).

66 A heart MRI has minimal risk, as well as few, if any, side effects.

67 Increasing evidence suggests that at least some of the unexplained incidence of cardiovascular disease (i.e., 10-25 percent) may be attributed to the adverse effects of psychosocial stressors.

68 The predominant cause of type 2 diabetes (the most prevalent form) is insufficient insulin secretion from the pancreas, or an inability of cells to utilize the insulin, called insulin resistance, most often seen in obese people.

69 Metabolic syndrome is defined by a clustering of risk factors that appear to promote the development of atherosclerotic cardiovascular disease.

70 According to the CDC, more than 29 million Americans have diabetes (a major risk factor for heart disease), and 86 million people have prediabetes (i.e., they're on the road to having diabetes).

71 Approximately 1.65 million cardiovascular-related deaths per-year can be attributed to sodium consumption levels above the recommended guidelines.

72 The hallmark of diabetes is high blood glucose levels that, over time, damage blood vessels, organs, and nerves.

73 About 610,000 people die of heart disease in the United States every year.

74 Pericarditis is inflammation of the pericardium—the two thin layers of sac-like tissue that surrounds the heart, holds it in place, and helps it work.

75 Pericarditis affects individuals of all ages, but males 25 to 50 years old are greatest at risk for developing it.

76 The specific cause of pericarditis is often unknown, although a viral infection is a common cause.

77 As a rule, pericarditis is mild and clears up on its own with rest or simple treatment; on occasion, more intense treatment is needed to prevent complications.

78 Trans fats raise a person's "bad" low-density lipoprotein cholesterol (LDL) and a subcomponent of LDL cholesterol (lipoprotein (a)), which is identified as another cardiac risk factor.

79 People who routinely work 11 or more hours per day have a significantly higher risk for heart-related problems, including fatal heart attacks and anginal chest pain, as compared with individuals who maintain a conventional eight-hour work day.

80 Heart disease is the biggest killer of both men and women.

81 Varicose veins are the most common cardiovascular disease manifestation, exceeding the incidence of heart disease, peripheral artery disease, and stroke combined.

82 The emerging use of chemotherapeutics for treating cancer patients, although effective, has an undeniable cardiovascular risk.

83 Psychological stressors that increase sympathetic neural activity also have the potential to trigger acute cardiovascular events.

84 A clot in the vein, a condition known as venous thromboembolism, can be deadly.

85 Snow shoveling can be a significant hazard to individuals with known or occult coronary heart disease.

86 Coffee consumption is not associated with an increased incidence of cardiovascular disease—in fact, it may actually have cardioprotective effects.

87 One of the first steps in successfully adopting a healthy lifestyle change is to be ready to make it.

88 Unhealthy dietary habits have been linked to the development of heart disease and the risk factors for it, including obesity, hypertension, hypercholesterolemia, and diabetes.

89 Obesity increases the risk for heart disease, type 2 diabetes, high cholesterol, high blood pressure, and stroke, among other conditions.

90 By the time children reach adolescence, subclinical heart disease may already be apparent.

91 A higher intake of magnesium (e.g., nuts and seeds) is associated with a lower incidence of type 2 diabetes, as well as a lower risk of stroke and heart disease.

92 Every hour per day spent watching television is associated with an increased risk of dying from heart disease, stroke, or cancer.

93 Sleep-deprived individuals may be more likely to develop obesity, diabetes, high blood pressure, and cardiovascular disease.

94 No increase in cardiovascular risk exists immediately after being vaccinated for the flu, whereas individuals who contract the flu are at increased risk for cardiac events.

95 Cardiovascular events and mortality peak in the winter months, with the seasonal increase following one to two weeks after the spread of flu in the community.

96 It appears that owning a pet can have a positive influence on decreasing some cardiovascular risk factors.

97 Among the physical benefits of practicing yoga is a reduction of both heart rate and blood pressure.

98 Heart patients who take care of themselves and develop the mind-set necessary to deal with the challenges of heart disease tend to live longer.

99 Obesity, diabetes, hypertension, physical inactivity, high cholesterol, and cigarette smoking are among the most predictive of future cardiovascular events.

100 Currently, the standard treatment for more severe degrees of aortic stenosis is open-   heart surgery to replace the aortic valve.

101 The best way to treat heart disease is to keep it from developing in the first place.

EDITORS

Barry A. Franklin, Ph.D., FACSM, MAACVPR, FAHA

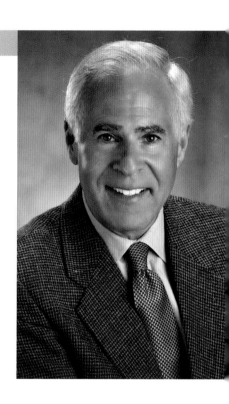

Dr. Barry Franklin serves as the Director of Preventive Cardiology and Cardiac Rehabilitation at William Beaumont Hospital in Royal Oak, Michigan. He also holds faculty appointments as Professor of Physiology, Wayne State University School of Medicine, and Professor of Internal Medicine and Biomedical Engineering, Oakland University William Beaumont School of Medicine.

Dr. Franklin's research over the past four decades combines exercise physiology, cardiac rehabilitation, preventive cardiology, and lifestyle medicine. In the process, he and his associates have studied the cardiorespiratory and hemodynamic responses to snow removal, lawn mowing, and deer hunting.

Dr. Franklin is a past editor-in-chief of both the *Journal of Cardiopulmonary Rehabilitation and Prevention* and *The American Journal of Medicine and Sports*, as well as a past president of the American Association of Cardiovascular and Pulmonary Rehabilitation (AACVPR, 1988) and the American College of Sports Medicine (ACSM, 1999). In addition, he has held multiple leadership positions with the American Heart Association (AHA), at the local, regional, and national level, including appointments to the national AHA Board of Trustees, as well as a member of the Administrative Cabinet. He is also a past chair of the AHA's Council on Nutrition, Physical Activity, and Metabolism, as well as its Advocacy Committee. In 1995, he served as a member of the expert Cardiac Rehabilitation Guideline Panel, convened by the National Heart, Lung, and Blood Institute. Dr. Franklin's professional accomplishments have been recognized through a number of honors and awards, including the Award of Excellence (AACVPR); the Pollock Established Investigator Award (AACVPR); the Award of Meritorious Achievement (AHA); the Outstanding Medical Research Award (William Beaumont Hospital); and both the Citation and Honor Awards (ACSM).

Currently, Dr. Franklin serves on the editorial boards of 15 scientific and clinical journals, including the *American Journal of Cardiology; Sports Medicine, Physician and Sportsmedicine; American Journal of Lifestyle Medicine; Journal of Cardiopulmonary Rehabilitation* and *Prevention; American Journal of Health Promotion;* and *BottomLine Health*. He has written or edited nearly 600 publications, including 481 papers, 85 book chapters, and 26 books. In addition, he has given over 1,000 invited presentations to state, national and international, medical, and lay audiences. In 2015, he was listed by Thomson Reuters among the World's Most Influential Scientific Minds (Clinical Medicine).

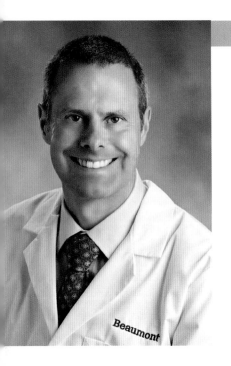

Simon R. Dixon, MBChB, FACC, FRACP

Dr. Simon R. Dixon received his medical training at the University of Auckland School of Medicine in Auckland, New Zealand. After completing fellowships in cardiology and interventional cardiology at Greenlane Hospital in Auckland, he moved to Beaumont Hospital Royal Oak in 1999 to further his interventional training. He has been on the academic faculty at Beaumont since 2001 and currently serves as the chair of the Department of Cardiovascular Medicine. He is also a Professor of Medicine at Oakland University School of Medicine.

Dr. Dixon specializes in the treatment of complex coronary artery disease and is nationally regarded for his research contributions in acute myocardial infarction, cardiogenic shock, percutaneous circulatory support devices, and coronary atherosclerosis. In 2015, he was awarded the inaugural Dorothy Susan Timmis Endowed Chair of Cardiology.